Human Disease In Color

Human Disease In Color

By Chandler Smith, M.D.

Medical Economics Company Book Division
Oradell, New Jersey 07649

Cover design by Penny G. Seldin

ISBN 0-87489-188-4

Medical Economics Company
Oradell, New Jersey 07649

Printed in the United States of America

CONTENTS

Cardiovascular System

Respiratory System

Digestive System

Genitourinary System

Lymphopoietic System

Endocrine System

Craniospinal System

PREFACE

Most medical students intend to practice medicine rather than devote their careers to research or teaching. However, most students also tend to specialize in their practices. This creates a divergence of goals for the students and a problem for the teachers of pathology. For example, the specialist in diseases of the aged need not know the fine details of the pathologic changes that occur in infants, whereas the pediatrician cannot function without this knowledge. The neurologist needs to know much about diseases of the brain, whereas this information is of scant use to the obstetrician. There are countless examples of these differences of interest. Thus a detailed knowledge of special pathology is excessive for the needs of all students, while those who limit their practices to a particular speciality must have a comprehension that exceeds the coverage provided by most general courses. It is therefore evident that the beginning general course in pathology must provide for the main features of the principal lesions in the various anatomical systems, and the details of the various specialties must be provided later in separate courses devoted entirely to those particular interests.

This book is intended to be helpful in meeting the first of these objectives, i.e., a preparation for the practice of general medicine and a background for specialization. Thus the book is a compilation of clinical cases selected to illustrate the morphologic features of the principal lesions that occur in the major anatomical systems. Since time for study is limited, text is brief, and only a characteristic example of each condition is given. Since pictures are more descriptive than words, photographs are abundant. Since gross pathology is difficult to demonstrate, gross aspects are emphasized. Microphotographs are taken at low magnification because it is more important for the student to have a grasp of the general structure of a lesion than to have a fine knowledge of the cytoplasmic or nuclear details of individual cells. The microphotographs are consistently taken from the sections of the gross lesions shown. Captions emphasize what the student should notice. A clinical account of each illness is given, and every case includes a brief review of the condition depicted.

The source of specific cases may be identified through their Clinical Account numbers. Cases with four numbers are from George Washington University Hospital, Washington, D.C.; case numbers preceded by SLH are from St. Luke's Hospital, Saginaw, Michigan; and those preceded by one letter or with fewer than four digits are from Mulago Hospital of Makerere University, Kampala, Uganda.

This format, structured around concise description and color illustration, covers the principal abnormalities seen in medical practice. It associates clinical manifestation with pathologic change. It covers the core of information all students should have. It encourages the student to study further, and it improves his understanding of didactic presentations. It inserts reality into what might otherwise appear abstract. It brings the key findings of the autopsy examination to his attention. It thus mobilizes the subject so that the student can see and understand and enjoy and apply. These goals are sufficient for a supplement to standard texts.

> *"The knowledge a man can use is the only real knowledge, the only knowledge which has life and growth in it and converts itself into practical power. The rest . . . dries like raindrops off the stones."*
> William Osler

Chandler Smith, M.D.

ACKNOWLEDGMENTS

Several helpful persons made the preparation of this book possible. Chief among them were my colleagues in the Department of Pathology at the George Washington University School of Medicine; uncomplainingly they allowed me to "interfere" with their case work. Special thanks are also due, of course, to Dr. Thomas M. Peery, then Chairman, who generously provided me with photographic equipment, time from my other duties for these indulgences, and permission to be away from the Department for the collection of unusual specimens. Gratitude is also expressed to Professor Raphael Owor, Chairman of the Department of Pathology at the School of Medicine, Kampala, Uganda. He and his staff were most helpful not only in selecting suitable specimens but also in encouraging the photographic registration of them. Dr. Robert W. Jones III was invaluable; he granted a travel fellowship from the World Health Organization without which the examples of specimens of tropical medicine could not have been obtained. The typing and retyping of the text was patiently and willingly performed by my office associates, Mrs. Lillian Strait, Miss Sue Kendrick, and Miss Roberta Garland. All of these persons in their several roles made essential contributions to this enterprise, and without their help the work could not have been completed. To all of them my enduring and heartfelt thanks.

C.S.

PUBLISHER'S NOTES

About the author

Chandler Smith, M.D., is Professor and Chairman of the Department of Pathology, Truman Medical Center, University of Missouri—Kansas City. He received his medical education at the University of Oregon School of Medicine and is certified by the American Board of Pathologic Anatomy and the American Board of Clinical Pathology.

Dr. Smith is a member of several professional societies, including the American Medical Association, the American Association for the Advancement of Science, the American Association of Pathologists and Bacteriologists, the International Academy of Pathologists, the American Society for Experimental Pathology, and the Radiation Research Society. He has twice received the Golden Appie award from George Washington University and is a member of Alpha Omega Alpha and Sigma Xi.

Dr. Smith is the author of more than 100 papers and has participated in numerous clinicopathologic conferences.

GLOSSARY

A

ACHLORHYDRIA: The absence of hydrochloric acid from the stomach.
ACHOLIA: The absence of bile.
ACHOLIC: Free from bile.
ACINIC: Glandular.
ADENOMA: Benign tumor of internal glandular structure.
ADIPOSE: Fatty or composed of fat tissue.
ADVENTITIA: The outer layer of a structure, especially a blood vessel.
AFEBRILE: Without fever.
ALVEOLI: Air sacs of lungs.
AMYLOIDOSIS: Accumulation of amyloid, an abnormal protein, between cells.
ANAPLASIA: Histologic properties of cancer, i.e., increased mitotic figures, hyperchromatism, variation in nuclear size, abnormal mitotic figures.
ANASARCA: Whole-body swelling due to increased fluid in tissues.
ANASTOMOSIS: Connection between hollow structures.
ANEURYSM: Localized outward bulging of a structure.
ANGINA PECTORIS: Pain in chest due to reduced oxygenation of cardiac muscle.
ANGIOCARDIOGRAPHY: Examination of vessels of heart, usually by injection of radiopaque substance.
ANGIOMA: Benign tumor composed of blood vessels.
ANOREXIA: Loss of appetite.

ANTHRACOSIS: Deposition of coal dust in the lungs; see Clinical Account 6121.
ANTICOAGULANTS: Substances that inhibit blood clotting.
ANURIA: Absence of urine.
AORTIC CUSP: One of three cusps of aortic valve.
APHASIA: Inability to speak.
APICAL: At or adjacent to apex.
ARTERIOLITIS: Inflammation of arterioles.
ASCHOFF BODIES: Granulomas characteristic of rheumatic fever.
ASCITES: Fluid accumulation in peritoneal (abdominal) cavity.
ATELECTASIS: Collapse of pulmonary tissue.
ATHEROSCLEROSIS: Deposition of lipids in arterial walls.
ATRIA: Two of the four cardiac chambers.
ATRIOVENTRICULAR GROOVE: Transverse groove of heart lying between atria above and ventricles below.
ATRIOVENTRICULAR NODE: Relay point of cardiac impulse, located at top of interventricular septum.
AUSCULTATION: The act of listening, usually with stethoscope.
AUTOLYSIS: Self-digestion of tissue that takes place after death.
AVASCULAR: Lacking blood vessels.
AXILLA: Armpit.
AZOTEMIA: Elevated blood levels of urea nitrogen.
AZYGOS VEIN: Internal vein of chest draining into superior vena cava.

B

BACTERIAL ENDOCARDITIS: Bacterial infection of heart valves.
BASOPHILIC: Dark blue staining.
BIFURCATION: A branching.
BRADYCARDIA: Slow heart rate.
BRONCHIECTASIS: Inflammation and dilatation of bronchi.
BRUIT: Sound heard by listening, usually with stethoscope.
BUCCAL: Pertaining to a lining, especially of the cheek.
BUCCAL MEMBRANE: Surface of oral cavity.
BULLAE: Giant blisters.

C

CACHEXIA: Pronounced wasting; malnourishment.
CALVARIUM: The domelike superior portion of the skull.
CALYCES: Cavities within kidney that connect to ureter.
CANDIDIASIS: Infestation with yeastlike fungus, *Candida albicans.*

CAPILLARIES: Smallest blood vessels lying between arteries and veins and connecting them.
CARDIAC ARREST: Cessation of heart beat.
CARDIAC TAMPONADE: Pressure within pericardial sac preventing ventricular filling in diastole.
CARINA: Region of bifurcation of trachea into bronchi.
CAROTID: An artery of the neck that extends to the brain.
CECUM: The pouchlike first portion of the colon.
CELLULITIS: Inflammation of tissue that is poorly demarcated.
CEREBROSPINAL FLUID: Clear fluid bathing brain and spinal cord.
CEREBROVASCULAR: Pertaining to the blood vessels of the brain.
CHIASM: A decussation or X-shaped crossing, e.g., the optic chiasm.
CHOLANGITIS: Inflammation of bile ducts.
CHOLECYSTITIS: Inflammation of gall bladder.
CHORDA TENDINEAE: Fibrous cords that connect heart valves to ventricular muscle.
CICATRIZATION: Scar formation.
CILIATED: Covered with cilia, i.e., fine 'hairs.'
CIRRHOSIS: Chronic inflammation of liver producing small or large nodules bounded by fibrous connective tissue throughout the whole organ.
CIRSOID: Of elongated oval shape.
CLONUS: Involuntary, usually rapid contractions of skeletal muscle.
COLLAGEN: The tough protein substance of fibrous connective tissue.
COMMISSURES: Site of union of corresponding parts, e.g., adjoining site of two cusps of a heart valve.
CONGESTIVE FAILURE: Consequences of inadequate pumping action of heart.
CONJUNCTIVA: Surface of eyeball.
CONUS: Cone-shaped structure, e.g., pulmonary conus.
COR PULMONALE: Right heart failure with thickening of right ventricle.
CORONARY SINUS: Large vessel delivering cardiac venous blood to right atrium of heart.
CORTICAL: Pertaining to the outside or cortex as opposed to the center or medulla.
COSTOPHRENIC: Pertaining to the junction of ribs (costo-) with diaphragm (-phrenic).
CREATININE CLEARANCE: A measure of renal function.
CREPITATION: Bubbles felt on palpation of tissue.
CYANOSIS: Blue discoloration of skin due to lack of oxygen.
CYTOPLASM: The extranuclear portion of a cell.

D

DECEREBRATE RIGIDITY: Fixed extension of limbs associated with cessation of cerebral function.
DECORTICATION: Procedure that removes surface tissue from an organ.
DEHYDROGENASE: Enzyme measurable in serum.
DIAPHORESIS: Increased perspiration.
DIASTOLIC: Pertaining to the relaxation phase of heart beat.
DIGITALIS: Drug that stimulates heart beat and slows heart rate.
DIPLOPIA: Double vision.
DIVERTICULUM: Focal outpouching of wall, especially of blood vessels and portions of intestines.
DUODENUM: Portion of intestine between stomach and jejunum; it measures about 12 fingerbreadths in length.
DYSARTHRIA: Difficulty in speaking, as with stammering.
DYSPHAGIA: Discomfort or difficulty in swallowing.
DYSPNEA: Shortness of breath.
DYSURIA: Discomfort or pain on urination.

E

ECCHYMOSES: Patchy hemorrhages of skin.
ECTOPIC: Displaced from normal anatomical site.
EFFUSION: Accumulation of fluid, e.g., pleural effusion.
ELECTROCARDIOGRAM: Tracing of electrical impulses of the heart beat.
EMBOLUS: Abnormal particulate matter floating in blood current.
EMPHYSEMA: Dilatation of air sacs of lung; see Clinical Accounts.
EMPYEMA: Pus in a pleural cavity.
ENDOCARDIAL SURFACE: Lining of heart chambers.
ENDOCARDITIS: Inflammation of lining of heart.
ENDOMETRIUM: Internal lining of the uterus.
ENDOTHELIUM: The cell layer lining the inside of blood vessels and body cavities.
EOSIN: A red tissue stain.
EPENDYMA: The lining surface of the ventricles of the brain.
EPIGASTRIUM: Upper midabdomen.
EPITHELIUM: The cell layer covering skin, respiratory, digestive, and urinary systems.
ERYTHROCYTIC: Pertaining to red blood cells, or erythrocytes.
EXSANGUINATION: Total blood loss.

F

FALX: Sickle-shaped structure.
F. CEREBELLI: The connective tissue membrane that separates the cerebellar hemispheres.
F. CEREBRI: The connective tissue membrane that separates the cerebral hemispheres.
FASCIA: A band of fibrous tissue such as lies deep to the skin or forms an investment for muscles and various body organs.
FECALITHS: Concretions of inspissated fecal material.
FIBRILLATION: Rapid, uncontrolled contractions as of the heart.
FIBROSIS: Scar tissue formation.
FILARIA: A tropical parasite.
FISTULA: An abnormal channel between two hollow structures or between a hollow structure and the skin surface.
FLOCCULATION: Precipitation of fine, solid masses out of solution.
FONTANELLE: A soft spot, as in the membrane-covered spaces between the occipital bones in the incompletely ossified skull.
FORAMEN: An opening.
F. MAGNUM: Opening in the skull to allow for passage of cranial nerves.
FRIABLE: Soft, lacking structure, easily broken.
FULMINANT: Overwhelming and rapidly progressive.

G

GALLOP RHYTHM: Extra heart sound producing auscultatory resemblance to galloping horse.
GLIAL: Pertaining to glia, the connective tissue cells of the brain.
GLIOBLASTOMA: A highly malignant brain tumor.
GLIOSIS: Increase of glial tissue, especially in the brain, as a response to injury.
GLYCOGEN: A storage form of carbohydrate that is converted into glucose for metabolic needs.
GLYCOSURIA: Presence of sugar (glucose) in the urine.
GRUMOUS: Clotted or lumpy.
GUAIAC: A gum that changes color in the presence of blood.
GUMMA: Localized tissue granuloma caused by late (tertiary) stage of syphilis.
GYNECOMASTIA: Enlargement of male breasts.

H

HEMATEMESIS: Vomiting of blood.
HEMATOCRIT: Per cent of blood volume occupied by red blood cells.
HEMATOXYLIN: A blue tissue stain.
HEMATURIA: Blood in urine.
HEMIPLEGIA: Paralysis of one side of body.
HEMITHORAX: Half of the chest.
HEMOGLOBIN: The oxygen-carrying pigment of the red blood cells.
HEMOPERICARDIUM: Blood in pericardial sac.
HEMOPOIESIS: Formation of new blood.
HEMOPTYSIS: Expectoration of blood.
HEMOSIDERIN: Pigment from ruptured red blood cells.
HEPATOMEGALY: Enlargement of liver.
HEPATOSPLENOMEGALY: Enlargement of liver and spleen.
HETEROZYGOUS: Having unlike pairs of genes.
HILAR SHADOW: X-ray shadow at root of lung.
HILUM: The root or attachment of an organ.
HOMOZYGOUS: Having identical pairs of genes.
HYALINIZATION: Conversion of connective tissue into firm, tough, acellular substance, as in scar formation.
HYPERCHOLESTEROLEMIA: Abnormally high blood cholesterol.
HYPERCHROMATISM: Excessive staining capacity of cells, especially their nuclei, characteristic of anaplasia.
HYPEREMIA: Engorgement of vessels with blood.
HYPERGLYCEMIA: Increased sugar (glucose) in the blood.
HYPERPLASIA: Increased number of cells.
HYPERTENSION: High blood pressure; normal is about 110 systolic, 70 diastolic in mm. of mercury (Hg).
HYPERTROPHY: Enlargement of cells due to demands of increased function.
HYPOCHONDRIUM: Region of abdomen under the lower rib margin.
HYPOGASTRIC PAIN: Pain in pit of stomach.
HYPOPLASIA: Failure to grow to normal adult size.

I

ICTERUS: Bile pigment in the skin, i.e., jaundice.
ILIAC VEINS: Large veins of groin.
INFARCTION: Localized death of tissue due to vascular obstruction.
INGUINAL: Pertaining to the groin.
INSPISSATED: Hardened by loss of water.
INTERCOSTAL SPACE: Space between ribs.

INTERVENTRICULAR SEPTUM: Muscle layer of heart that separates the right and left ventricles.
INTIMA: Internal lining surface of blood vessels.
INTUSSUSCEPTION: Slipping of one part of intestine into the lumen of an adjoining part.
ISCHEMIA: Local deoxygenation of tissue, usually from obstruction of blood supply.

J

JAUNDICE: Yellow discoloration of skin due to retention of bile.
JEJUNUM: The second portion of the small intestine, extending from the duodenum to the ileum.

K

KARYOTYPE: Chromosomal make-up of an individual cell.
KERATINIZATION: Development of keratin, usually of skin. The process of becoming hard or horny.
KYPHOSCOLIOSIS: Humpback condition with lateral curvature of the spine.

L

LAVAGE: Cleansing of a cavity by copious washing.
LDH: Abbreviation for lactic dehydrogenase.
LEUKOCYTE: White blood cell.
LIGATURE: A thread or wire for tying a vessel or strangulating a part.
LUMEN: The inside of a hollow chamber.
LYMPHADENOPATHY: Enlargement of lymph nodes, usually inflammatory.
LYMPHATICS: Vessels that permeate tissues, collect extravascular tissue fluid, and empty into large veins.
LYMPHEDEMA: Swelling from increased fluid in a body part.
LYMPHOBLAST: Formative cell of the lymphocyte series of leukocytes.

M

MACROPHAGES: Scavenger cells of blood and tissue.
MALABSORPTION SYNDROME: Failure to absorb ingested food, characterized by malnutrition and stools that are yellow, copious, greasy, foul, and floating.

MASTECTOMY: Surgical removal of breast.
MEDIASTINUM: Tissue between lungs.
MEDULLA: The center of a structure.
MELENA: Black, viscous stool due to bleeding into bowel.
MENINGES: Delicate membranes that cover the brain and spinal cord.
MENTATION: The process of thinking.
MESENCHYMAL: Pertaining to cells and structures of connective tissue origin.
MESENTERY: Fibroadipose attachment of intestine to body wall.
METAPLASIA: Conversion of adult cells in a tissue to a form which is not normal for that tissue.
METASTASES: Deposits of cancer away from site of origin.
MICTURITION: The act of urination.
MIDCLAVICULAR LINE: Vertical line equidistant from ends of clavicles.
MILIARY: Tiny and usually widely disseminated.
MITOCHONDRIA: Intracellular organelles that generate energy by adenosine triphosphate (ATP) synthesis from cell nutrients.
MITOSIS: A process of cell division.
MORPHOLOGY: The science of shape and structure.
MURAL THROMBUS: Thrombus on wall of a chamber, such as a cardiac ventricle.
MUSCULARIS: A layer of muscle, as in the intestinal tract.
MYOCARDIAL INFARCTION: Localized death of cardiac muscle.
MYOCARDIUM: Muscle of heart.
MYOFIBRILS: Individual muscle cells or filaments.
MYOMETRIUM: Muscle of the uterus.

N

NECROSIS: Localized tissue death.
NEUTROPHILIA: Increase in granular leukocytes (white blood cells).
NUCHAL: Pertaining to the neck, as in nuchal rigidity (stiff neck).
NYSTAGMUS: An involuntary, rapid movement of the eyeballs up and down, laterally, or some combination of directions.

O

OLIGURIA: Decreased secretion of urine.
OMENTUM: A fold of tissue hanging from the stomach over the abdominal organs.
ORTHOPNEA: Shortness of breath except in upright position.
OS: An opening.

OSTEOPOROSIS: Increased porosity of bone marrow.
OVOID: Nearly oval.

P

PACEMAKER, CARDIAC: Sino-atrial node.
PANCYTOPENIA: Decrease in cellular elements of the blood—red cells, leukocytes, and platelets.
PAPILLARY MUSCLE: Muscle that prevents eversion of cardiac valve (tricuspid and mitral) leaflets.
PAPILLEDEMA: Swelling (edema) of the optic nerve head in the back of the eye.
PARADOXICAL PULSATION: Pulse that diminishes with inspiration.
PARENCHYMA: The essential elements of an organ in contrast to its framework (stroma).
PARESTHESIA: Abnormal skin sensation, such as burning or prickling.
PEDUNCULATED: Connected by a narrow, elongated attachment.
PERICARDIAL EFFUSION: Fluid collection in pericardial sac.
PERICARDIUM: Smooth sac in which the heart lies.
PETECHIAE: Multiple, minute, punctate hemorrhages in skin.
PHLEBOTHROMBOSIS: Noninflammatory thrombus formation in veins.
PHONATION: Sound production through larynx.
PIA MATER: Innermost of three membranes covering the brain and spinal cord.
PLEURA: Smooth surface of lungs and chest cavities.
PLICATION: A folding of a layer; usually a surgical procedure.
POLYARTERITIS NODOSA: Segmental arterial inflammation of unknown cause.
POLYCYTHEMIA: An increased concentration of red blood cells usually circulating in an increased volume of blood.
POLYPOID: Globular in shape.
PONS: A portion of the brain between the cerebral peduncles and the medulla.
PONTINE: Pertaining to the pons.
PRECORDIAL THRILL: Vibration felt with hand over precordium.
PRECORDIUM: Area of chest over heart.
PRETIBIAL: In front of the tibia, the large bone in the lower leg.
PRIAPISM: Persistent, abnormal penile erection without sexual stimulation.
PROPTOSIS: Protrusion of the eyeballs.

PROTHROMBIN: Blood clotting factor II, a blood protein involved in thrombin formation.
PSAMMOMA: Pertaining to flecks of calcium, especially in tumors of the ovary and brain.
PTOSIS: Drooping or downward displacement of a part, as in drooping of an eyelid.
PULMONARY EDEMA: Fluid in lungs.
PYLORUS: The distal opening of the stomach.

R

RALES: Abnormal respiratory sound heard on auscultation, due to fluid in lungs.
RAPHE: A seam delineating a line of union of two parts.
RECTUM: Last portion of colon extending from sigmoid to anus.
RENAL FAILURE: Failure of kidneys to produce urine.
RETICULUM: A network, especially a protoplasmic network in cells.
RETROPERITONEUM: The space behind the peritoneum, the membrane lining the abdominal cavity.
RHONCHI: Extremely coarse breath sounds often due to excessive mucus in bronchi.
RIBONUCLEASE: An enzyme that breaks down ribonucleic acid (RNA).

S

SCALENE: Pertaining to a muscle of the anterior neck or a region adjacent to this muscle.
SCIRRHOUS: Hard in texture.
SCLERODERMA: A systemic disease causing hardening of connective tissues of any part of the body.
SCLEROSING MEDIASTINITIS: Fibrosis of mediastinum.
SENSORIUM: Parts of brain involved in consciousness or mental clarity.
SEROSA: Membrane lining of a body cavity, e.g., pleura, pericardium, peritoneum.
SERPIGINOUS: Spreading gradually or creeping along an irregular margin.
SESSILE: Flat with broad attachment at base.
SGOT: Abbreviation for serum glutamic-oxaloacetic transaminase.
SINOATRIAL NODE: Point of origin of heart beat, located in atrium.
SINUSOID: Resembling a sinus. A small vascular lake, especially in liver or spleen.

SMEGMA: A thick, cheesy, ill-smelling secretion of desquamated epithelial cells, found chiefly about the external genitals.
SQUAMOUS: Pertaining to flat-surfaced cells as on skin, mouth, esophagus, vagina, external cervix.
STEATOSIS: Infiltration with fat.
STEROID THERAPY: Treatment with adrenocorticoid steroids.
STRABISMUS: Deviation of the eye which the patient cannot overcome.
STROMA: Supporting framework of an organ.
SUBARACHNOID: Pertaining to a membrane covering the brain.
SUBSTERNAL: Underneath breast bone.
SUBUNGUAL: Under finger or toe nail.
S. HEMORRHAGE: Hemorrhage under finger nails.
SUBXIPHOID: Beneath the xiphoid, the lower end of the sternum or breast bone.
SULCUS: A crease or groove.
SUPRACLAVICULAR LYMPH NODE: Lymph node above the clavicle.
SYNCOPE: Fainting.
SYSTOLIC: Pertaining to the contraction phase of heart beat.
S. MURMUR: Heart murmur coinciding with heart contraction.

T

TACHYCARDIA: Increased heart rate.
TACHYPNEA: Increased rate of breathing.
TAMPONADE: Acute compression, especially of heart due to filling of pericardial sac with fluid, usually blood.
TENESMUS: Straining at stool.
THENAR: Pertaining to the palm.
T. EMINENCE: Fleshy mound at base of thumb.
THORACENTESIS: Aspiration of fluid from chest cavity.
THROMBOEMBOLISM: Blocking of a blood vessel by a migrating thrombus.
THROMBOSIS: Process of clot formation within blood vessel.
TRABECULATED: Crisscrossed with supporting fibers or bony spicules.
TRANSAMINASE: Enzyme measurable in serum.
TRANSMURAL: Across the total thickness of a wall.
TRIGONE: A triangular space, especially at the base of the urinary bladder.
TUBERCLE: Small granuloma, especially one due to *Mycobacterium tuberculosis.*

TUBERCULOUS ENDOCARDITIS: Inflammation of endocardium due to tubercle bacillus.

V

VARICES: Dilatation of veins.
VASA VASORUM: Minute blood vessels that nourish the walls of large blood vessels such as the aorta.
VASOPRESSOR: Substance that contracts vessels and raises blood pressure.
VENA CAVA: Major vein that empties into right atrium of heart.
VENTRICLE: Chamber, especially of heart or brain.
VENTRICULAR FIBRILLATION: Ineffective and uncoordinated contraction of separate muscle bundles of the heart ventricles.

X

XANTHOCHROMIA: Yellow discoloration.

NORMAL HEART

CLINICAL ACCOUNT 6166

The patient was a white female 61 years old who developed an epidermoid carcinoma of the floor of the mouth one year before admission to the hospital. This was treated, first surgically and later by irradiation. The tumor recurred and gradually involved the right side of the face. Five days before admission, swelling of the ankles was noted. In the last two days the left foot became red, warm, and painful.

The temperature was 96.8 degrees F., respirations 18, pulse 120, and blood pressure 96/70 mm. Hg. The right jaw and neck were disfigured by recurrent tumor. The heart and lungs were not remarkable. There was slight ankle edema, and the left calf and foot were tender, warm, and red. The hemoglobin was 12.1 Gm., the hematocrit was 38, and the leukocytes numbered 7,900, with 63 neutrophiles, 35 band cells, and 2 lymphocytes. The total protein was slightly decreased. The clinical impression was recurrent tumor of the mouth and acute cellulitis of the left leg. On the day after admission the patient was unexpectedly found to be comatose; she died one hour later.

Autopsy examination revealed a thrombo-embolus of the right lung, a cellulitis of both lower legs, and a recurrent carcinoma of the mouth and neck. Additional diagnoses were incidental. The heart weighed 240 Gms.

THE ENTITY

The normal heart contracts about 70 times per minute and moves about 70 ml. of blood through each of its chambers with each beat. The beat is involuntary, originates in the sinoatrial node (pacemaker), and is conveyed to the atrioventricular node and thence to the ventricles over specialized muscle cells that constitute a conduction system. The myocardium is nourished by two coronary arteries; the left, which consists of an anterior descending and left circumflex branch, and the right, which consists of a marginal and posterior descending branch. Anastomoses between branches exist and may become large. They are endomural, retrocardiac, transepicardial, and intercoronary. The last are the most important and connect adjacent main vessels. Stimuli to their development include hypoxia and anemia (1). The capillaries of the distal vessels empty into the ventricles directly through the Thebesian veins, and into veins that merge to form the coronary sinus, which lies in the atrioventricular groove and empties into the right atrium. Small arteries extend through the ventricular wall to empty directly into the ventricular lumen (arterioluminal vessels). Retrograde flow through these vessels may alleviate myocardial ischemia. Lymphatics converge to form a single main channel at the base that traverses the arch of the pulmonary artery and conveys lymph to extra-cardiac veins.

1. Bloor, C.M. Functional significance of the coronary collateral circulation. Am. J. Path. 76: 562-586, 1974.

NORMAL HEART

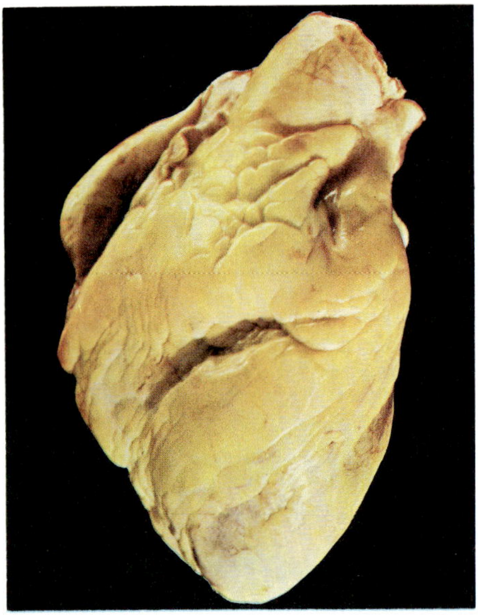

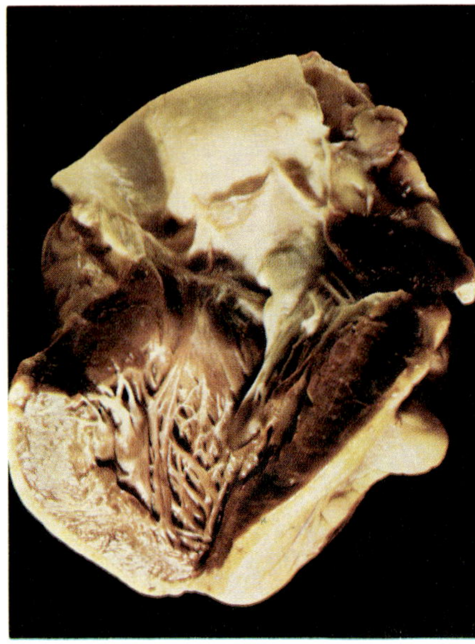

Left: The epicardium is smooth and glistening, the contour is normal, and the weight is not excessive. A weight of more than 400 gm. is abnormal for men; a weight in excess of 350 gm. is abnormal for women. **Right:** On section the endocardium is smooth, the muscle is brownish red, and the interface with subepicardial adipose tissue is sharply delineated.

Left: The mitral valve is composed of two leaflets that are smooth and avascular. Each is attached to the ventricular muscle by chordae tendineae that are delicate and discrete. The columnae carneae and papillary muscles are robust. **Right:** The aortic valve is composed of three cusps that are thin, translucent, and avascular. The commissures at the points of aortic attachment are free of adhesions.

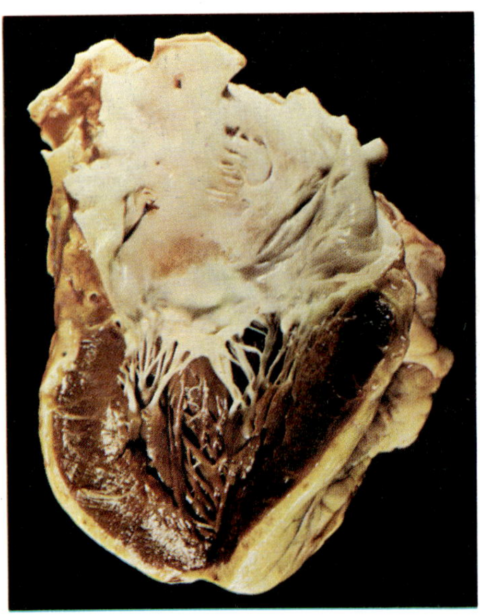

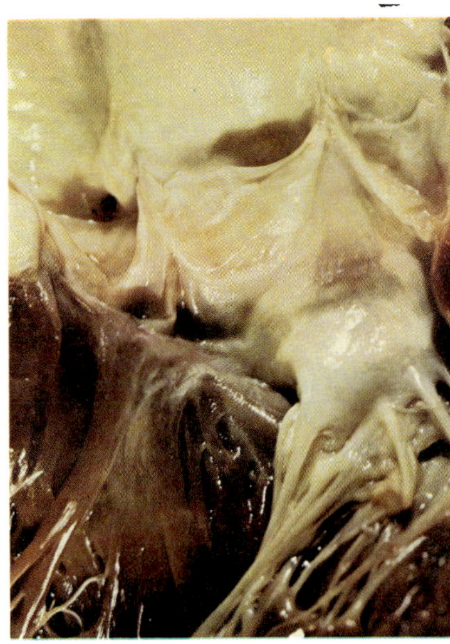

RECENT INFARCT OF MYOCARDIUM

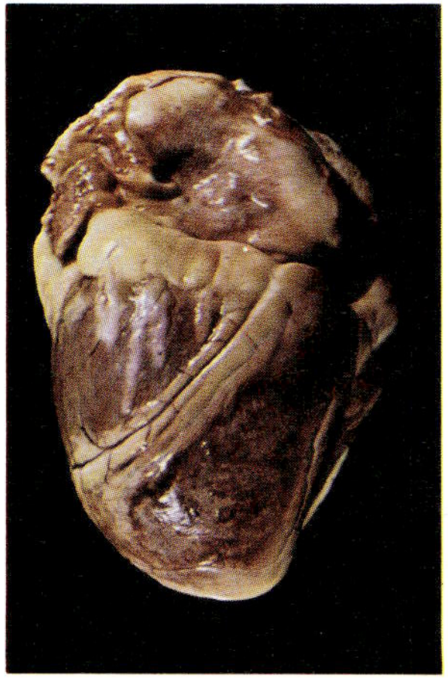

The posterior surface of the heart is shown. The epicardium, in the right lower portion of the photograph, is mottled with pale gray areas; it is roughened with fibrin, and discolored by foci of recent hemorrhage.

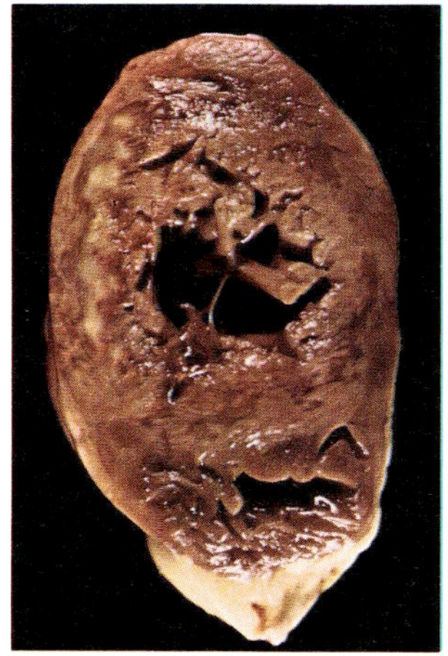

Section reveals a large focus of pale yellowish-gray discoloration in the central portion of the left ventricle. This is the principal site of the recent infarct. Foci of hemorrhage discolor the interventricular septum.

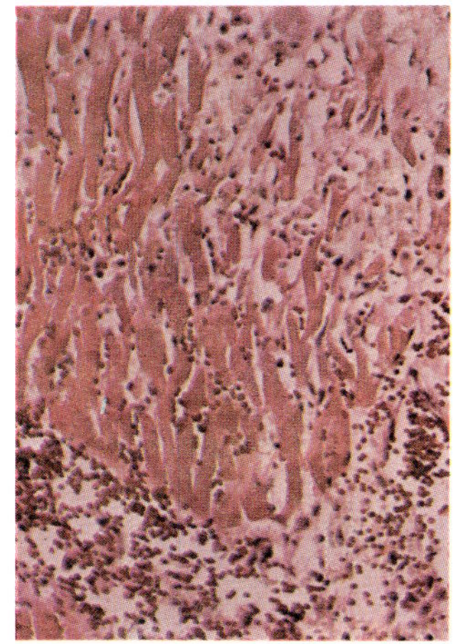

Histologic examination reveals necrotic muscle with myofibrils separated by intervening hemorrhage. Capillaries are forming and connective tissue infiltrates the margins of the infarct.

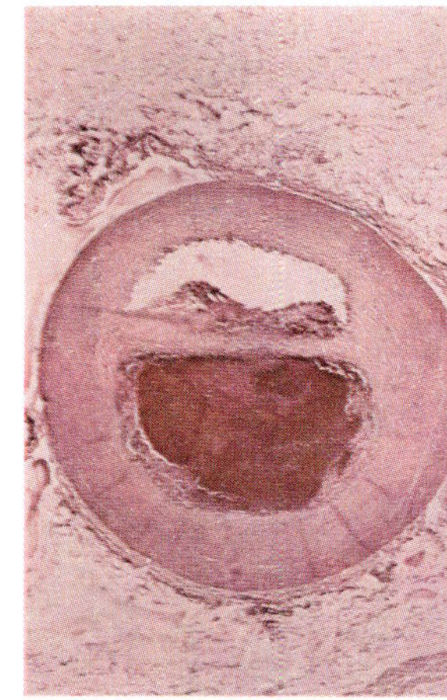

Histologic examination of the right main coronary artery reveals a recent thrombus (lower portion) and an empty space (upper portion) where the embedding process dissolved out lipids in the atherosclerotic wall.

RECENT INFARCT OF MYOCARDIUM

CLINICAL ACCOUNT 6136

The patient was a white male 56 years old who was admitted to the hospital because of severe chest pain. The pain began in the morning of the day of admission and was substernal in location with radiation to the back, neck, and left arm. It was accompanied by apprehension, diaphoresis, and a feeling of weakness. The patient had had several episodes of severe angina pectoris in the year prior to the present illness but had otherwise been well.

The temperature was 97.4 degrees F., respirations 22, pulse 108, and blood pressure 100/70 mm Hg. The neck veins were not distended. Fine rales were heard over both lung bases. The pulse was regular, the heart was not enlarged, and no murmurs were heard.

The patient was unable to void. The hemoglobin was 16.8 Gm., hematocrit 52, and leukocytes 15,400, with a moderate neutrophilia. The blood cholesterol was 275 mg., the serum glutamic transaminase was 60 u/100 ml. A chest x-ray showed no cardiac enlargement and slight pulmonary congestion. An electrocardiogram revealed a posterior myocardial infarct.

On the second hospital day the serum glutamic and lactic dehydrogenase enzymes rose to 242 and 2040 units, respectively. The patient was nauseated and vomited. The pain persisted; a pacemaker was inserted. His condition regressed; death occurred after the patient had been hospitalized for five days.

Autopsy examination revealed a recent thrombus of the right coronary artery and a massive recent infarct of the left ventricle. An old infarct of the posterior wall of the left ventricle was also present.

THE ENTITY

Myocardial infarction occurs more often in Caucasians than Negroes, more often in men than premenopausal women, and more often in the 35 to 70 year age group than younger or older persons. Patients with obesity, hypertension, and hypercholesterolemia are especially susceptible. The clinical feature is sudden sharp pain in the chest that is usually substernal and is often referred to the left arm, the left shoulder, or the left side of the neck. This is accompanied by apprehension, often nausea and vomiting, occasionally shock, and less frequently cyanosis and dyspnea. The leukocyte level and sedimentation rate are increased, and these increases are followed by fever and elevation of serum enzymes (SGOT, LDH). The electrocardiogram provides the most reliable evidence of the diagnosis.

Infarction of the myocardium is due to thrombosis of a coronary artery. The thrombi tend to occur in the first portions of the main vessels. The infarct almost always occurs in the left ventricle or interventricular septum. The lesion is not grossly evident in the first 12 hours, foci of hemorrhage become apparent in the period of two to four days, and yellow discoloration due to fat droplets in the necrotic muscle becomes most noticeable in the fourth to the tenth day. After ten days, marginal granulation tissue is well formed, a scar develops in six weeks, and this scar hyalinizes in succeeding months.

Complications include mural thrombus of the endocardium, thrombo-embolism, ventricular aneurysm, rupture of the interventricular septum, rupture of a papillary muscle with fulminant heart failure, and rupture of the left ventricle with cardiac tamponade. Death is most commonly due to ventricular fibrillation with cardiac arrest, congestive failure, thrombo-embolism especially to the brain, and phlebothrombosis of the leg veins with pulmonary embolism.

ANEURYSM OF LEFT VENTRICLE

CLINICAL ACCOUNT 5981

The patient was a Negro female 42 years old who lost consciousness, had a convulsion, and was admitted to the hospital. The informant stated that she had been hypertensive for the past five years and that she had recovered from a myocardial infarction. The date of this was not given.

Physical examination disclosed decerebrate rigidity and indicated a recent cerebrovascular accident. The cerebrospinal fluid was blood-tinged. An electrocardiogram was consistent with an old myocardial infarction. A chest x-ray was suggestive of an aneurysm of the left ventricle. On the day after admission the patient died.

Autopsy examination revealed acute fibrinous pericarditis, hypertrophy of the heart (475 Gm.), and an aneurysm of the left ventricle filled with mural thrombus. There were also a recent thrombus of the right internal carotid artery, a recent infarct of the cerebrum, and a terminal bronchopneumonia of the right and left lungs.

THE ENTITY

A complication of transmural infarction of the myocardium is aneurysm formation. An aneurysm may be defined as an outpouching of the external surface of the heart accompanied by a corresponding protrusion of the endocardial surface. Such aneurysms occur in males more often than females (4:1); they occur in the left ventricle almost exclusively, and their incidence is about 3.5 per cent of patients with myocardial infarctions (1). The clinical diagnosis is indicated by the x-ray outline of the heart, paradoxical pulsation on fluoroscopy (ventricle enlarges at systole), and angiocardiographic studies in a patient with a history of recent infarction.

The average size is about 5 cm. in diameter. The wall of the aneurysm measures 0.1 to 0.6 cm. in thickness and is composed of fibrous tissue, often with residual bundles of muscle, and occasionally with foci of calcification. In over half of the cases the external surface is roughened by fibrous adhesions, and the internal surface is covered by mural thrombus. The complications of ventricular aneurysms, in order of decreasing frequency, are recurrent infarction, congestive failure, thrombo-embolism, and rupture with cardiac tamponade. While excision of aneurysms has been performed, a conservative view has been recommended because of the considerable risk of the surgical procedure and the observation that the survival of patients with aneurysm is not significantly different from the survival of all patients with myocardial infarction (2).

1. Dubnow, M.H., Burchell, H.B., and Titus, J.L. Postinfarction ventricular aneurysm. Am. Heart J. 70:753, 1965.
2. Abrams, D.L., Edelist, A., Luria, M.H., and Miller, A.J. Ventricular aneurysm. Circulation 37:164, 1963.

ANEURYSM OF LEFT VENTRICLE

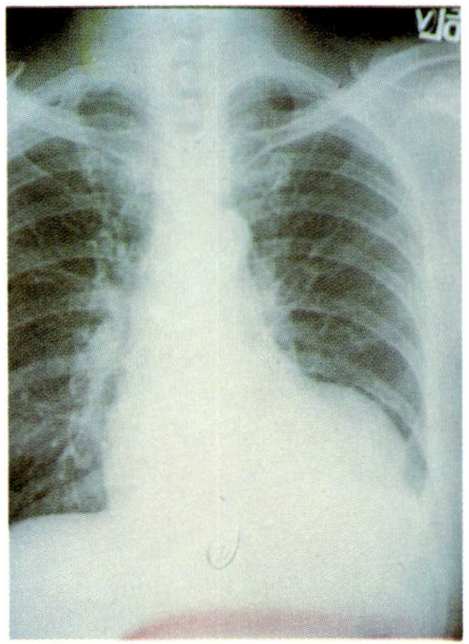

The chest x-ray had shown a conspicuous bulge of the ventricular outline to the left. This "boot-shaped" heart is consistent with pronounced hypertrophy of the left ventricle due to aortic stenosis, or with infarct of the myocardium with aneurysm formation.

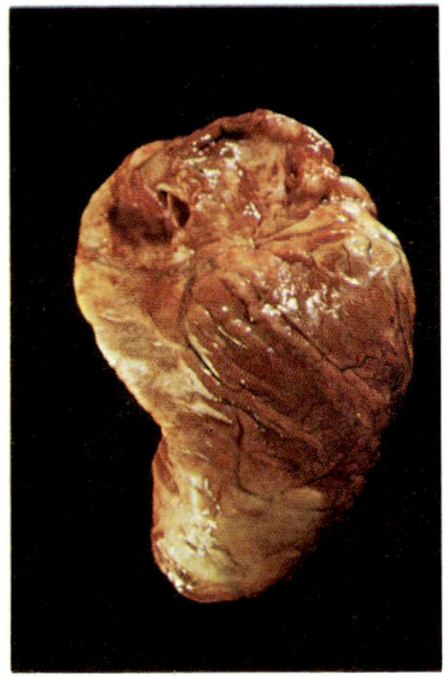

The anterior surface of the unopened heart shows elongation of the ventricular contour suggestive of aneurysm.

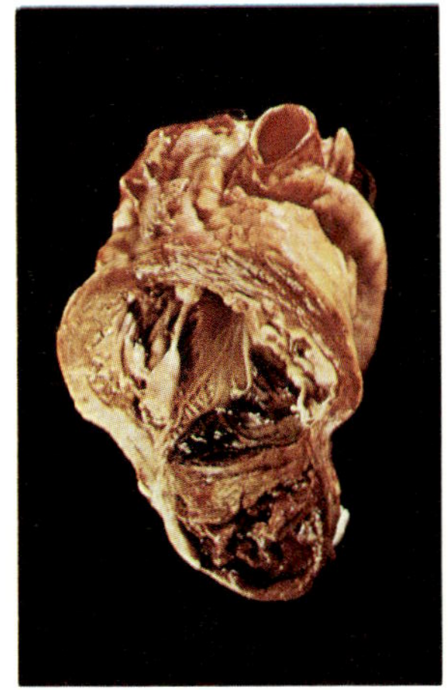

Section of the left ventricle reveals the aneurysm. It is filled with a laminated mural thrombus undergoing central degeneration. The ventricular wall overlying the aneurysm is extremely thin.

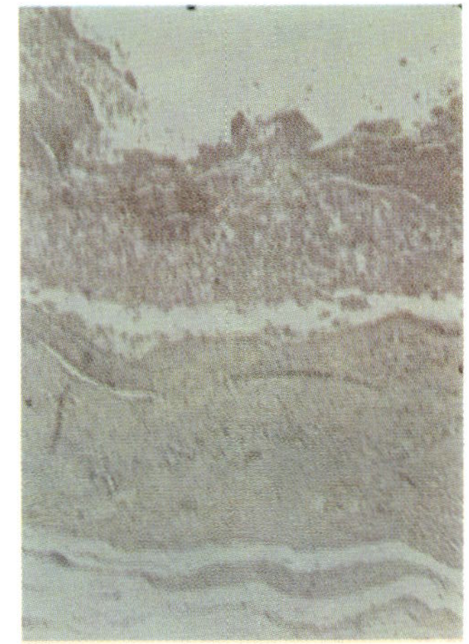

A microsection of the aneurysmal wall shows that it is composed only of a thin layer of dense fibrous connective tissue. The internal surface is covered by a mural thrombus; the external surface is roughened by fibrous adhesions.

RUPTURE OF PAPILLARY MUSCLE

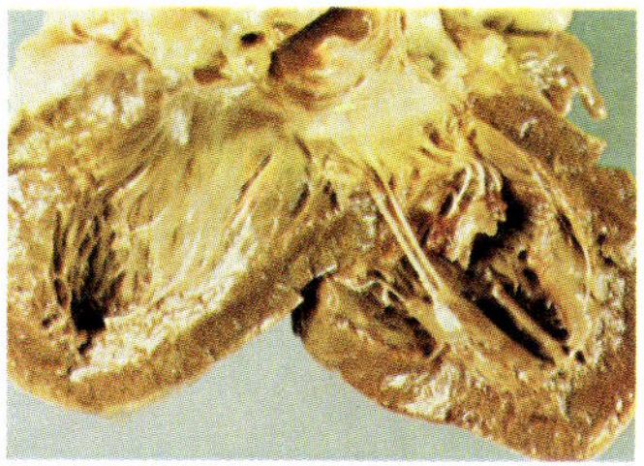

The left anterior papillary muscle is ruptured and a large muscle fragment lies free in the ventricle except for the attached chordae tendineae.

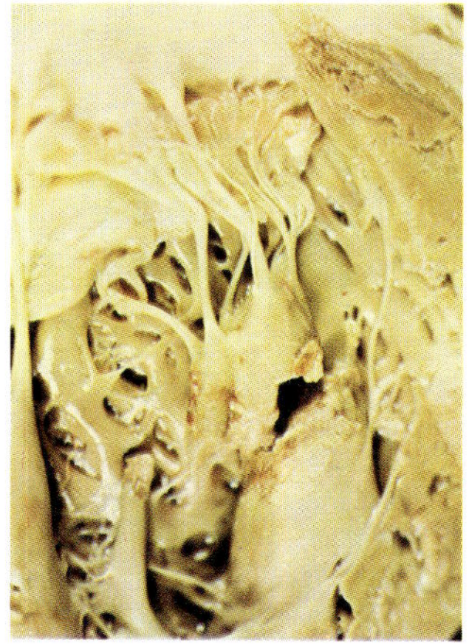

A closer view shows the margin of separation, the loosened fragment above, and the main belly of the muscle below.

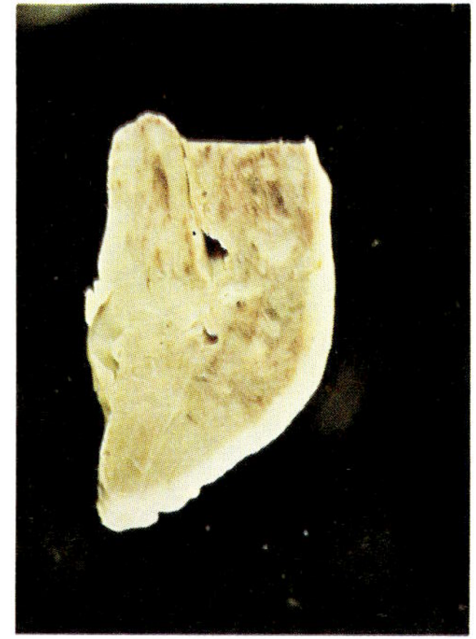

A cut surface discloses the left ventricle on the right with the attached lower portion of the papillary muscle projecting upward on the left. Necrosis extends through the ventricular wall and into the papillary muscle.

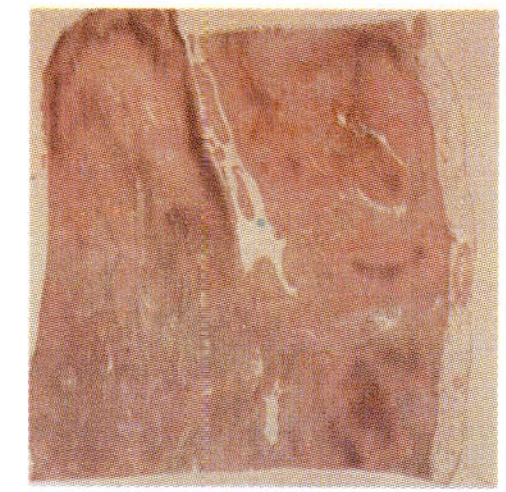

Histologic section reveals the necrosis of recent infarction as it affects the papillary muscle and the ventricular wall.

RUPTURE OF PAPILLARY MUSCLE

CLINICAL ACCOUNT 5771

The patient was a white male 76 years old who experienced severe pain of sudden onset in the left anterior chest that radiated to both shoulders and both arms. The pulse was 72 and the blood pressure was 120/80 mm. Hg. An electrocardiogram indicated a recent infarction of the left ventricle. The serum glutamic transaminase was 220 units per 100 ml., and the serum lactic dehydrogenase was 2800 units per 100 ml. Anticoagulants and digitalis were given.

On the day after admission the patient became markedly agitated and short of breath. A chest x-ray indicated pulmonary edema. Cyanosis developed, the blood pressure dropped, the pulse rate increased, and a convulsion occurred. Oxygen, vasopressors, and assisted respiration failed to lessen this distress; the patient died.

Autopsy examination revealed a recent infarct of the myocardium with rupture of the anterior papillary muscle of the left ventricle. A recent thrombus was present in the circumflex branch of the left coronary artery.

THE ENTITY

Rupture of a papillary muscle is uncommon. The lesion occurs in the left ventricle, and the posterior muscle is more frequently affected than the anterior. The common cause is infarction of the myocardium. Rare causes include bacterial endocarditis, tuberculous endocarditis, trauma, syphilis, and polyarteritis nodosa (1).

The signs and symptoms begin with myocardial infarction. If the patient dies immediately the clinical diagnosis is precluded. If the patient lives, the diagnosis is suggested by a sudden change; i.e. the severity of the angina increases, a harsh systolic apical murmur appears, and profound shock develops. The patient ordinarily dies within 24 hours of this change.

The lesion must be distinguished from rupture of an aortic cusp, rupture of the chordae tendineae, rupture of the interventricular septum, and rupture of the left ventricle. Aortic cusp rupture is characterized by a high pulse pressure. Rupture of the chordae tendineae is usually antedated by bacterial endocarditis, and death is not sudden. Rupture of the interventricular septum is attended by an undilated left atrium and a precordial thrill that is transmitted chiefly to the right. Rupture of the left ventricle is immediately fatal if large; if small, cardiac tamponade gradually develops so that the neck veins are distended, the pulse pressure is low, and the heart sounds are suppressed.

The diagnosis is suggested by clinical evidence of a recent myocardial infarct, followed by a pronounced increase in the severity of the chest pain of sudden onset that is associated with profound shock, and a harsh apical systolic murmur that was not previously present.

1. Smith, J.C. Rupture of a papillary muscle of the heart: Report of two cases. Circulation 1:766-711, 1950.

RUPTURE OF LEFT VENTRICLE

CLINICAL ACCOUNT 6138

The patient was a white male 67 years old who experienced chest pain of sudden onset on the morning of the day of admission. The pain was severe and radiated into both arms and to the epigastrium. Nausea, chilliness, and a "cold sweat" were associated. He had previously been well.

The patient was afebrile. The pulse was 68, respirations 24, and blood pressure 120/90 mm. Hg. The neck veins were not distended, the lungs were clear, and the heart sounds were faint. No murmurs were heard. There was no edema or cyanosis. An electrocardiogram revealed a recent anterior infarct of the myocardium. Nausea, vomiting, and shortness of breath developed. The patient died six hours after being admitted.

Autopsy examination revealed a thrombus of the anterior descending branch of the left coronary artery, a recent infarct of the myocardium, and a rupture of the left ventricle. The pericardial sac contained 250 ml. of clotted blood.

THE ENTITY

Cardiac rupture occurs in 7 to 14 per cent of autopsy cases of recent myocardial infarction (1). The sites of the rupture are the apex and the free walls of the left ventricle with the anterior being twice as common as the posterior. The disorder occurs after the age of 40 years unless hypertension is present. Although myocardial infarction is nearly 5 times more common in males, rupture in females is equal to males in frequency. The rupture occurs at sites of recent infarction and may occur before the infarct is sufficiently well developed to be grossly discernible. Although the average time of rupture is 7.4 days after the clinical onset of the infarct, 8 of 11 cases reported by Sigler occurred within 4 days of the myocardial infarction (1). The mechanism of the rupture is based on the inability of the necrotic muscle to contract. With each systole the ventricle bulges at the necrotic site. This stretches the small vessels which break and form dissecting hematomas. As these coalesce an irregular channel is formed and the epicardium is eventually reached and perforated. Hemopericardium follows and cardiac tamponade causes death. Hypertension is a predisposing condition because the muscle is hypertrophic, the vascularity of the ventricular wall is reduced, and the vulnerability of the tissue is increased. Ventricular rupture after myocardial infarction is 3 times more common in hypertensives than normotensives.

1. Sigler, L.H. Sudden death due to cardiac rupture in myocardial ischemia and infarction. New York State J. Med. 69:794, 1969.

RUPTURE OF LEFT VENTRICLE

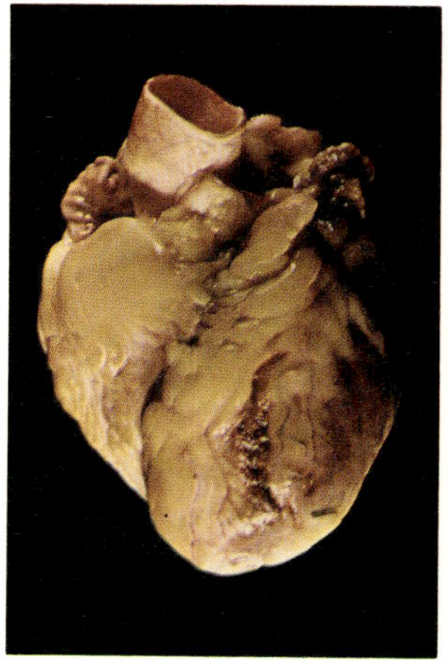

A laceration is present over the anterior surface of the left ventricle. The adjacent muscle is soft; elsewhere it is firm.

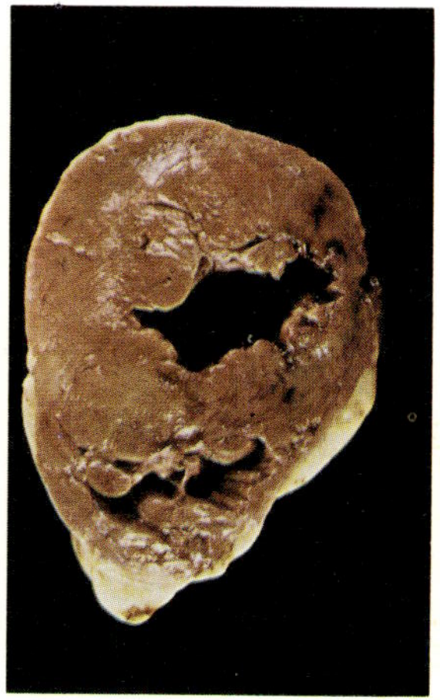

The cut surface discloses a recent infarct of the left ventricle, pronounced atrophy at that site, and hemorrhages in the wall that on serial section connected the ventricular chamber with the pericardial sac.

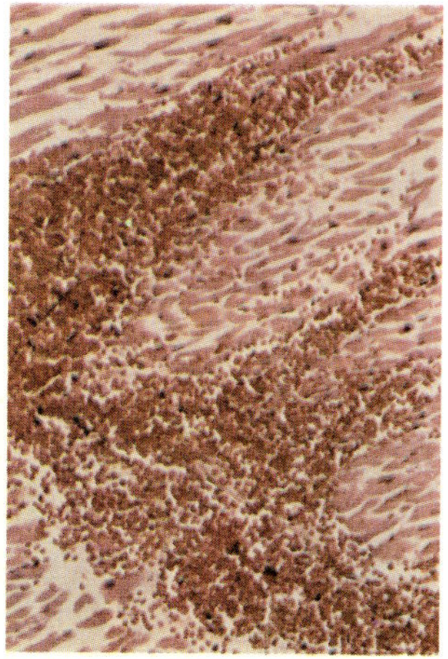

Histologic examination of the myocardium discloses necrotic muscle fibers and evidence of extensive recent hemorrhage.

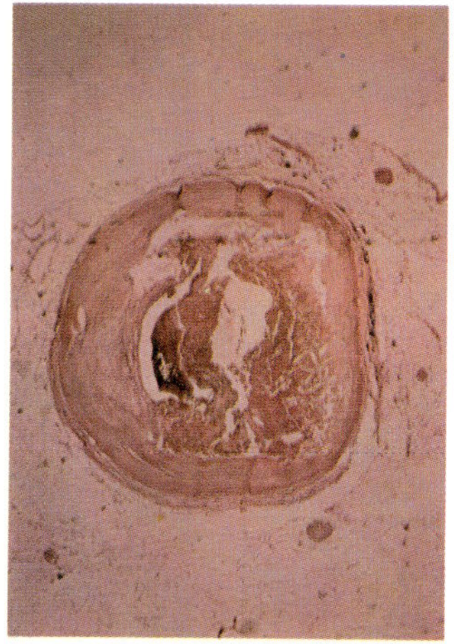

Histologic examination reveals that the anterior descending branch of the left coronary artery is obstructed by a recent thrombus. Atherosclerosis markedly narrows the lumen. The patient died of hemopericardium with cardiac tamponade.

PAPILLARY MUSCLE DYSFUNCTION

Foci of yellow and red discolor the cut surface of the opened papillary muscle. The heart weighed 450 Gm. Only a slight arteriosclerosis was present in the coronary arteries and no thrombi were found.

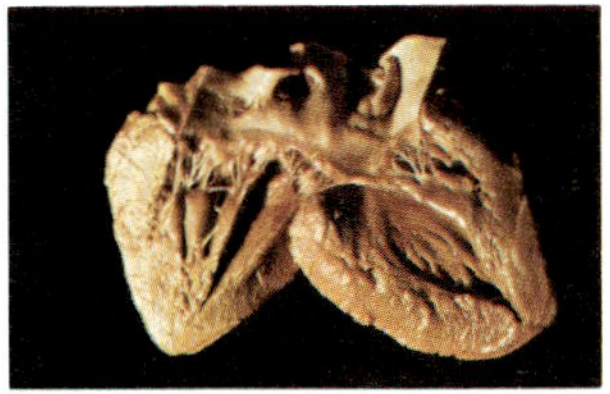

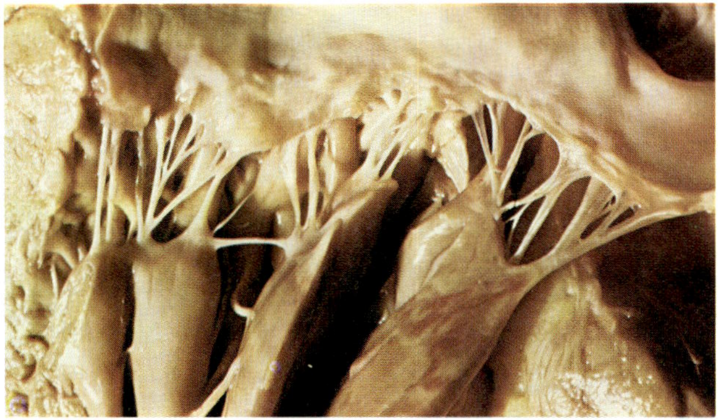

Closer examination reveals the discoloration of the necrotic papillary muscle. The mitral leaflets are not remarkable and the chordae tendineae are delicate and discrete.

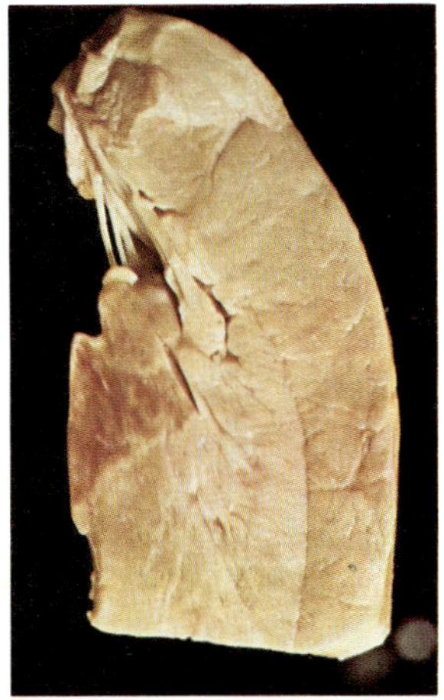

On section the necrosis and discoloration may be seen limited to the upper portion and tip of the papillary muscle.

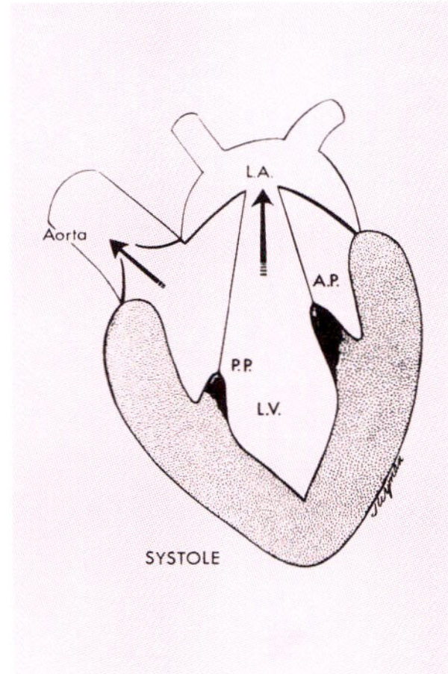

The diagram reveals the nature of the functional disturbance that arises when infarction disallows systolic contraction and mitral regurgitation follows as the result.

PAPILLARY MUSCLE DYSFUNCTION

CLINICAL ACCOUNT 6153

The patient was a white female 52 years old who had experienced chronic renal failure for the past two years. The nature of the renal disease was uncertain. Her treatment consisted of diuretics and a low sodium, low protein diet. Two months before admission her blood pressure was 250/115 mm. Hg., and her creatinine clearance was 15 ml. per minute (normal 90-120 ml. per min.). On the day before admission shortness of breath began and became pronounced on the following day.

The temperature was 98.6 degrees F., pulse 82, respirations 12, and blood pressure 230/140 mm. Hg. Coarse bubbly rales were heard over both lung fields. The heart was not remarkable. The bowel sounds were normal. The lower legs disclosed 3-plus pitting edema. The neurologic function was physiologic.

The urine was alkaline and cloudy, with a specific gravity of 1.009. There was a trace of protein and sugar, and the sediment revealed a few epithelial cells and 5 to 9 leukocytes per high power field. The hemoglobin was 8.4 Gm., hematocrit 25, and leukocytes 15,000 with a normal differential count. The blood sugar was 218 mg., urea nitrogen 57 mg., and serum creatinine 8.2 mg. per 100 ml. The blood carbon dioxide exceeded 40 meq./L., and the serum glutamic transaminase and lactic dehydrogenase were normal. An x-ray of the chest revealed pulmonary congestion and cardiac enlargement. An electrocardiogram disclosed "ST changes of uncertain significance." On the day after admission the lactic dehydrogenase was 2490 units per 100 ml. (normal under 550 u.). On the next day the patient died.

Autopsy examination revealed recent infarcts of the papillary muscles of the left ventricle, hypertrophy of the heart, edema of the lungs, pleural effusions (500 ml., right, 500 ml., left), and marked chronic pyelonephritis. There were also recent infarcts of the liver, ascites (1000 ml.), focal hemorrhagic necrosis of the colon, and cortical necrosis of the kidneys with calcification of the renal papillae.

THE ENTITY

When the left ventricle contracts, it is necessary for the papillary muscles to contract also; if they don't the mitral leaflets evert into the left atrium and blood regurgitates into that chamber during systole. Papillary muscle dysfunction, or failure to contract, is due, in part, to coronary artery disease, which causes infarction of that tissue. It is also due to dilatation of the left ventricle, which displaces the papillary muscles and renders their contraction less effective. The postero-medial muscle is affected more often than the antero-lateral muscle because it is situated farther from its coronary blood supply. Clinical manifestations are those of coronary heart disease, i.e., angina pectoris, infarction of the myocardium, and congestive failure. The physical feature is a "diamond shaped" apical systolic murmur. The abrupt onset of such a murmur after myocardial infarction is much more often due to papillary muscle dysfunction than to rupture of a papillary muscle or rupture of the interventricular septum (1).

1. Burch, G.E., DePasquale, N.P., and Phillips, J.H. The syndrome of papillary muscle dysfunction. Am. Heart J. 75:399 1968.

ENDOMYOCARDIAL FIBROSIS

CLINICAL ACCOUNT 454

The patient was a Ugandan female 24 years old who developed exertional dyspnea 3 months before hospital admission. This progressed, orthopnea developed, and the legs became markedly swollen. The temperature was 98.9 degrees F., pulse 116, respirations 22, and blood pressure 100/70 mm. Hg. Rales were present, the heart was slightly enlarged, and a soft systolic murmur was heard. The fingers were clubbed. The patient suddenly died.

Autopsy examination revealed endomyocardial fibrosis with a mural thrombus of the left ventricle, superimposed acute bacterial endocarditis, bronchopneumonia, pleural effusions of 500 ml. on each side, and pronounced passive hyperemia of the liver. The heart weighed 360 Gms., lungs 880 and 770 Gms., liver 2700 Gms., and spleen 520 Gms.

THE ENTITY

Endomyocardial fibrosis is a common cause of heart failure in Uganda although it occurs throughout Africa; it is less common in Indonesia, Southern India, and South America (1). It affects all ages and both sexes but is noticeably frequent in young adults. Onset may be heralded by transient pericardial effusion after which fever and relentlessly progressive heart failure develop. The functional effects include mitral regurgitation which is manifested by right and left ventricular failure, and obstruction of the right ventricle which is evidenced clinically by ascites and edema without dyspnea. Digitalis and steroid therapy are not helpful.

The lesion is a pearly white plaque of endocardial fibrosis that occurs in one or both ventricles and measures 2 to 5 mm. in thickness. The surface is often covered by superimposed reddish brown mural thrombus. The process extends to the posterior papillary muscle and attached chorda tendineae which become buried in the scar tissue. On this account the posterior leaflet of the mitral valve becomes immobilized and later fuses to the wall of the left ventricle. An unrelenting mitral insufficiency follows. The process may extend into the left atrium. On the right, the tricuspid leaflets may be affected and the endocardial mass may be so great as to fill that chamber. Contraction of this scar indents the right ventricle to produce a cardiac outline resembling the map of Africa. This radiographic configuration is known as "the Heart of Africa."

Microsections reveal a superficial zone of clear hyalinized tissue, an intermediate zone of loose fibrous connective tissue, and a deep zone of richly vascularized granulation tissue that extends into the myocardium. The muscle fibers at this junction reveal atrophy and degeneration. A light infiltration with lymphocytes and macrophages is present. Granules of calcium are frequent in

1. Davies, J.N.P., and Ball, J.D. The pathology of endomyocardial fibrosis in Uganda. Brit. Heart J. 17: 337-359, 1955.

ENDOMYOCARDIAL FIBROSIS

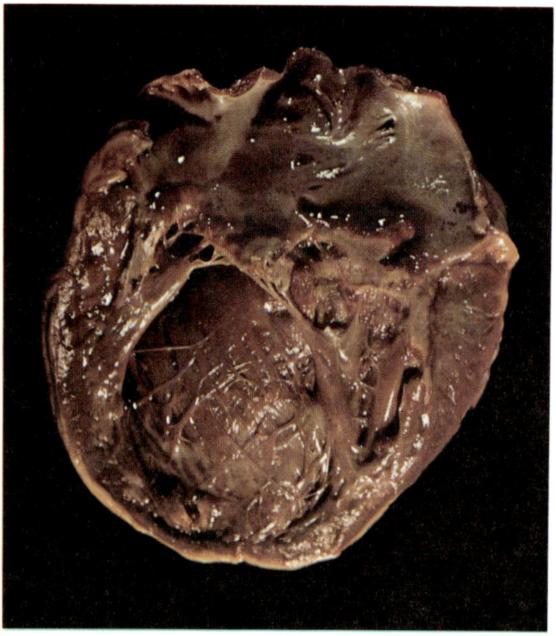

The heart is opened, showing the left atrium above and the left ventricle below. A thick layer of pale yellow exudate extends from the endocardium at the base of the chamber to affect both leaflets of the mitral valve. At the apex of the left ventricle there is a mural thrombus composed of similar exudate, and a subendocardial gray scar that is smooth and glistening.

The cut surfaces of the left ventricle reveal exudate and necrotic tissue that have extended into a papillary muscle on the left and into the myocardium of the wall on the right.

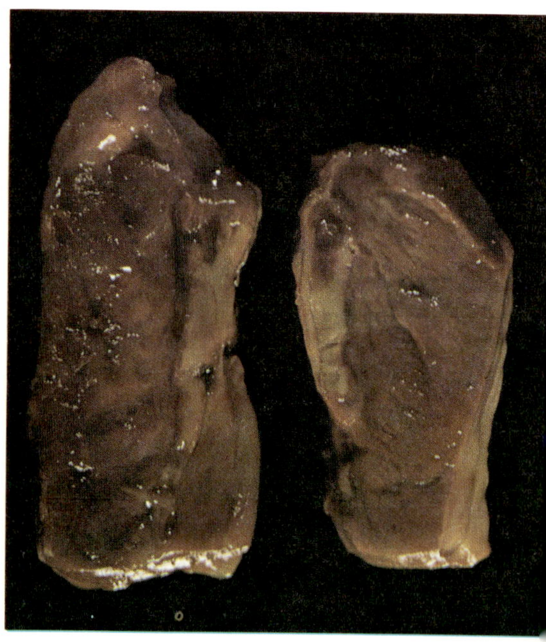

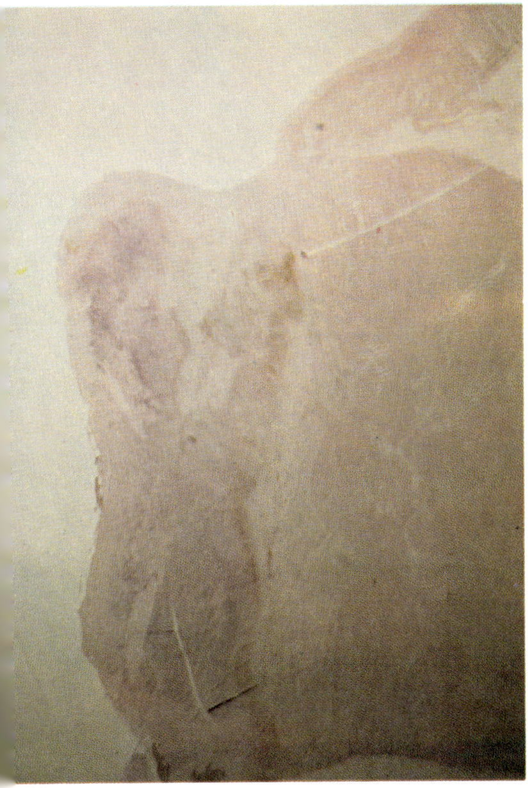

The unmagnified histologic section shows the atrial wall above and the ventricular wall below within the endocardial surface on the left. Necrosis and inflammation bind the mitral leaflet to the endocardial surface and render it nonfunctional.

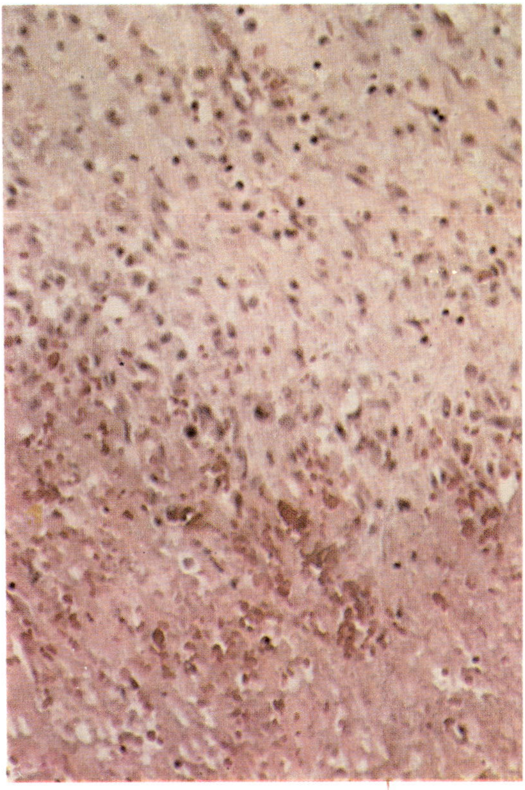

The microsection of the lesion reveals fibrin, cellular debris, and necrotic muscle with a thick organizing margin composed of granulation tissue.

the scar. This structure suggests injury to the subendocardial muscle, overlying thrombus formation, organization, obstruction of arterioluminal vessels, immobilization of the wall, and extension to the adjacent chorda tendineae and valve leaflets. The heart may be atrophic, normal, or hypertrophic.

The cause is unknown. The aortic and pulmonic valves are unaffected. Superimposed bacterial endocarditis is uncommon. Blood cultures are negative. Murmurs are inconspicuous and the electrocardiogram is non-specific. Syphilis and malnutrition are not more common in these patients. Extracardiac lesions are attributable to congestive failure or terminal infection. There is no resemblance to rheumatic disease. The progress of the failure is irreversible; death occurs within a few weeks or months of the onset.

BACTERIAL ENDOCARDITIS, MITRAL

CLINICAL ACCOUNT 6131

The patient was a white female 80 years old who noted a small mass in the right upper quadrant of her abdomen one year before hospital admission. This mass gradually enlarged and was associated with anorexia, weight loss, weakness, and a constant dull pain. She had also experienced dyspnea on exertion and paroxysms of nocturnal dyspnea during the past year.

The vital signs were normal. The heart was enlarged to the left, an aortic systolic and an apical diastolic murmur were heard, and the abdominal mass was pulsatile. Laboratory data were not helpful. An x-ray of the abdomen disclosed calcification in the region of the abdominal mass. Aortography revealed an aneurysm of the lower aorta. An exploratory operation was performed, but the aneurysm was not resected.

Recovery was uneventful until the eleventh post-operative day when the temperature rose to 100.8 degrees F. On the next day the temperature was 104.0 degrees F., the blood pressure fell to 70/50 mm. Hg., and the patient became unresponsive and died.

The heart weighed 400 Gm. and revealed bacterial endocarditis of the mitral valve and abscesses of the myocardium. In addition, there were septic emboli in the lungs with infarction of the pulmonary tissue and abscess formation. Recent infarcts were identified in both kidneys and in one papillary muscle of the left ventricle. Old infarcts were present in the myocardium and spleen.

THE ENTITY

Bacterial endocarditis occurs in children with congenital heart disease, in young adults with rheumatic heart disease, in middle aged adults with no heart disease, and in the elderly with such lesions as calcific disease of the mitral ring or aortic valve (1). The main congenital conditions include interventricular septal defect, bicuspid aortic valve, patent ductus arteriosus, coarctation of the aorta, and the tetralogy of Fallot. These and rheumatic lesions alter hemodynamics so that high pressure jets damage endothelial sites and predispose to infection.

While many organisms may be causal, *Streptococcus viridans* (alpha hemolytic) is most often associated with subacute disease while acute endocarditis is caused mainly by virulent staphylococci and enterococci. Pre-existing conditions associated with transient bacteremia include gingivitis, poor oral hygiene, minor dental procedures, tonsillectomy, and viral pneumonitis. Enterococcal organisms may similarly be associated with prostatitis, catheterization, parturition, and especially septic abortion. Staphylococcal endocarditis may arise from subcutaneous furuncles, wound infections, and osteomyelitis.

The clinical features are protracted fever associated with a heart murmur and evidence of embolization. The fever tends to be slight, irregular, and intermittent. The murmur is apical and sys-

1. Pomerance, A. Pathology and valvular heart disease. Brit. Heart J. 34: 437, 1972.

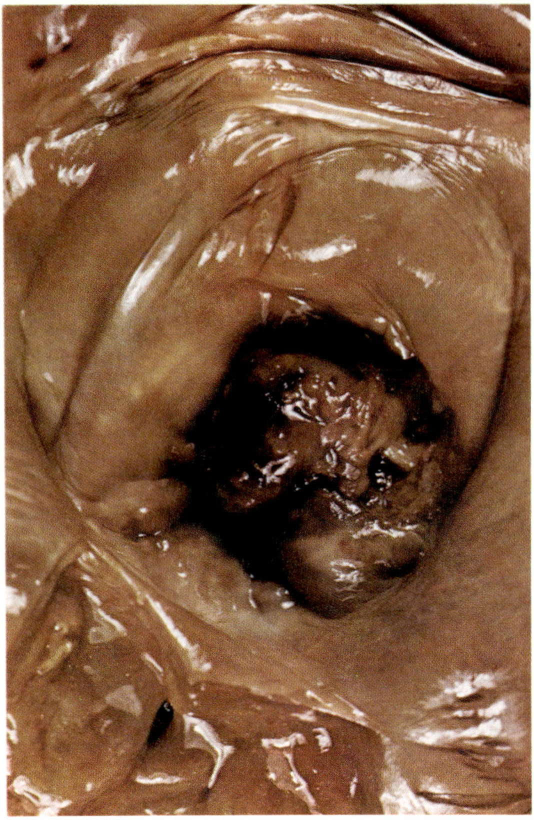

BACTERIAL ENDOCARDITIS, MITRAL

The unopened mitral valve viewed from above, reveals a large, friable, dark-red vegetation that is attached to the atrial surface of the posterior leaflet.

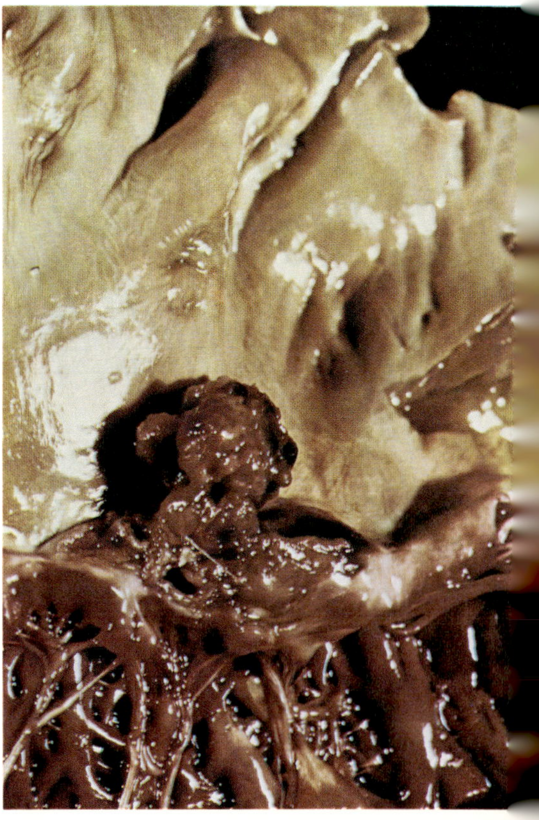

The opened valve discloses the vegetation. The leaflet adjacent to the base of the vegetation is perforated.

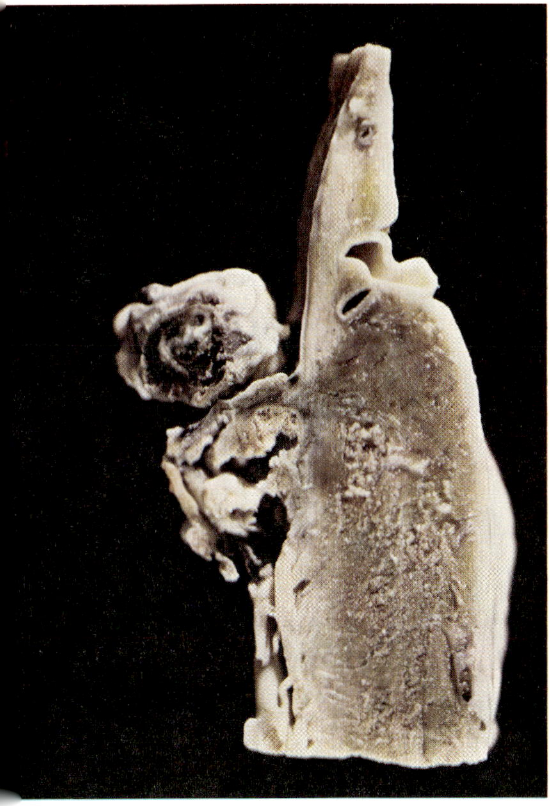

The fixed cut surface reveals the atrial wall (upper right), ventricular wall (lower right), and mitral leaflet projecting to the left. The large bulky vegetation lies on top of the leaflet and penetrates through it so that a septic mass also lies underneath the leaflet at the endocardial junction. An abscess is apparent in the myocardium just below the level of the mitral valve ring. Note the coronary vessels in the atrioventricular sulcus.

Microsection reveals the septic vegetation and the inflamed and focally necrotic valve leaflet.

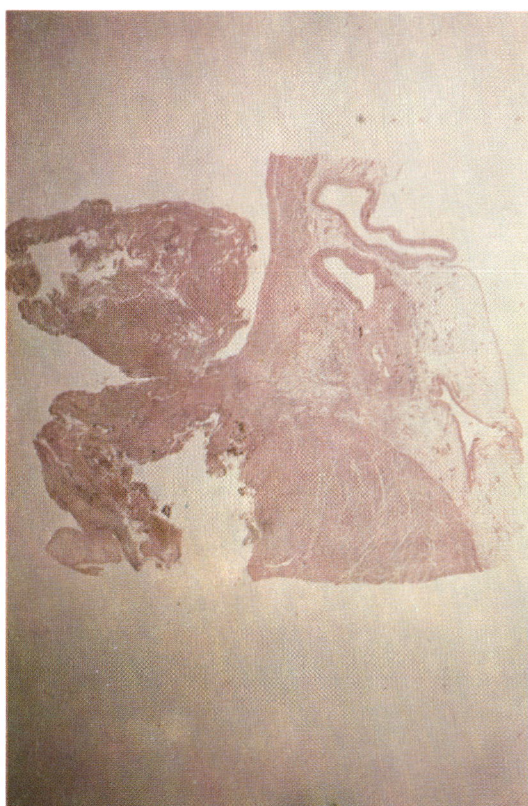

tolic and may be regarded as insignificant. Fever lasting more than a week, however, associated with a murmur, should suggest the diagnosis. Embolization is often indicated by showers of petechiae that are especially noticeable on the skin, in the retinae, over the sclerae, and under the fingernails. Positive blood cultures tend to confirm the diagnosis.

The mitral and aortic valves are most often affected. The vegetations tend to be large, bulky, friable, and attached to the free borders of the valves. The vegetations are composed of strands of fibrin, masses of platelets, necrotic tissue, erythrocytic debris, degenerated leukocytes, and colonies of bacteria. Extension of the process causes erosion of the valves with perforation, rupture of the chorda tendineae, and abscess formation in the myocardium. Complications include pericarditis, myocarditis, and septic embolization. The consequences of the septic emboli include mycotic aneurysms, disseminated abscesses, acute pleuritis, mesenteric occlusion, sudden hemiparesis, splenic infarcts, renal failure, acute arthritis, and debilitation associated with progressive anemia.

The condition is curable with antibiotic therapy but the mortality remains high because medical attention is delayed and disseminated infection or intractable heart failure is already in progress. Death is usually attributable to congestive failure, renal failure, uncontrolled infection or hemorrhage from rupture of an arterial aneurysm.

RHEUMATIC MITRAL STENOSIS

CLINICAL ACCOUNT 6271

The patient was a Chinese female 63 years old who entered the hospital because of extreme shortness of breath. She had had rheumatic fever at age 17, "heart trouble" at age 22, and congestive failure requiring hospitalization at ages 56, 59, and 61. At the time of hospitalization she was able to walk only 8 to 10 steps to the bathroom and had pronounced orthopnea and frequent paroxysms of nocturnal dyspnea.

The systolic blood pressure was 100 mm. Hg.; the diastolic pressure was not audible. The pulse rate was 90. The neck veins filled from below at 45 degrees recumbency. Rales were audible over both lung fields. The precordium was pulsatile; the point of maximum impulse was in the epigastrium. Harsh systolic and diastolic murmurs over the precordium radiated to the neck and axilla. The liver was both enlarged and tender.

The blood and urine were normal. A chest x-ray revealed marked dilatation of the heart and pronounced hyperemia of the lungs. Digitalis, diuretics, salt-free diet, and nasal oxygen were given. Her shortness of breath increased in severity, and she died after 49 days in the hospital.

Autopsy examination revealed hypertrophy of the heart (425 Gm.), chronic rheumatic endocarditis of the mitral valve with slight stenosis and marked regurgitation, and centrilobular fibrosis of the liver. There were also edema of the lungs, sclerosis of the pulmonary arteries, an adenoma of the thyroid, and a polyp of the endometrium.

THE ENTITY

The cause of mitral stenosis is rheumatic disease. The mitral leaflets undergo fibrosis, thickening, retraction, and fusion of the commissures. The process extends to the chordae tendineae, which thicken, fuse, and contract. These changes, often with calcification, reduce the mitral opening to a small fixed "button hole" aperture that can neither open widely in diastole nor close completely in systole. The stenosis is compensated for by dilatation and hypertrophy of the left atrium for long periods. When this fails, the hydrostatic pressure in the lungs increases, and dilatation and hypertrophy of the right ventricle take place. Mitral stenosis causes a diastolic murmur. X-rays reveal dilatation of the left atrium and fullness of the pulmonary conus. Prolonged hyperemia of the lungs causes diffuse fibrosis and hemosiderin deposition, known as brown induration, that is associated with cough, rust colored sputum, and hemoptysis. As the tricuspid valve ring dilates, the passive hyperemia escapes the pulmonary circuit and becomes generalized.

With mitral insufficiency the murmur is systolic and the left ventricle also dilates. Compensatory capacity is large, however, and the physiologic disturbance tends to be slight until the regurgitation is pronounced. Therefore, atrial dilatation and pulmonic hypertension tend to be less in degree and later in time than with mitral stenosis. The two conditions, stenosis and insufficiency, tend to occur together.

RHEUMATIC MITRAL STENOSIS

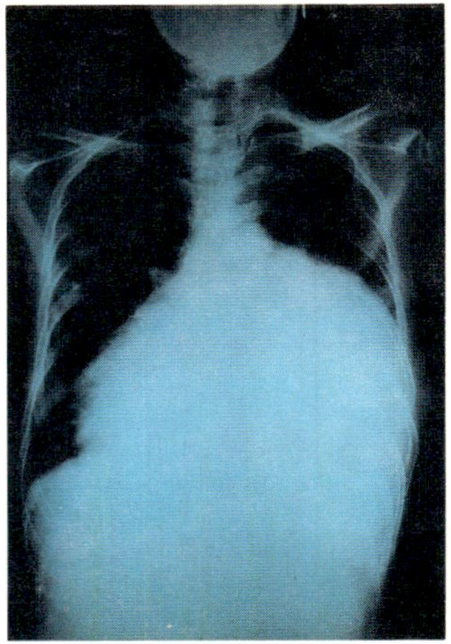

The chest x-ray revealed extreme enlargement of the cardiac outline and pronounced hyperemia of the lungs.

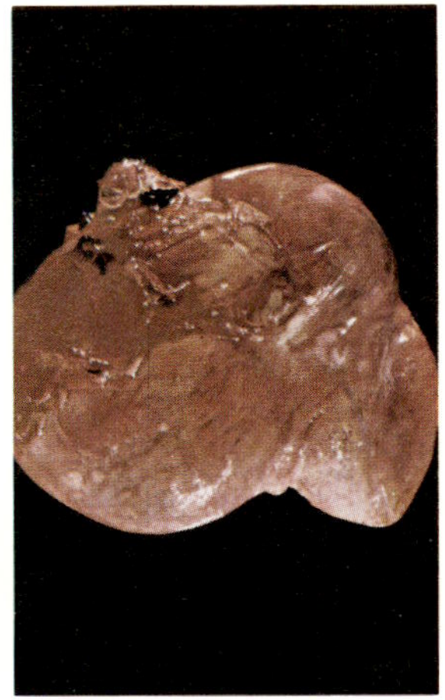

The photograph shows the posterior surface of the heart with an enormously enlarged left atrium projecting to the left as an ovoid mass, and the ventricles projecting downward to a blunt point on the right. It can be foreseen that this degree of left atrial enlargement might distort the cardiac outline, compress the lung, and push the esophagus to one side.

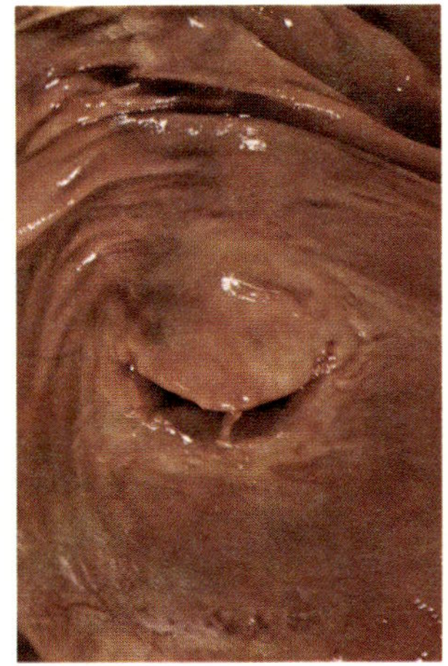

The mitral valve reveals thickening, fibrosis, and commissural adhesions. The aperture is stenosed. The consequence is to cause dilatation of the left atrium, passive hyperemia of the lungs, hypertrophy of the right ventricle, and eventually right ventricular failure.

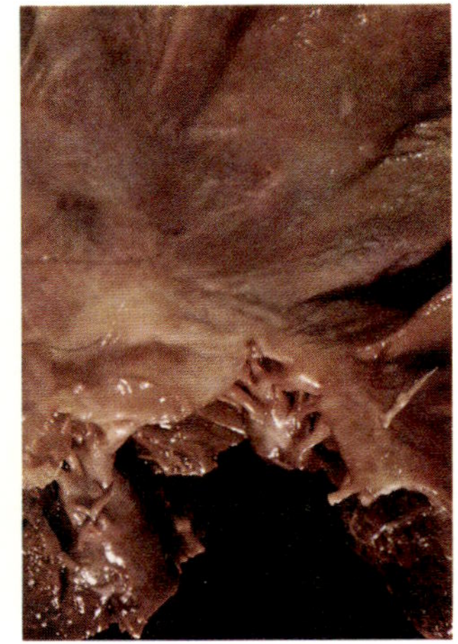

The opened valve shows the leaflet to be thick and stiff, the chordae fused and short, and the structure nonpliable and rigid. These changes, plus a fine vascularity that is often grossly evident over the atrial surface of the leaflet, are the characteristic gross changes that are caused by rheumatic mitral disease.

CALCIFICATION OF MITRAL ANNULUS

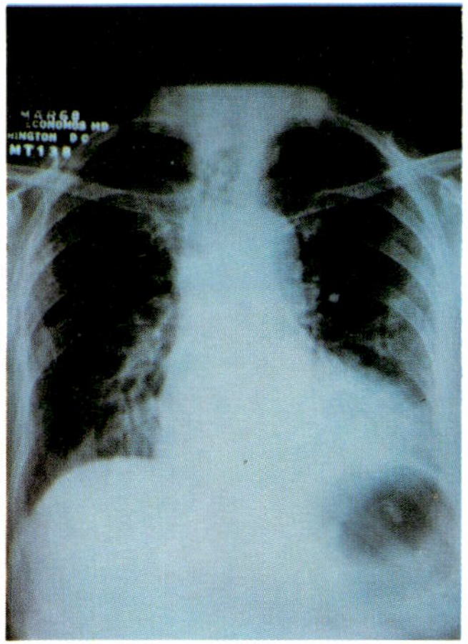

The chest x-ray disclosed blunting of the costophrenic angle on the left, a finding indicative of pleural effusion. The prominent bulge of the left ventricle suggests cardiac hypertrophy. The lung fields are clear. Calcification of the mitral annulus is not visible here.

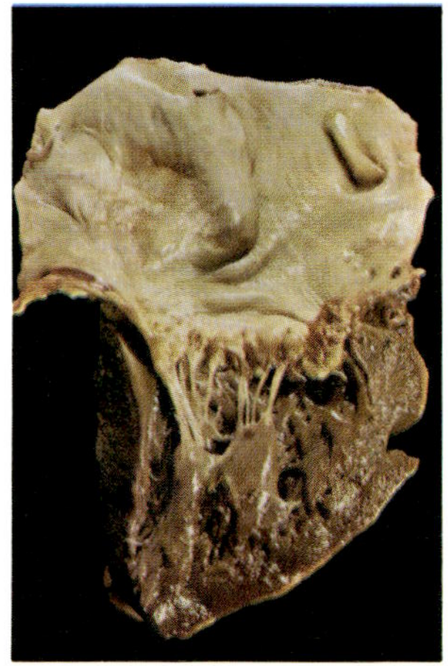

The atrium, ventricle, papillary muscles, and chordae tendineae are normal. The mitral valve is smooth and overlies a thick ring of calcified tissue that bulges upward underneath the leaflets.

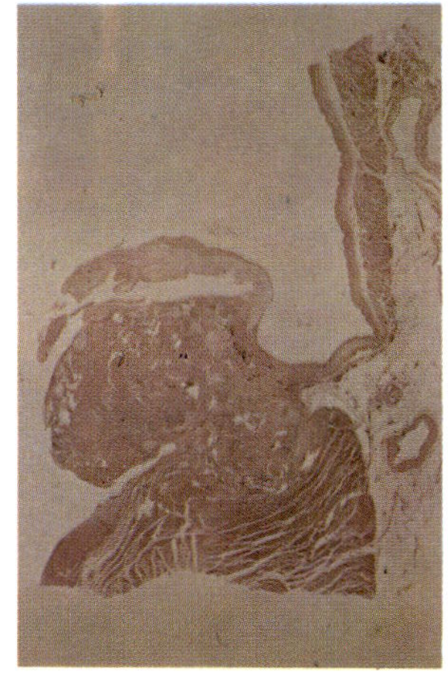

On histologic section the free valve can be seen overlying the subjacent calcified mass. The ventricular muscle is below, and the left atrium is to the right and above.

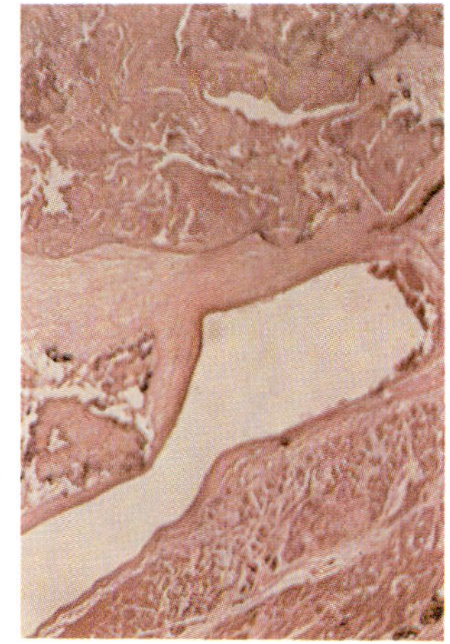

The smooth, sharply delineated and uninflamed margin of the calcified annulus with the adjacent ventricular muscle is shown.

CALCIFICATION OF MITRAL ANNULUS

CLINICAL ACCOUNT 5813

The patient was a white female 92 years old who was admitted to the hospital because of dyspnea. Shortness of breath had been pronounced on several occasions during the past three years. The patient had never been in congestive failure, she had never taken digitalis, and she had never been hypertensive. She had been diabetic for the past eight years, and a right radical mastectomy had been performed twenty years previously. She was thin, undernourished, confused, and markedly short of breath. Rales and rhonchi were present over both lung fields. A chest x-ray was interpreted as showing pulmonary edema. The heart was not enlarged, the rhythm was regular, and no murmurs were heard. She was treated with penicillin, aminophylline, digitalis and a diuretic. Her condition steadily worsened and she died after three days in the hospital.

Autopsy examination revealed interstitial fibrosis of the lungs, pleural effusions, (500 ml., right, 600 ml., left), pulmonary hyperemia, arteriolar nephrosclerosis, and calcification of the annulus of the mitral valve.

THE ENTITY

Calcification of the mitral annulus is common in women; the average age is 70 years, and the lesion is rare under 50. Some part of the mitral annulus is calcified in 10 per cent of adult autopsies, although massive calcification is seen in less than 1 per cent (1). The latter consists of a shelf of calcium that projects into the left ventricle just beneath the peripheral attachment of the mitral leaflets. Marked functional disturbance is uncommon, although both mitral stenosis and insufficiency occur (2). Mitral insufficiency is caused by loss of the sphincteric action of the annulus and by elevation of the leaflets, which tightens the chordae tendineae and pulls the free margins downward so that closure is impaired. Mitral stenosis is caused by projection of the calcified shelf into the ventricle so that the orifice is narrowed and by fixation of the leaflets so that they are transformed into rigid projections. Auscultation reveals a loud, harsh, or musical systolic murmur at the apex. X-rays disclose a J, U, or oval-shaped density within the cardiac outline. These findings in an elderly female with no history of rheumatic disease suggest the diagnosis.

The condition is regarded as an end stage of a degenerative process. It is distinguished from healed rheumatic disease by mitral leaflets that have thin free margins and by chordae tendineae that are delicate and discrete. The condition is not infrequently associated with calcific stenosis of the aortic valve.

1. Simon, M.A., and Liu, S.F. Calcification of the mitral valve annulus and its relation to functional valve disturbance. Am. Heart J. 48:497, 1954.
2. Korn, D., De Sanctis, R.W., and Sell, S. Massive calcification of the mitral annulus. New Eng. J. Med. 267:900. 1962.

BACTERIAL ENDOCARDITIS, AORTIC

CLINICAL ACCOUNT 5832

The patient was a Negro woman 39 years old who complained of cough, fever, and dyspnea of seven weeks' duration. Vigorous antibiotic therapy, begun four weeks after the onset, provided only partial relief. Later, weakness, anorexia, and swelling of the ankles developed. The dyspnea and ankle swelling became progressively worse, and swelling of the abdomen followed. Fluid accumulated in the chest, and four thoracenteses were performed; cultures were negative. The patient had not been previously ill, although a miscarriage occurred one month prior to the present illness. Pelvic instrumentation was denied.

The temperature was 99.0 degrees F., pulse rate 150, respiratory rate 60, and blood pressure 170/20 mm. Hg. The neck veins were distended. Fluid was percussed in both pleural spaces. The heart was enlarged, and a harsh systolic murmur was heard over the left upper sternal border. The abdomen was distended; a fluid wave was present. Pitting edema of the legs was pronounced. The hemoglobin was 7.6 Gm., the hematocrit was 25 per cent, and the leukocytes numbered 10,800, with 84 segmented granulocytes, 7 band cells, 8 lymphocytes, and 1 monocyte. She was treated with digoxin, diuretics, antibiotics, oxygen, and ethacrynic acid. She died of respiratory failure on the second hospital day.

Autopsy examination revealed bacterial endocarditis of the aortic valve, nonbacterial thrombotic endocardiosis of the tricuspid valve, acute fibrinous and organizing pericarditis, pericardial effusion (750 ml.), recent infarcts of the spleen and both kidneys, and acute necrotizing endometritis. Cultures of blood, pericardial fluid, and endometrium revealed enterococci.

THE ENTITY

Bacterial endocarditis occurs in children with congenital heart disease, in young adults with rheumatic heart disease, in middle aged adults with no heart disease, and in the elderly with such lesions as calcific disease of the mitral ring or aortic valve (1). The main congenital conditions include interventricular septal defect, bicuspid aortic valve, patent ductus arteriosus, coarctation of the aorta, and the tetralogy of Fallot. These and rheumatic lesions alter hemodynamics so that high pressure jets damage endothelial sites and predispose to infection.

While many organisms may be causal, *Streptococcus viridans,* (alpha hemolytic) is most often associated with subacute disease while acute endocarditis is caused mainly by virulent staphylococci and enterococci. Pre-existing conditions associated with transient bacteremia include gingivitis, poor oral hygiene, minor dental procedures, tonsillectomy, and viral pneumonitis. Enterococcal organisms may similarly be associated with prostatitis, catheterization, parturition, and especially septic abortion. Staphylococcal endocarditis may arise from subcutaneous furuncles, wound infections, and osteomyelitis.

The clinical features are protracted fever associated with a heart murmur and evidence of embolization. The fever tends to be

1. Pomerance, A. Pathology and valvular heart disease. Brit. Heart J. 34: 437, 1972.

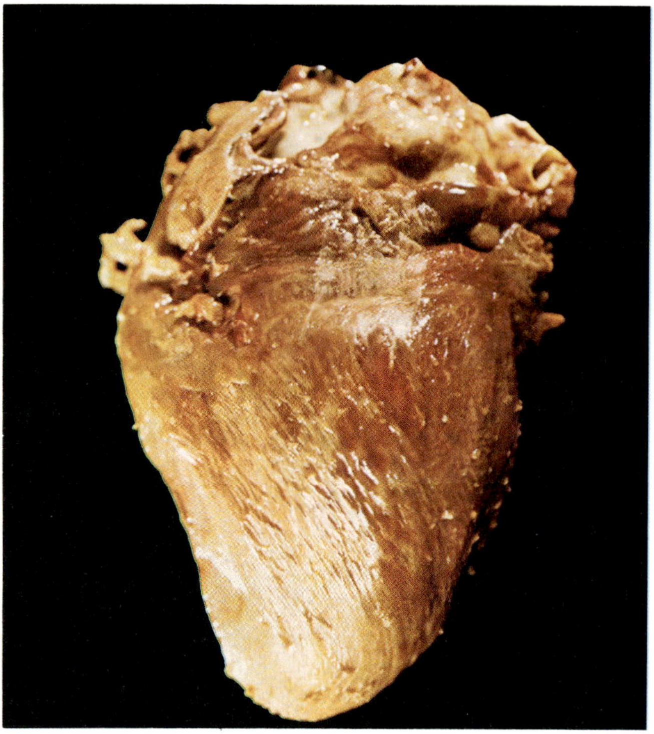

The epicardium is roughened by granulation tissue and acute fibrinous adhesions.

BACTERIAL ENDOCARDITIS, AORTIC

Opposite page, left:
The unopened aortic valve, viewed from above, reveals a large friable and hemorrhagic vegetation attached to the free border of one cusp.

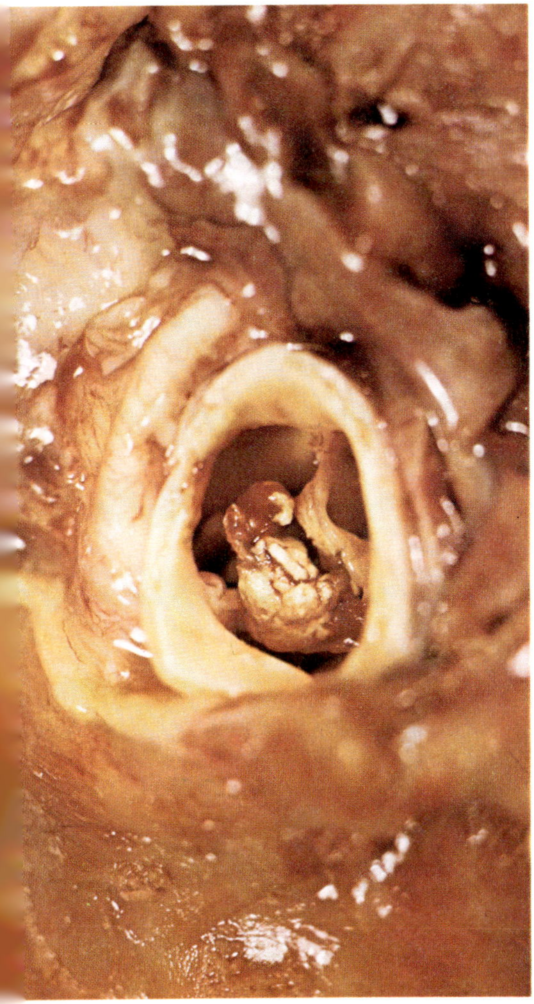

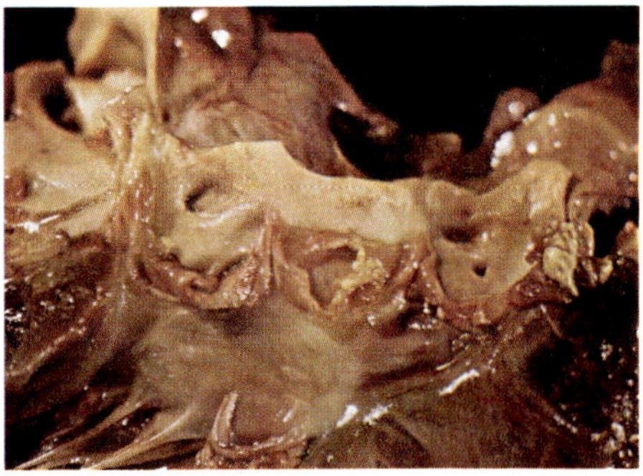

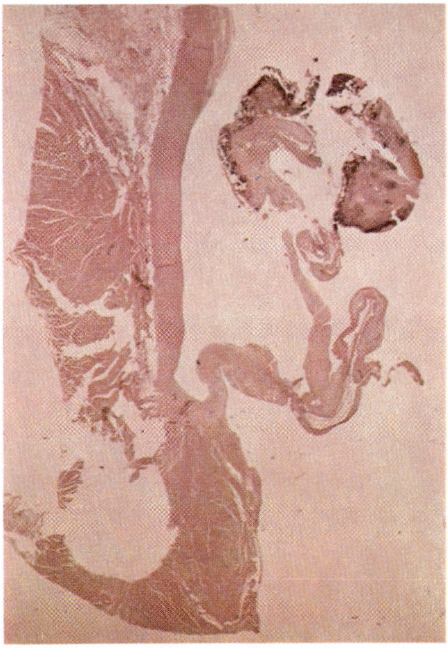

Right, upper photo:
The opened aortic valve discloses rupture or perforation of all three cusps. The vegetation, also shown in the preceding photograph, is attached to a ruptured cusp at one side of the opened valve. The reason for the patient's low diastolic pressure, recent infarcts of kidneys and spleen, and fulminant cardiac failure is now evident.

Right, lower photo:
The histologic section reveals the aortic cusp (right), aortic wall (center), and ventricular muscle (below). The vegetation is situated on top of the cusp; it is composed of fibrin, bacterial colonies, erythrocytes, leukocytes, and masses of platelets. Failure of antibacterial agents to penetrate this avascular structure can be understood. The mechanism of septic embolization is also clear.

slight, irregular, and intermittent. The murmur is apical and systolic and may be regarded as insignificant. Fever lasting more than a week, however, associated with a murmur, should suggest the diagnosis. Embolization is often indicated by showers of petechiae that are especially noticeable on the skin, in the retinae, over the sclerae, and under the fingernails. Positive blood cultures tend to confirm the diagnosis.

The mitral and aortic valves are most often affected. The vegetations tend to be large, bulky, friable, and attached to the free borders of the valves. The vegetations are composed of strands of fibrin, masses of platelets, necrotic tissue, erythrocytic debris, degenerated leukocytes, and colonies of bacteria. Extension of the process causes erosion of the valves with perforation, rupture of the chorda tendineae, and abscess formation in the myocardium. Complications include pericarditis, myocarditis, and septic embolization. The consequences of the septic emboli include mycotic aneurysms, disseminated abscesses, acute pleuritis, mesenteric occlusion, sudden hemiparesis, splenic infarcts, renal failure, acute arthritis, and debilitation associated with progressive anemia.

The condition is curable with antibiotic therapy but the mortality remains high because medical attention is delayed and disseminated infection or intractable heart failure is already in progress. Death is usually attributable to congestive failure, renal failure, uncontrolled infection or hemorrhage from rupture of an arterial aneurysm.

RHEUMATIC AORTIC STENOSIS

CLINICAL ACCOUNT 6196

The patient was a white female 75 years old who had had rheumatic fever at age 15, "heart flutter" at age 61, hypertension since age 65, and angina pectoris since age 70. For the past three months there had been dyspnea on exertion, orthopnea, and recurring edema of the ankles. On the day before admission a severe pain developed in the precordium that radiated to both shoulders and was not relieved by treatment with nitroglycerin.

The blood pressure was 92/60 mm. Hg. Rales were audible over the lower chest, the heart was enlarged to the left, a systolic murmur was heard over the aortic area, and a diastolic gallop was detected. The ankles displayed slight edema.

The urine was loaded with leukocytes. The hemoglobin was 12.9 Gm., hematocrit 41, and leukocytes 9,000, with a normal differential count. The serum glutamic transaminase and lactic dehydrogenase were normal. An electrocardiogram failed to reveal a recent infarct. A chest x-ray disclosed pleural effusions and left ventricular enlargement. Although digitalis and diuretics were given, the shortness of breath progressed and the patient died after fourteen days in the hospital.

Autopsy examination revealed rheumatic disease of the aortic valve with stenosis and calcification. The heart weighed 475 Gm. The epicardium was roughened with fibrous adhesions and the myocardium disclosed extensive focal fibrosis and an old infarct of the left ventricle. Additional diagnoses included hyperemia of the lungs and liver, a bilateral pleural effusion of 400 and 350 ml., arteriolar nephrosclerosis, a small primary carcinoma of the right breast, and a cortical adenoma of the left adrenal. No recent infarct of myocardium was found.

THE ENTITY

Rheumatic carditis is the most crippling heart disease of youth and early middle age. It causes pericarditis, myocarditis with Aschoff bodies, endocarditis of the left atrium, and inflammation of the heart valves. As the inflammation subsides, fibrosis develops, especially in the valves. The mitral valve is affected most often, the mitral and aortic valves together next most often, and the aortic valve alone least often. Tricuspid and pulmonic valve involvement is uncommon.

The aortic cusps become thick, stiff, and fused to one another at the commissures. Microscopically the fibrosis is pronounced, hyalinization is frequent, lymphocytic infiltration is regular, and vascularization with minute musculo-elastic arteries is constant. Rigidity of the cusps prevents flattening with systole and closure with diastole. Stenosis and insufficiency result. Aortic stenosis causes a prolongation of systole, a lowering of systolic pressure, a systolic murmur transmitted to the neck, a thrill over the aortic area, dilatation and hypertrophy of the left ventricle, and congestive failure. The failure is badly tolerated, and death may be abrupt. With insufficiency, the murmur is diastolic, the pulse pressure is wide, and the subungual capillaries and retinal arterioles show an exaggerated "dancing" pulsation. The two conditions often occur together.

RHEUMATIC AORTIC STENOSIS

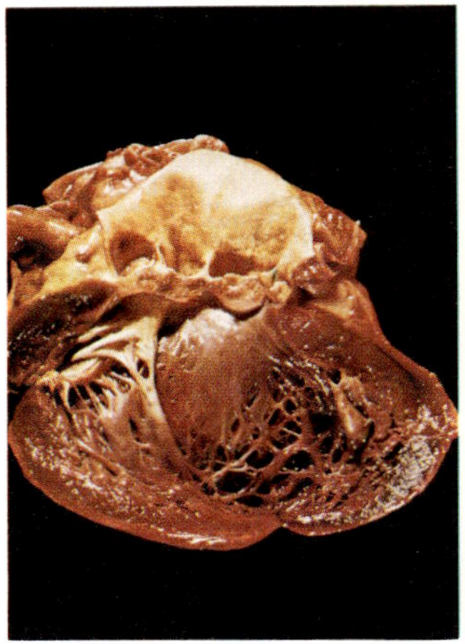

The opened left ventricle reveals the aortic valve in which the cusps are fused along their margins of closure. This fusion prevented retraction during systole and induced a work hypertrophy on the part of the ventricular muscle.

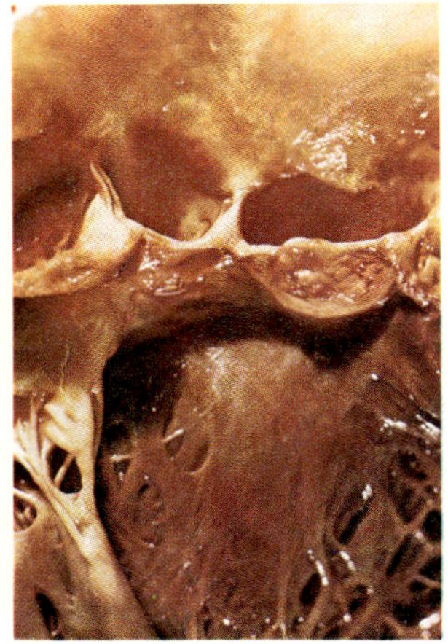

Rheumatic disease first affects the cusps along their margins of closure which lie just below the free borders. Along those margins fibrosis takes place so that adjacent cusps are sealed together. This process forms a rigid shelf that projects into the aortic outlet and causes a permanent stenosis of that channel. Note the fibrosis of the cusps in this specimen.

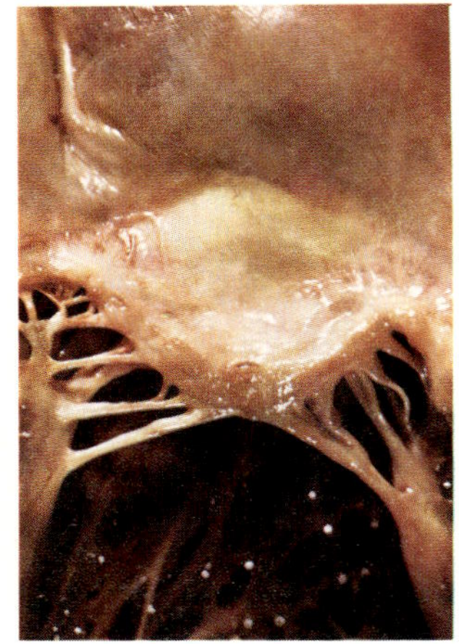

The mitral valve also discloses rheumatic scarring although the degree is slight. The leaflet is thick and stiff and opaque rather than thin, pliable, and translucent. In addition, the chordae tendineae are thickened and fused rather than delicate and discrete. Both of these changes are characteristic features of rheumatic disease.

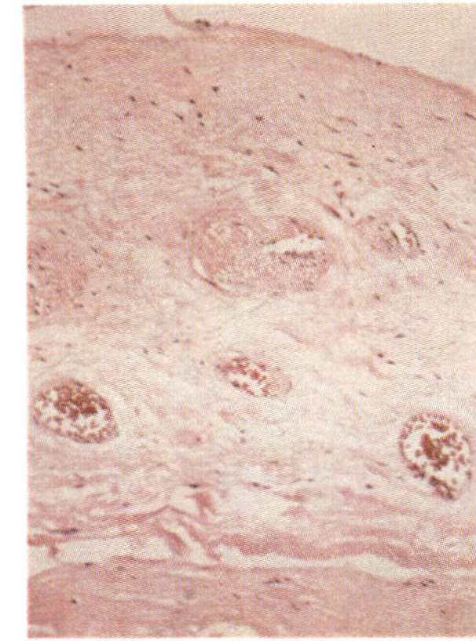

This microsection of mitral valve reveals vascularization and fibrous thickening. While the leaflet is normally without vessels, the vascularization of rheumatic disease is unique in that both capillaries and musculoelastic arteries form. In the photograph, the capillaries are deep and contain blood while the thick-walled small arteries are near the upper surface and are empty.

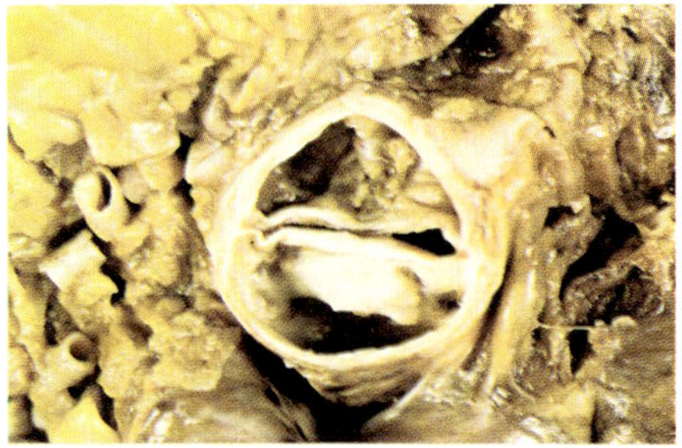

The right and left coronary cusps are at the top of the photograph; the raphe between them is calcified and broken down.

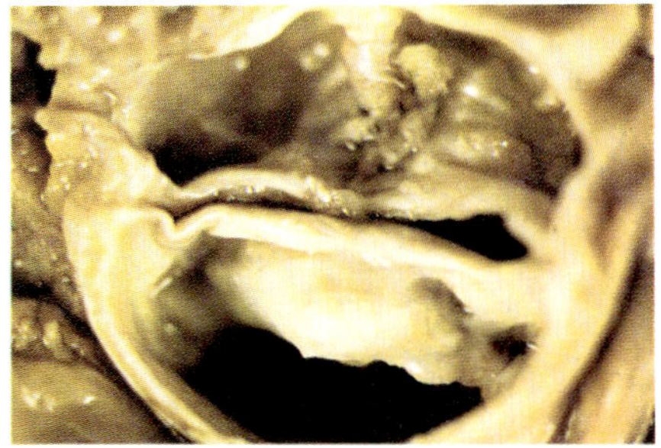

A close-up of the aortic valve reveals the two coronary arteries emerging from the fused upper cusps. A rigid transverse cleft is the only opening of the valve.

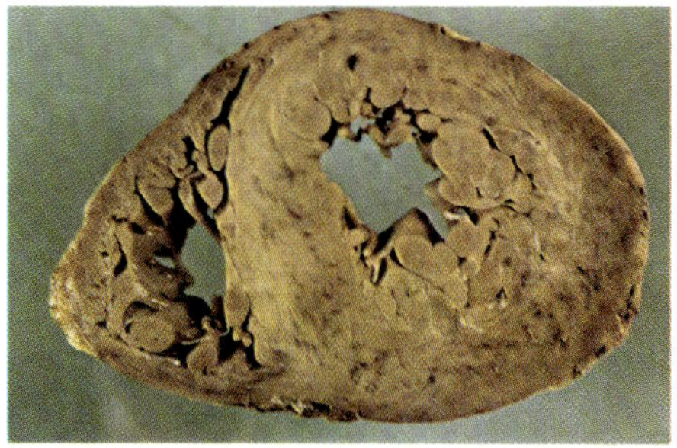

The cut surface of the myocardium shows pronounced thickening of the left ventricle.

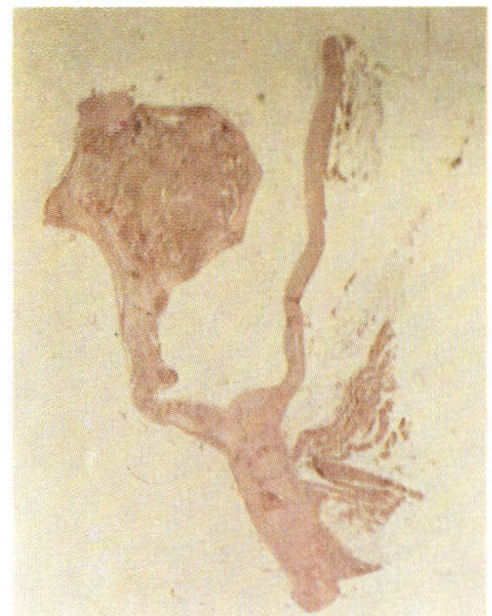

The unmagnified histologic section is from the lower noncoronary cusp; it reveals that the smooth calcified mass seen in the previous photograph is located within the sinus of Valsalva just below the free border of the cusp.

CALCIFIC AORTIC STENOSIS

CALCIFIC AORTIC STENOSIS

CLINICAL ACCOUNT 7259

The patient was a white female 82 years old who had experienced episodes of congestive heart failure at irregular intervals over the past twelve years. At these times she noted paroxysms of nocturnal dyspnea, dyspnea on exertion, edema of the ankles, and orthopnea requiring three pillows for relief. During the past six months the dyspnea and orthopnea increased, and weakness and fatigue developed. During the two weeks before admission there had been a 5-pound gain of weight. There had been no chest pain or history of myocardial infarction. The blood pressure was 100/70 mm. Hg. Respiratory distress was moderate, the jugular veins were distended to the mandibles, and basilar rales were heard over both lower lung fields. The heart was not enlarged, the rhythm was regular, and no murmurs were heard. The liver edge was palpated 10 cm. below the right costal margin. The extremities revealed pronounced subcutaneous edema without clubbing or cyanosis. On the day of admission the patient became cyanotic, tachypneic, and diaphoretic; coma developed and death occurred that evening.

Autopsy examination revealed calcific disease of the aortic valve, hypertrophy of the myocardium, pulmonary emphysema, and a pulmonary embolus with infarction of the lower lobe of right lung. The heart weighed 550 Gms. The mitral, tricuspid, and pulmonic valves were normal.

THE ENTITY

Calcific disease of the aortic valve occurs more often in men than women and three times more often after the age of 50 years than before. It is uncommon in blacks. The patients complain of anginal pain and exertional dyspnea; they may also experience palpitation, dizziness, and syncope. Physical signs include a weak pulse, a cardiac outline enlarged to the left, a harsh systolic murmur, an aortic thrill, and a diminished aortic second sound. X-rays disclose left ventricular predominance and a "dancing shadow" at the base of the heart. Despite these characteristics, however, the left ventricle is sometimes not enlarged, the aortic murmur is often absent, and the aortic thrill occurs in only a fourth of cases (1).

The process appears to begin by fusion of the right and left coronary cusps at the commissure to form a bicuspid valve with a raphe that later calcifies. Less often all three commissures are equally affected. The fused cusps become rigid, and the calcification in them becomes nodular, extensive, and pronounced within the cusps and often on the ventricular aspects as well. Ulceration of the endocardium is rare. Coronary atherosclerosis is not lessened by the aortic calcification. With symptoms the outlook is poor, i.e., only half survive a period of two years. Without surgical replacement of the valve, death may be sudden but most often occurs with congestive failure.

The cause is controversial; Karsner and Koletsky found stigmata of rheumatic disease in most hearts with calcific aortic stenosis, while Roberts presumes most to be congenital bicuspid valves that later calcify because of aging and degenerative change (2). Peery makes the case for Brucella endocarditis as the initiating event (3).

1. Karsner, H.T., and Koletsky, S. Calcific Disease of the Aortic Valve. J.B. Lippincott Co., 1947.
2. Roberts, W.C. Anatomically isolated aortic valvular disease. Am. J. Med. 49:151-159, 1970.
3. Peery, T.M. Brucellosis and heart disease. Etiology of calcific aortic stenosis. J.A.M.A. 166:1123-1127, 1958.

SUPERIOR CAVAL SYNDROME

CLINICAL ACCOUNT 5940

The patient was a Negro male 45 years old who entered the hospital because of increasing shortness of breath. For the past six years he had had dyspnea on exertion, nocturnal paroxysms of dyspnea, and slight pain in the chest. The pain was especially prominent over the right hemithorax. For the past six months pain had also been present over the left side of the chest. The patient was a chronic alcoholic and had been hypertensive for the past 23 years.

The blood pressure was 140/110 mm. Hg. The conjunctivae were flushed and the buccal membranes were cyanotic. The right optic disc was blurred. The subcutaneous tissues of the face and neck were full and thick. The neck veins were distended and firm. A venous pattern over the chest was not described. The abdomen was distended; the remainder of the examination was not remarkable. An x-ray of the chest disclosed an enlarged right hilar shadow. Biopsy of a bronchus and a right supraclavicular lymph node revealed undifferentiated carcinoma at both sites. The patient died after two weeks in the hospital.

Autopsy examination revealed an undifferentiated carcinoma of the right main bronchus that metastasized widely and extended into the superior vena cava causing stenosis of that vessel. Additional significant diagnoses were hypertrophy of the heart, bronchopneumonia, and bronchiectasis of the right lung.

THE ENTITY

Superior vena caval obstruction has three principal causes: carcinoma of a bronchus, Hodgkin's disease of the mediastinum, aneurysm of the aorta. Less frequent are localized phlebitis and sclerosing mediastinitis (1). Clinical features include vertigo and throbbing headache that are accentuated by bending over. Physical signs include ruddy discoloration or cyanosis of the head, neck, and upper extremities, subcutaneous edema of the same parts, and elevation of the venous pressure of the upper extremities only. Dilated capillaries in the skin over the lower chest signify obstruction of the superior vena cava above the entrance of the azygos vein (2). Obstruction that is below or includes the azygos vein ostium is characterized by reversal of flow in dilated veins over the abdomen as blood passes through the superior epigastric veins to enter the external iliac veins and thence the inferior vena cava. The clinical course varies with the cause of the obstruction. Since most of the common causes are serious or progressive, the outlook is ordinarily grave.

1. McIntyre, F.T., and Sykes, E.M., Jr. Obstruction of the superior vena cava: A review of the literature and report of two personal cases. Ann. Int. Med. 30:925, 1949.
2. Schlecter, M.M. The superior vena cava syndrome. Am. J. Med. Sci. 227: 46, 1954.

SUPERIOR CAVAL SYNDROME

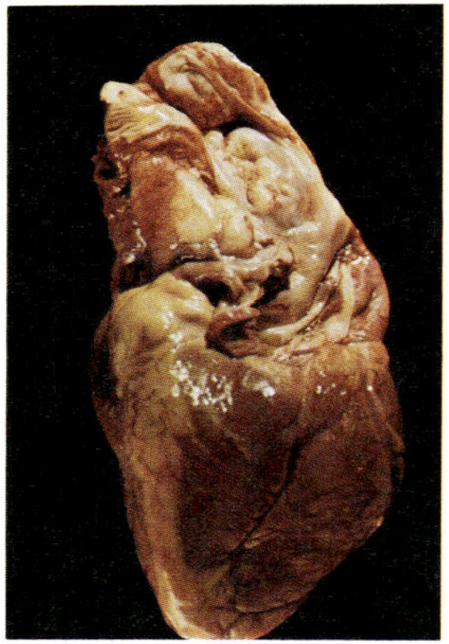

In this photograph of the posterior surface of the heart, the upper portion reveals the opened superior vena cava. The coarsely corrugated, pale gray, nodular mass in that vessel is a tumor that fixes the wall and causes stenosis of the lumen.

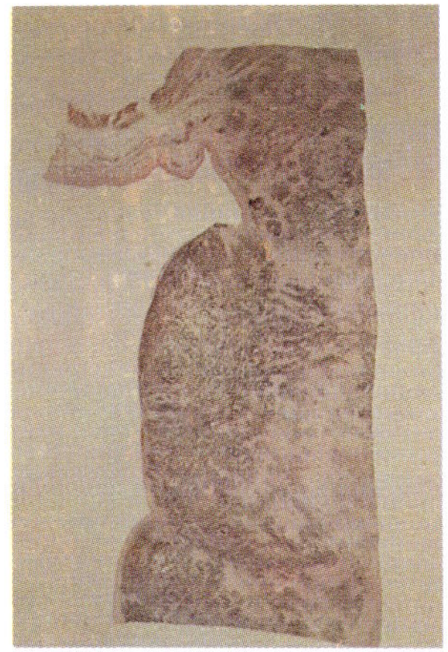

A low power magnification of the superior vena cava shows the extension of basophilic tumor through the wall of that vessel. Emboli from this surface may have contributed to the extremely wide distribution of metastases.

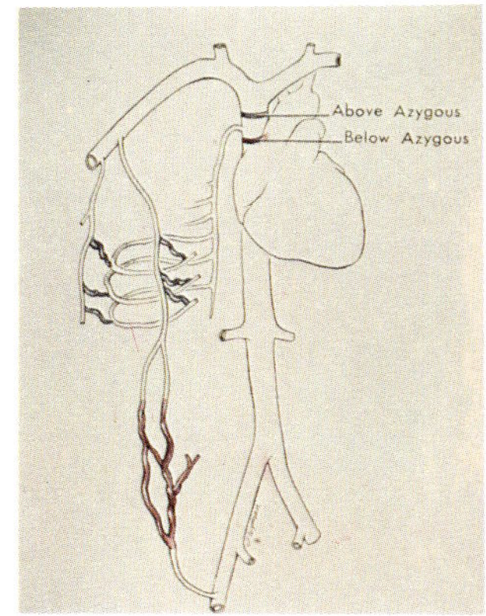

This diagram of the superior vena cava demonstrates the effects of superior caval obstruction above and below the ostium of the azygos vein. When the obstruction is above the azygos ostium, a wide band of dilated veins extends transversely over the lower chest. When the obstruction is below the azygos ostium, the epigastric veins are dilated over the abdomen as they carry blood downward to the iliac vessels and inferior vena cava.

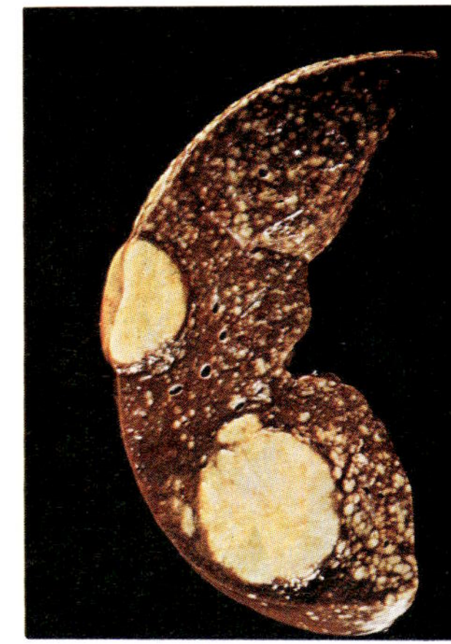

The liver at autopsy reveals widespread metastases. A central depression in the large serosal mass, called "umbilication," is characteristic of metastatic tumor in the liver. Umbilication is said to be occasionally palpable through the abdominal wall.

MEDIASTINOPERICARDITIS

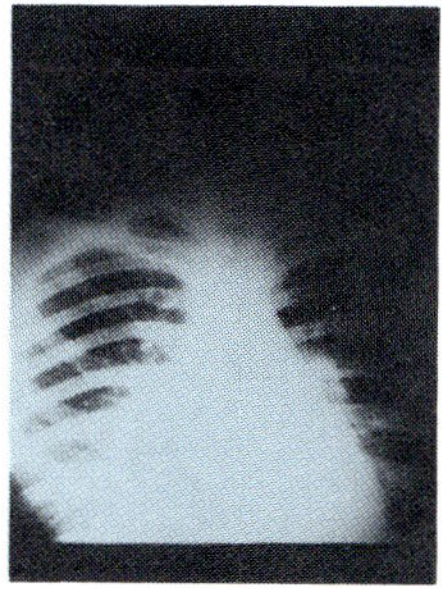

Chest x-ray of patient at age 24 revealed cardiac enlargement. At this age dyspnea developed; some time later weakness and edema of the ankles were noted.

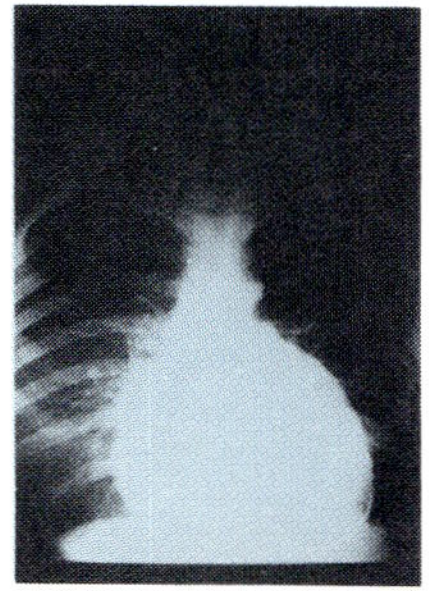

Chest x-ray of patient at age 30 disclosed further cardiac enlargement. A rim of calcium is visible in the region of the apex on the patient's left.

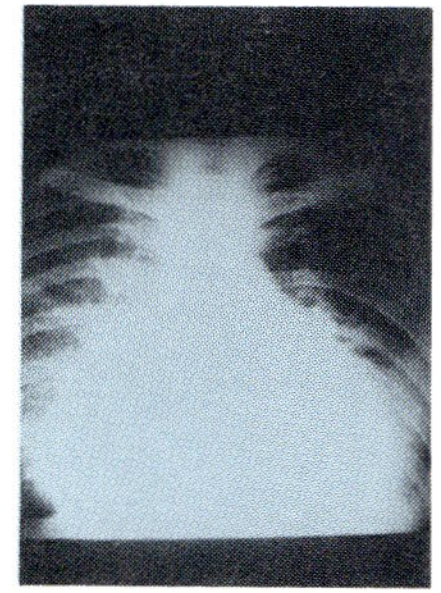

Chest x-ray of patient at age 41, three weeks before death, showed massive cardiac enlargement. This was manifested clinically by progressive heart failure. Instead of a "small quiet heart" which is characteristic of constrictive pericarditis, the patient had a "large noisy heart."

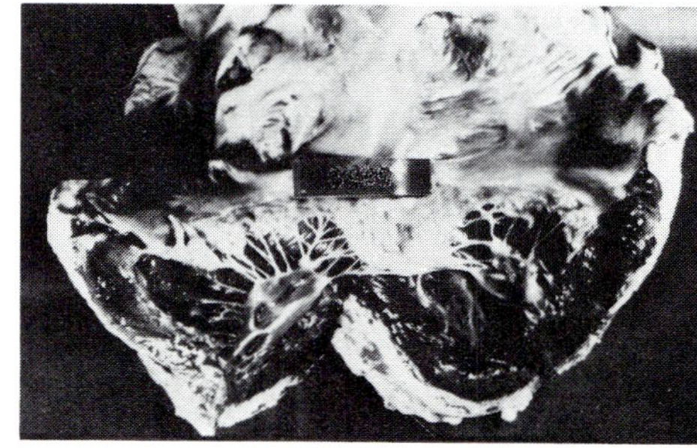

The opened heart reveals dilated valve rings and normal valves. The massive hypertrophy was due to the tugging of the myocardium against this fixed coating of attached connective tissue.

MEDIASTINOPERICARDITIS

CLINICAL ACCOUNT 5859

The patient was a white man 41 years old who developed dyspnea at age 24. An x-ray disclosed enlargement of the heart and calcification of the pericardium. A pericardiectomy of the right ventricle was performed. Congestive failure was unrelieved, and decortication of the left ventricle was performed two years later. No tubercles or Aschoff bodies were found in either specimen. Bouts of gradually progressive congestive failure occurred over the ensuing fifteen years.

Temperature was 99.6 degrees F., pulse rate 84, respiratory rate 22, and blood pressure 120/60 mm. Hg. The neck veins were pulsating. The heart was markedly enlarged, the rate was irregular, and loud systolic and diastolic murmurs were heard. The abdomen was distended, and shifting dullness was detected. The liver was not enlarged. Pitting edema was present to the knees.

The laboratory data were not remarkable. An x-ray revealed pronounced cardiac enlargement, calcification of the pericardium, and pulmonary vascular engorgement. An electrocardiogram disclosed atrial fibrillation and right axis deviation. Treatment included digoxin, diuretics, bed rest, and a low salt diet. The patient improved, was discharged after ten days, and died unexpectedly three months later.

Autopsy examination revealed chronic mediastinopericarditis, hypertrophy of the myocardium (1.025 Gm.), and passive hyperemia of the lungs. The pericardium was thick, extensively calcified, and attached to the heart on the inner surface, and to the lungs, mediastinum, diaphragm, and retrosternum on the outer surface. The cardiac chambers were markedly dilated, and the valves were structurally normal. The murmurs were attributed to dilatation of the valve rings with insufficiency. Cause of pericardial fibrosis not discerned.

THE ENTITY

There are four forms of pericarditis. The first is acute fibrinous inflammation, often associated with uremia, that does not impair cardiac function and very likely subsides without sequelae. The second is fibrous pericarditis that obliterates the sac but does not constrict the heart. The third is constrictive pericarditis that binds the ventricles so that filling is reduced and hypertrophy is prevented. The clinical features are a small silent heart with a decreased stroke volume and a reduced pulse pressure. Frequently associated are hyperemic lungs, pulmonary edema, pleural effusions, and ascites. Pericardiectomy often provides marked improvement.

The fourth is mediastinopericarditis in which the connective tissue attaches to the mediastinal structures as well as the heart. With systole the muscle mass tugs at these structures and hence undergoes dilatation and hypertrophy. As the valve rings dilate, the valves become insufficient. Examination reveals a "large noisy heart" instead of a "small silent" one. The cardiac enlargement is often enormous, and the course may be especially long.

NORMAL AORTA

CLINICAL ACCOUNT 6208

The patient was a Negro male 43 years old who had been a chronic alcoholic for the past several years. He was found unconscious in the street and was brought to the hospital.

The blood pressure was 150/80 mm. Hg. The patient was comatose. He responded to painful stimuli. Neurologic examination was normal. The cerebrospinal fluid was grossly bloody. The patient died after sixteen hours in the hospital.

Autopsy examination revealed a recent intracerebral and subarachnoid hemorrhage. The circle of Willis was intact and no aneurysm was found. The brain weighed 1625 Gm. Additional diagnoses were pulmonary edema, atelectasis of both lungs, and fatty metamorphosis of the liver.

THE ENTITY

Arteries are composed of an innermost intima, an intervening media, and an outermost adventitia. Arteries are classified according to composition and size as elastic, muscular, and small. The last means less than 2 mm. in diameter and includes the arterioles. The aorta and its main branches are elastic arteries because of the abundance of elastic fibers in the media.

The aortic intima is smooth and consists of a thin layer of endothelium. As age progresses, this layer diffusely thickens, especially in the abdominal portion (1). The media is composed of elastic fibers and smooth muscle cells. This layer is thickest in middle age, decreasing thereafter as smooth muscle and elastic fibers are gradually replaced with connective tissue that later hyalinizes. The vessel consequently loses its elasticity. The adventitia is composed of fibrous tissue in which there are nerves and small vessels. The latter arise from large branches emerging from the aorta and deliver oxygenated blood to the outer media as vasa vasorum. The intima and inner media are nourished directly from blood within the aorta.

1. Movat, H.Z., More, R.H., and Haust, M.D. The diffuse intimal thickening of the human aorta with aging. Am. J. Path. 34:1023, 1958.

NORMAL AORTA

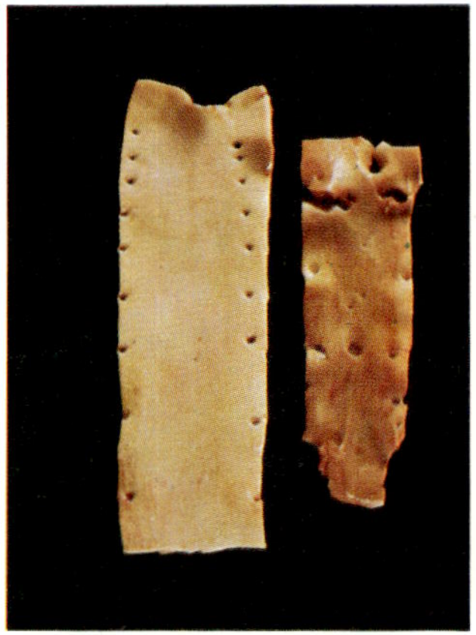

The aorta is divided with the thoracic portion on the left and the abdominal portion on the right. A very slight intimal streaking is present in both portions. Otherwise the intima is normal; this is especially noticeable within the abdominal segment where atherosclerosis is usually most pronounced.

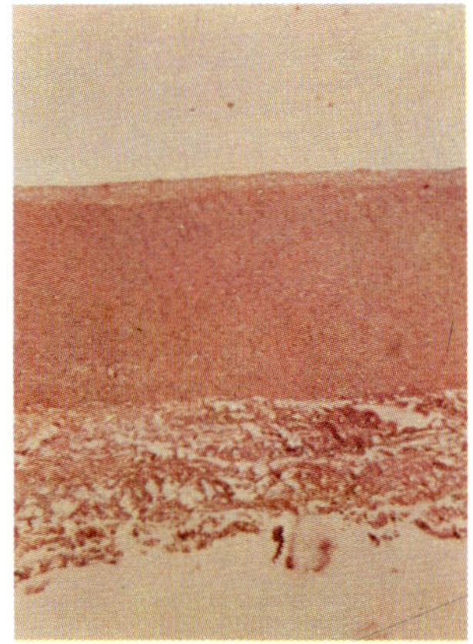

At low power magnification the intima is smooth, the media is uniform in composition, and the adventitia is loosely constructed and devoid of leukocytes.

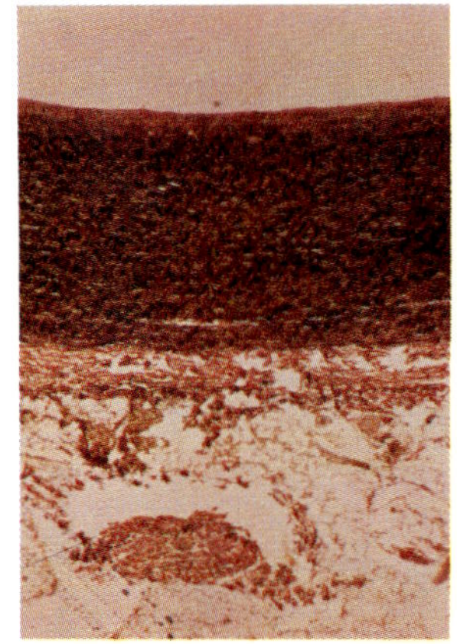

This microsection of the aorta stained with Verhoeff's solution reveals the evenly spaced elastic fibers of the media.

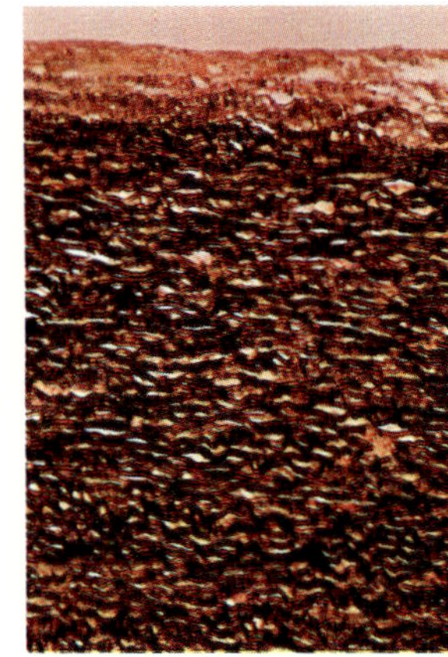

The distribution of elastic fibers is emphasized at higher power magnification. The sharp delineation of intima from media is evident at the top.

ATHEROSCLEROSIS OF AORTA

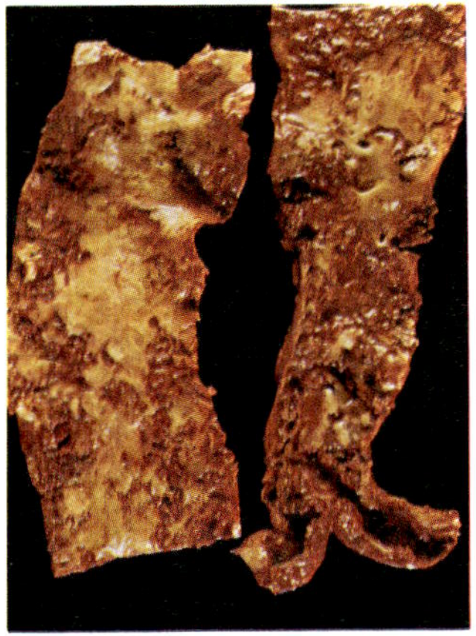

The aorta is bisected with the thoracic portion on the left, and the abdominal portion on the right. The intima is extensively ulcerated and the wall is focally calcified.

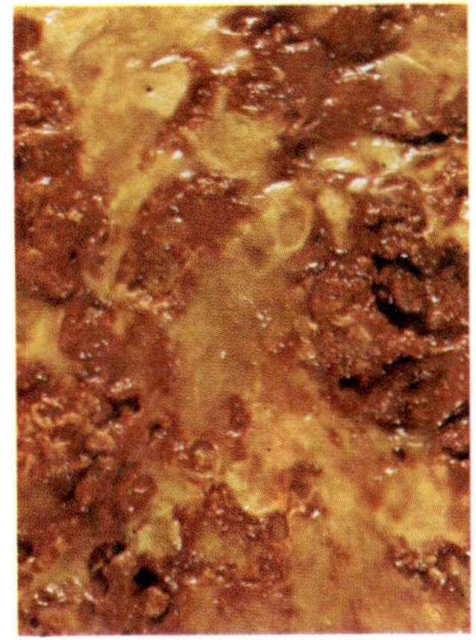

Widespread ulceration of the intima exposes the mushy reddish-yellow material of the atheromatous plaques. Mural thrombi often cover such ulcers. The pale gray, slightly raised portions of intact intima cover foci of fibrosis and calcification.

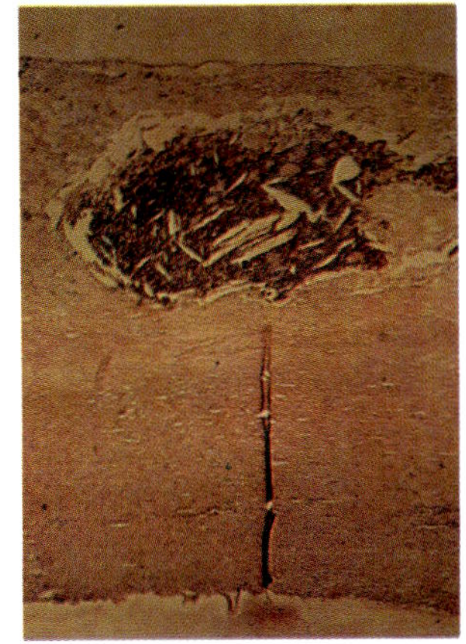

A grumous mass with recent hemorrhage lies in the upper portion of the wall. Cholesterol slits are present in this deposit. The overlying intima is intact and the subjacent media appears to be uninvolved.

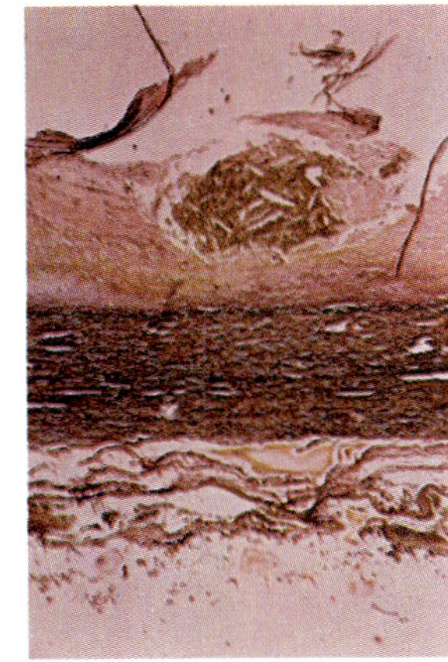

At another site, the grumous mass is exposed to the aortic lumen because of intimal ulceration. Cholesterol slits are again evident. Atheromatous emboli can be foreseen from such a lesion.

ATHEROSCLEROSIS OF AORTA

CLINICAL ACCOUNT 6205

The patient was a white male 89 years old who had been treated for obstructive uropathy, transient episodes of cerebral ischemia, and gall bladder disease. He had had hepatosplenomegaly which recently increased and was associated with ascites formation and a fever of 100 degrees F.

Although the vital signs were normal, the patient was incontinent of urine and stool. The chest was clear to auscultation. The heart was not remarkable. The abdomen was soft and the liver edge was firm, nontender, and 15 cm. below the right costal margin. The spleen was palpable.

The hemoglobin was 11.9 Gm., hematocrit 35, and leukocytes 15,200, with a normal distribution. The urine was normal. A chest x-ray revealed a dense infiltration in the upper lobe of the left lung that was suggestive of neoplastic disease. The patient died after nine days in the hospital.

Autopsy examination revealed a carcinoma of the left lung with metastases to liver, spine, and lymph nodes (bronchopulmonary and para-aortic). The hepatic metastases were extensive and the liver weighed 3050 Gm. The heart weighed 350 Gm. and revealed calcification of the mitral annulus. Additional diagnoses included pulmonary emphysema, a pleural effusion on the left (250 ml.), focal chronic pyelonephritis, and nodular hyperplasia of the prostate.

THE ENTITY

Arteriosclerosis is a generic term that encompasses atherosclerosis, medial sclerosis, and arteriolar sclerosis. Of these, the first is the most common and the most important. Atherosclerosis is a lipid change in the intima that progresses to involve the media and is associated with fibrosis and calcification of the wall. It begins with yellow streaking of the sub-intima that is due to macrophage-like cells distended with lipid rich in cholesterol. The lipid-laden cells increase, the "atheromas" enlarge and coalesce, fibrosis and calcification follow, and ulceration and thrombosis may develop. The wall of the aorta is weakened, dilatation occurs, and aneurysms form. The consequences are embolic phenomena from the intimal ulcerations, occlusion of the iliac bifurcation by saddle emboli, and exsanguination from rupture of the aneurysms.

The process occurs in middle-aged males and postmenopausal females, increasing in old age in both sexes. It is constant in the aortas of elderly well nourished Americans and is most pronounced in the abdominal portion. It is irregular, however, in the coronary, cerebral, mesenteric, and renal branches. At these sites, stenosis and thrombosis are the principal complications. The cause is unknown, but the process may be metabolic, due to an excess of lipid in the diet, or thrombogenic, due to the repair of fibrin thrombi of the intima.

SACCULAR ANEURYSM OF AORTA

CLINICAL ACCOUNT 6131

The patient was a white female 80 years old whose present illness began one year before admission to the hospital. At that time she noted a small, tender, gradually enlarging mass in the right upper quadrant of her abdomen. A dull constant ache was associated with the mass over the past six months. Anorexia and weight loss had become pronounced. There had been no nausea, vomiting, constipation, or melena.

The temperature was 98.6 degrees F., respirations 18, pulse 100, and blood pressure 120/70 mm. Hg. The lung fields were clear. A rough grade 2 systolic ejection murmur was heard in the right second intercostal space at the sternal margin. A soft grade 2 diastolic murmur was heard best at the apex. The abdomen was soft and flat except for a hard, pulsatile, slightly tender mass measuring 10 cm. in greatest dimension in the epigastrium and right upper quadrant. There was slight pedal edema. The blood and urine were normal. An x-ray revealed calcification in the region of the abdominal mass. A catheter was inserted into the femoral artery and advanced to the level of the second lumbar vertebra; 50 ml. of radio-opaque medium were injected, and an aneurysm extending to the iliac bifurcation was revealed. After abdominal incision the blood pressure fell and the patient was not deemed strong enough to undergo resection of the aneurysm. Postoperative recovery was uneventful until the eleventh day, when the temperature rose to 100.8 degrees F. On the next day the temperature was 104.0 degrees F., the blood pressure fell, and the patient became unresponsive and died.

Autopsy examination revealed a recent infarct of the left ventricle, a recent thrombus of the circumflex branch of the left coronary artery, an acute bacterial endocarditis of the mitral valve, recent infarcts of the kidneys and spleen, and a saccular aneurysm of the abdominal aorta.

THE ENTITY

Saccular aneurysms of the aorta tend to arise in the elderly, more commonly in men than women. They are almost always between the renal arteries and the iliac bifurcation. One fourth to one half of patients are unaware of such aneurysms until they rupture (1). The classical symptoms of rupture are sudden, often excruciating mid-abdominal or low-back pain that radiates into one or both groins. There may be nausea, vomiting, weakness, or fainting. Signs include shock and a tender pulsatile abdominal mass. There may be pallor, sweating, or tachycardia. Rupture occurs into the retroperitoneum, the peritoneal cavity, the inferior vena cava, or the duodenum. Retroperitoneal rupture is often accompanied by a period of relative cardiovascular stability before exsanguinating hemorrhage occurs. Rupture into the peritoneal cavity is attended by sudden unrelenting shock. Rupture into the vena cava is manifested by an abdominal bruit and congestive heart failure with edema and venous engorgement of the lower extremities. Rupture into the duodenum is evidenced by sudden hematemesis. The hematocrit is variable, leukocytosis is constant, and microscopic hematuria is frequent due to ureteral displacement. The diagnosis is urgent, since life depends on replacement of the dilated segment with a prosthetic device.

1. Mannick, J.A. Diagnosis of ruptured aneurysm of the abdominal aorta. Current Concepts. New Eng. J. Med. 176:1305, 1967.

SACCULAR ANEURYSM, AORTA

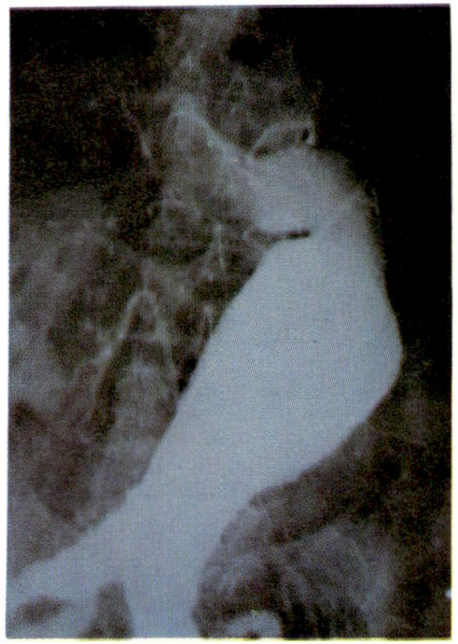

This aortogram showed the size and extent of the aneurysm which was in the abdominal portion.

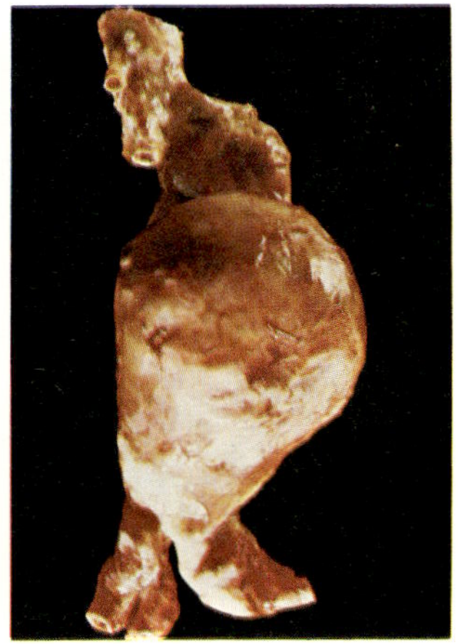

The gross specimen reveals the somewhat cirsoid shape of the aneurysm. It arises distal to the renal arteries, and extends to the iliac bifurcation.

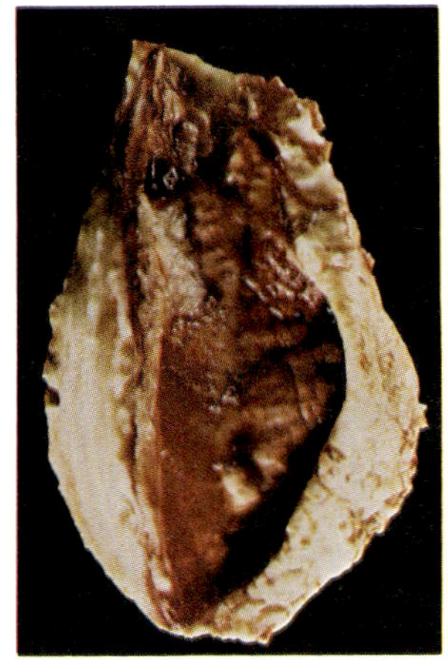

Section discloses a dilated lumen, a surface that has become covered with endothelium, and a thick wall composed of laminated thrombus.

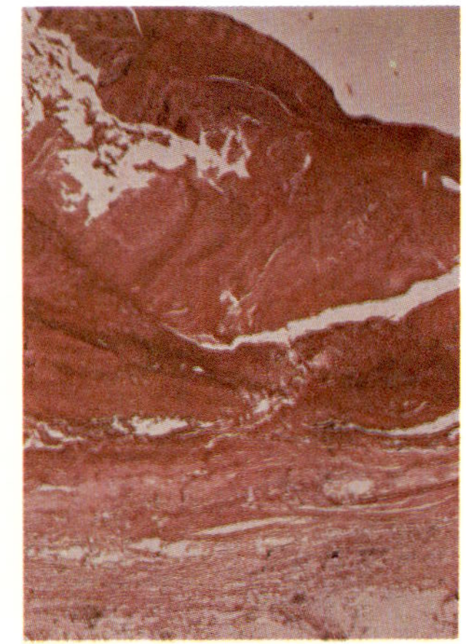

The microsection reveals that the wall consists mostly of thrombus; only thin layers of adventitia make up the external structure of the aorta.

DISSECTING ANEURYSM, AORTA

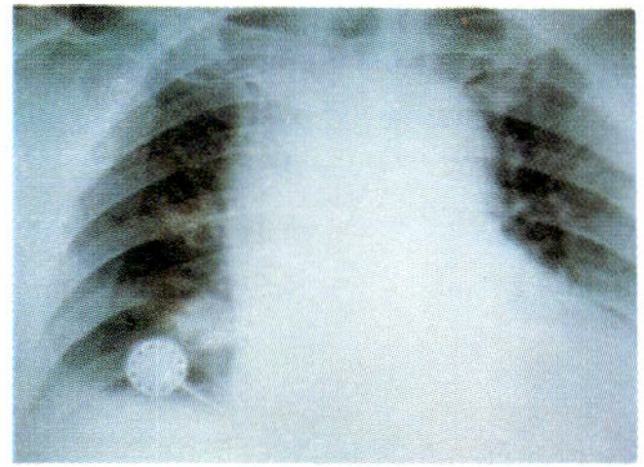

The chest x-ray disclosed widening of the mediastinum which is a cardinal diagnostic sign of dissecting aneurysm.

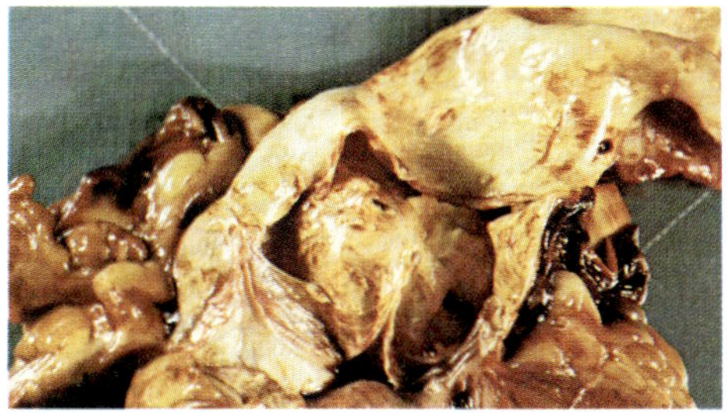

The heart and aorta reveal a thick left ventricle and a large transverse rent in the aorta just above the cusps of the aortic valve. The dissection progressed distally to the iliac bifurcation and proximally to the pericardium into which it then ruptured.

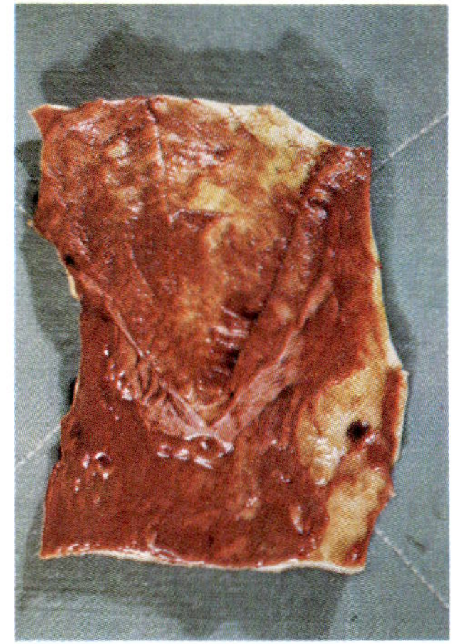

The aorta opened from the external surface (adventitia) shows the channel in which the dissection took place.

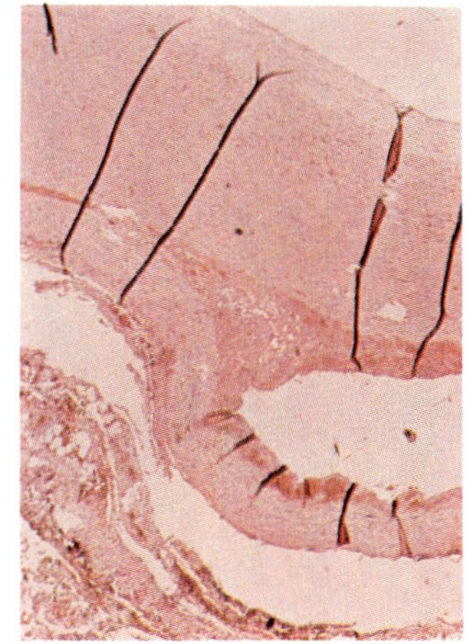

A histologic section of the aorta shows the media with the outer third split away from the inner two thirds. Hemorrhage is present within this channel. This is the portion of the wall in which the dissection usually takes place.

DISSECTING ANEURYSM OF AORTA

CLINICAL ACCOUNT 6049

The patient was a Negro male 46 years old who was well until 6:00 a.m. on the morning of admission. At that time he suddenly developed pain in the upper abdomen. This was moderately severe and was unassociated with cough, fever, digestive disturbance, or other history of recent illness. The patient was not diabetic and had no history of heart disease. The pulse was 80, respirations 22, and blood pressure 170/110 mm. Hg. The heart was not enlarged, no murmurs were heard, and the rhythm was regular. The lungs and abdomen were not remarkable. An electrocardiogram showed no "acute changes." The urine was normal. The hemoglobin was 13.2 gms. per 100 ml., hematocrit 42, and leukocyte count 10,300 per cmm. The patient suddenly felt weak and collapsed. He now stated that the pain was in his anterior chest and radiated to his left arm. Shortness of breath developed. The blood pressure was unobtainable, the respirations were 44 per minute, and the skin was cool, pallid, and moist. The neck veins were distended and the chest disclosed coarse rales throughout both lower lung fields. The abdomen was soft. The serum glutamic transaminase was 41 units per 100 ml., and the serum lactic dehydrogenase was 415 units per 100 ml. On the next day, an x-ray of the chest revealed "a very wide mediastinum." A second electrocardiogram revealed only premature ventricular beats. On the third day cyanosis developed and the patient died.

Autopsy examination revealed a dissecting aneurysm of the aorta that ruptured into the pericardium with hemopericardium (500 ml.) and cardiac tamponade.

THE ENTITY

Dissecting aneurysms are most frequent in hypertensive male adults (1). The lesion begins as a transverse tear at the base of the aorta, usually within 5 cm. of the aortic valve. The dissection proceeds for a variable distance and usually extends into the abdominal portion. The advancing dissection often compresses the carotid, celiac, renal, lumbar, or femoral arteries, and usually ruptures externally into the pericardium, pleura, mediastinum, or retroperitoneum. It uncommonly ruptures internally to produce a false aortic channel that endothelializes. In this event, the condition is compatible with a long survival.

The onset is sudden with severe stabbing pain in the chest that is attended by shock and collapse. The pain often radiates to the back, and frequently shifts as the dissection proceeds. The electrocardiogram is negative for infarct, the x-rays show widening of the mediastinum, and the blood pressures in the extremities are often asymmetrical. Extension of the dissection to the tributaries of the aorta may be associated with confusion, coma, hemiplegia, paralytic ileus, anuria, paresthesias, weakness, or paralysis. Death usually occurs within a few hours or days from rupture into the pericardium with cardiac tamponade, or rupture externally with massive hemorrhage.

1. Hirst, E.E., Jr., Johns, V.J., Jr., and Kime, S.W. Dissecting aneurysm of the aorta: A review of 505 cases. Medicine 37:217, 1958.

SYPHILITIC ANEURYSM OF AORTA

CLINICAL ACCOUNT SLH-113

The patient was a white male 60 years old who was well except for a chronic cough until six weeks before entering the hospital. At that time he experienced a sharp tearing pain in the right upper chest during an episode of coughing. The pain was replaced by a dull ache; it recurred, however, every two weeks or so and radiated down the right arm. The pain was not throbbing and not related to exertion, and the cough was not brassy. A penile chancre had been treated by excision 20 years previously (1936), and thereafter arsphenamine injections had been given. Subsequently the blood and spinal fluid serology were consistently negative.

The blood pressure was 150/80 mm. Hg. The trachea showed neither tug nor deviation. A heaving pulsation synchronous with systole was palpable over the right upper chest. Harsh systolic and diastolic murmurs were audible over the entire precordium. No other physical findings were significant. The urine and blood were normal. A chest x-ray revealed a large oval mass in the upper mediastinum on the right. The right leaf of the diaphragm was paralyzed; the lung fields were clear. The clinical diagnosis was syphilitic aortitis with aneurysm of the ascending aorta. The patient was given symptomatic treatment and discharged. He died elsewhere two months later.

Autopsy examination revealed a large saccular aneurysm of the ascending aorta that ruptured into the right pleural space. The aneurysm measured 18 cm. in diameter and impinged on the right brachial plexus. The aortic ring was dilated and the cusps revealed thickening, fibrosis, retraction, and separation of the commissures. Additional diagnosis included syphilitic aortic valvulitis with insufficiency, hypertrophy and dilatation of the heart (490 Gm.), syphilitic mesoaortitis, and chronic passive hyperemia of the lungs and liver.

THE ENTITY

The basic lesion of cardiovascular syphilis is aortitis. The condition requires ten to thirty years to develop and affects especially the ascending and transverse portions. At these sites fibrosis and hyalinization corrugate the intima in a characteristic way. Histologic examination reveals elastic fragmentation of the media, miliary gummas of the adventitia, and lymphocytic and plasma cell infiltrations of both. As this process moves proximalward, the ostia of the coronary arteries become narrowed; angina results. When the process reaches the valve ring, dilatation occurs and insufficiency develops. When the process extends into the valve cusps, the walls thicken, the margins retract, and the commissures separate. This increases the insufficiency so that the pulse pressure widens, diastolic murmurs become harsh, the left ventricle hypertrophies, and the peripheral arteries reveal a "pistol shot" or Corrigan pulse. Within the wall of the aorta, aneurysms form. They are saccular, measure up to 15 cm. in diameter, and bulge against the spine in back and the sternum in front. Impingement on the recurrent laryngeal nerve causes a brassy cough, on the bronchi a tracheal tug, on the trachea lateral deviation, and on the esophagus, dysphagia. Uncommonly syphilitic aneurysms occur in the abdominal aorta. They arise above the renal arteries and occur in younger patients (30-50 yrs.) than arteriosclerotic aneurysms. Ten to 15 per cent of patients with syphilitic aortitis have negative serologic tests for syphilis (1).

1. Kampmeier, R.H. The late manifestations of syphilis: skeletal, visceral and cardiovascular. Med. Clin. N. Am. 48:667, 1964.

SYPHILITIC ANEURYSM, AORTA

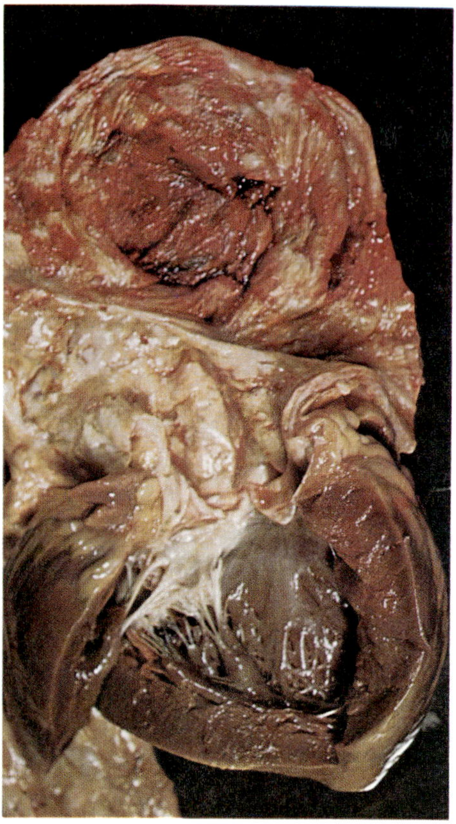

The photograph reveals the thin wall of the aneurysm, the fibrin-covered surface, and the dark red rent of perforation on the left. Although the commissural separation of the aortic cusps is not well seen, the pronounced thickness of the left ventricle is characteristic of aortic regurgitation.

This routine hematoxylin and eosin stain of a microsection of the aorta does not give convincing evidence of syphilitic disease, although vascular spaces are present just below the intima and leukocytes surround a small vessel in the adventitia.

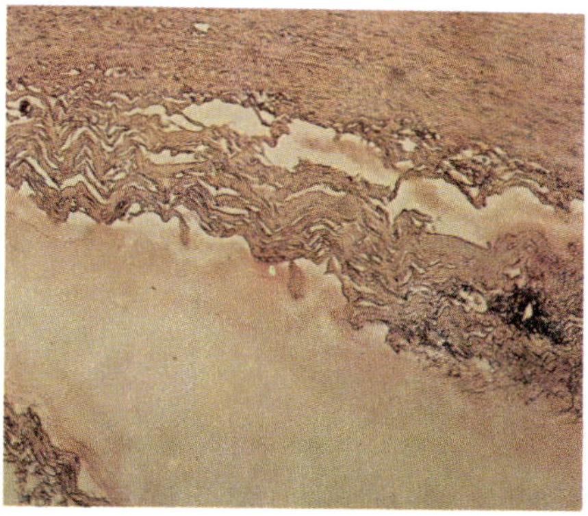

Below, left: This microsection of the aorta stained with Verhoeff's solution reveals extensive disruption and disappearance of the elastic fibers of the media. This finding in association with vascularization of the media, which is also present, is characteristic of syphilitic mesoaortitis. **Below, right:** The extensive disruption of elastic fibers is again evident at higher magnification.

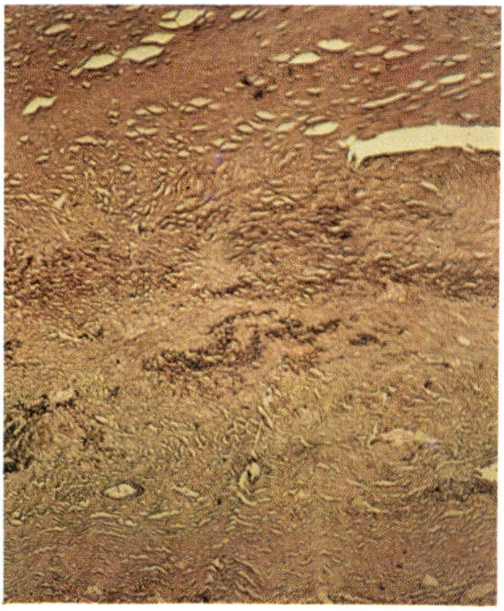

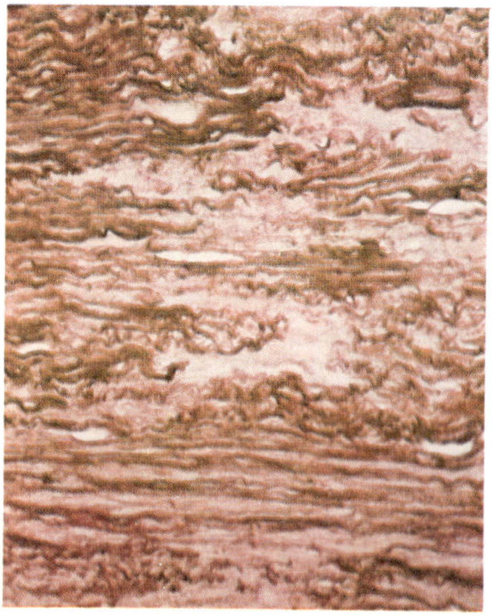

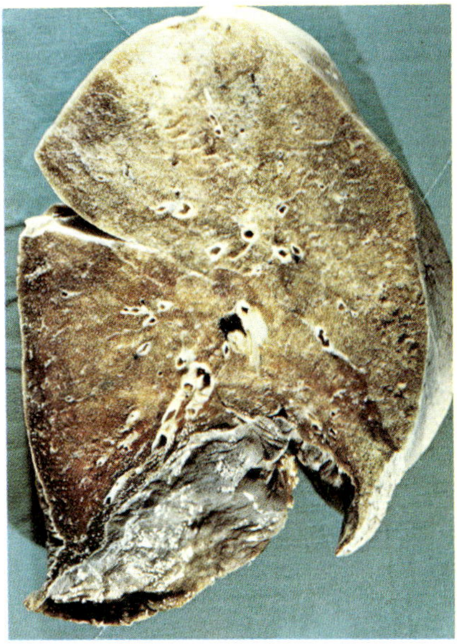

The cut surface of the fixed lung reveals a uniformly and finely porous pale grayish brown cut surface. Carbon pigment is present in lymphoid tissue adjacent to two central bronchi.

Alveolar walls consist of septal cells attached to connective tissue in which elastic fibers are abundant. The elastic fibers contribute to the expansibility of the tissue. Capillaries within the alveoli are lined by a single layer of endothelial cells. Gaseous diffusion thus takes place through two cell layers. Surfactant, a lipoprotein, alters surface tension so that alveolar stability and uniformity of ventilation are enhanced. Alveolar walls are perforated by the pores of Kohn. The pulmonary arterial pressure is only 1/8 of systemic arterial pressure. This low hydrostatic pressure with normal osmotic pressure protects the air sacs from fluid accumulation.

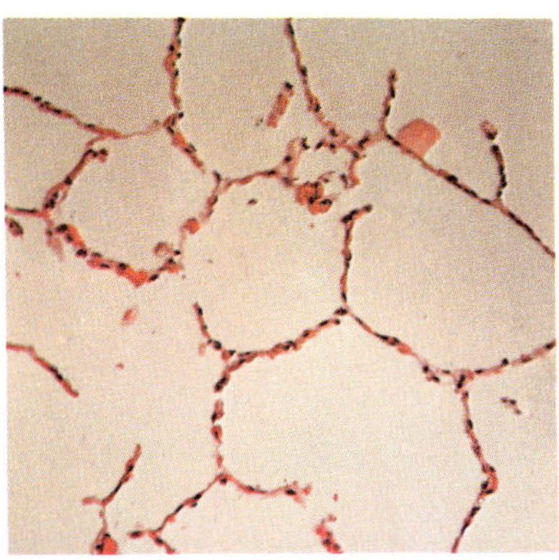

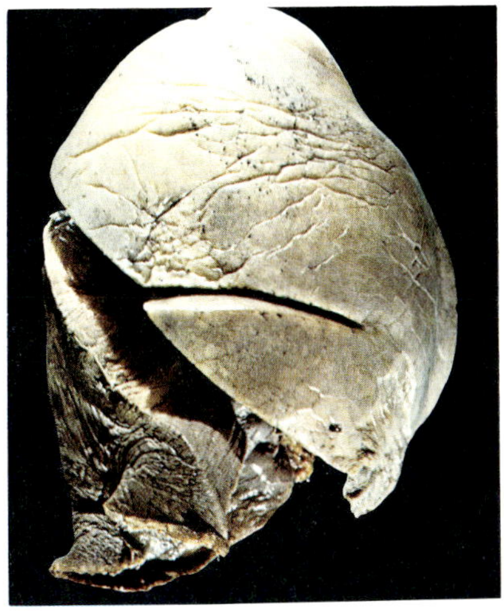

The formalin-inflated right lung discloses a smooth and glistening pleura. The lower lobe is failed to inflate and is dark grayish blue and atelectatic. The black flecks are anthracotic pigment, i.e., carbon particles from industrial effluence. These are noninflammatory and cause no adhesions. In urban dwellers such pigmentation is often pronounced. In each 24 hour period, 12,000 liters of air enter and leave the lungs.

NORMAL LUNG

The microsection of bronchial wall reveals a pseudostratified columnar mucosa in which the cells are ciliated. The detachment of this layer is artefact. Goblet cells are dispersed within this layer, and mucous glands are present in the submucosa. A thin pale pink basement membrane separates the epithelium from the subjacent tissue. In asthma the basement membrane undergoes conspicuous thickening and the mucous glands increase markedly in number.

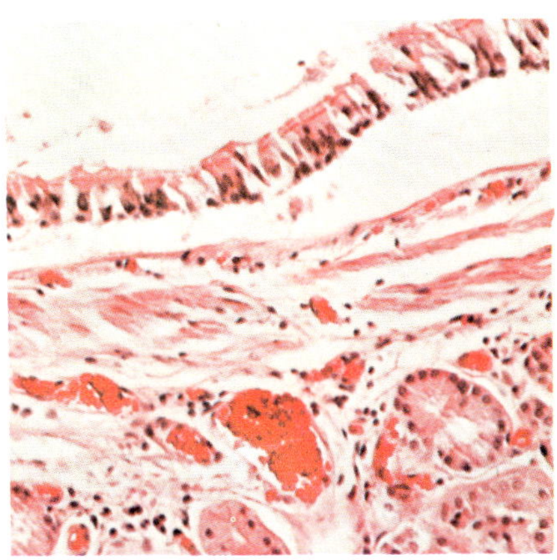

NORMAL LUNG

CLINICAL ACCOUNT 6121

The patient was a white female 67 years old who was admitted to the hospital because of severe pain in the upper abdomen that radiated to the back. The pain was intractable and had been present for the preceding week. She had been treated over the past three years for a myeloproliferative disorder characterized by anemia and thrombocytosis. Two courses of irradiation to the spine had been given for the control of pain. Physical examination revealed clear lungs, tenderness in the right upper quadrant of the abdomen, and edema of the feet and ankles. The urine was normal. The blood revealed anemia and leukopenia. A prefrontal lobotomy was performed for relief of pain, post-operative hemorrhage occurred, and coma supervened. An intracerebral blood clot was removed; the patient did not respond, and death occurred four days after the lobotomy.

The necropsy revealed recent hemorrhages of the frontal lobes of the cerebrum and cerebral edema. In addition, there were focal necrosis and atrophy of the liver, atrophy of the pancreas, diverticula of the sigmoid colon, and widespread osteoporosis. Right lung weighed 400 Gm.; the left 450 Gm.

THE ENTITY

Progressive branching reduces the bronchi to terminal bronchioles that are less than 1 mm. in diameter and devoid of cartilage. These are followed by respiratory bronchioles, alveolar ducts, and air sacs. Each lung is divided into broncho-pulmonary segments, a combined total of 18, in which pathologic processes tend to be localized because of separate bronchial, arterial, and venous connections. The lungs have a dual arterial supply, the pulmonary artery arising from the right ventricle, and the bronchial arteries arising from the thoracic aorta. In the absence of congestive failure, the bronchial arteries sustain the viability of the tissue even when the pulmonary artery is completely blocked.

The respiratory passages between the vocal cords and the alveolar ducts are lined by pseudo-stratified columnar epithelium that is ciliated. Goblet cells are interspersed on the mucosal surfaces. Inspired particulate debris clings to the mucus, and the cilia work the debris proximalward to be swallowed. This clearance function is aided by contractions of muscle fibers in the bronchial walls that alter both the length and the diameter of the channels.

Each inspiration carries about 500 ml. of air into the lungs (tidal volume). Forced inspiration brings in about 4,000 ml. (vital capacity). About 1200 ml. remains stationary in the tissue (residual volume). The partial pressure of oxygen in alveolar air is 100 mm. Hg., that of venous blood 40. This gradient favors inward diffusion of oxygen. The partial pressure of carbon dioxide in venous blood is 46 mm. Hg., that of alveolar air 40. This gradient favors outward diffusion. The permeability of the alveolar membrane is 20 times greater for carbon dioxide than for oxygen. While the pulmonary capillaries are extremely distensible, their total blood volume at any moment of rest is about 70 to 100 ml.

POLYP OF VOCAL CORD

CLINICAL ACCOUNT 6325

The patient was a white male 57 years old who entered the hospital because of a draining sinus of the perineum. Biopsy of the sinus revealed squamous cell carcinoma. The sinus tract, urinary bladder, prostate, and seminal vesicles were resected; the ureters were fixed to the abdominal wall and drained onto the skin. Infective post-operative complications developed, and the patient died after five weeks in the hospital. No mention was made of hoarseness or unusual phonation.

Autopsy examination revealed bronchopneumonia, pleural effusions (250 ml., each side), a recent infarct of the spleen, arteriolar nephrosclerosis, and recent thrombi of the right subclavian and left internal iliac veins.

THE ENTITY

Vocal nodules are discrete masses of connective tissue covered with intact mucosa that arise on the true vocal cords and cause abnormal phonation. They occur especially in singers, arise at the center of the membranous cord which is the point of maximum vibration, and cause vocal fatigue and "cracking" of the higher notes. They are related to pitch, being more common in males under 20 and in females than in basses or baritones (1). Hoarseness eventually develops, and complete aphonia may follow.

The nodules are soft and red at the outset, later becoming small, firm, and pale yellowish gray. The projections may become polypoid, with either a sessile or pedunculated base. A sensation of something in the throat, with constant attempts to clear it, may develop. The nodules are easily visualized. Surgical excision is curative. The central connective tissue on microscopic examination may show slight chronic inflammation, proliferation of numerous capillary vessels, recent hemorrhage, hemosiderin-laden macrophages from old hemorrhage, or hyalinization of the fibrous connective tissue. Nodules don't tend to become malignant.

1. Ballenger, J.J. Diseases of the Nose, Throat, and Ear. Eleventh Edition. Lea and Febiger, Philadelphia, 1969.

POLYP OF VOCAL CORD

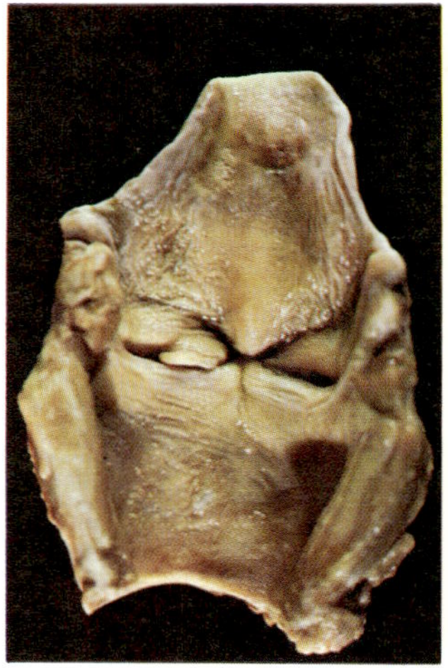

The photograph shows the larynx opened from the posterior surface and fixed in formalin. A polypoid mass projects from the ventricle between the vocal folds on the left.

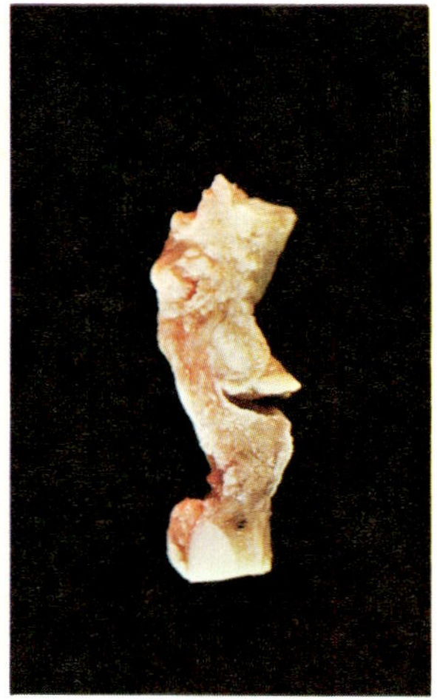

A vertical section shows the vocal cleft on the right; a polypoid mass projects into it from the upper cord.

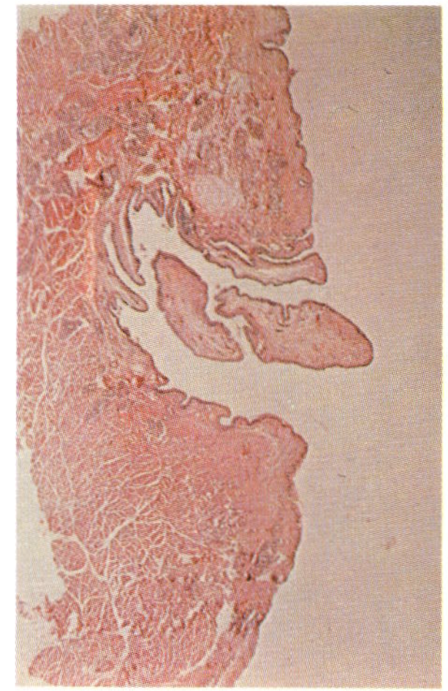

The polypoid mass can be seen projecting into the vocal cleft between the upper and lower cords.

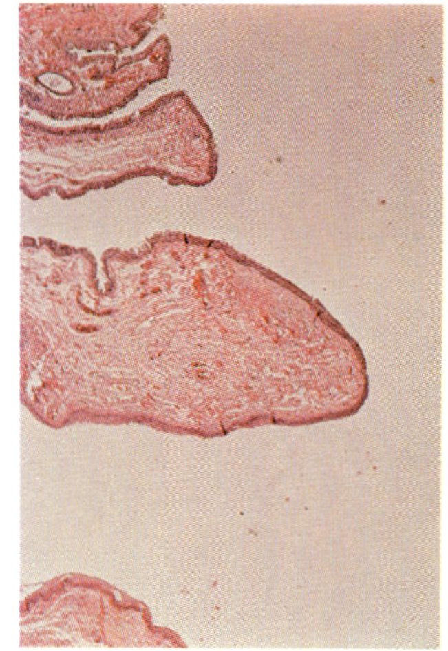

At higher power the polypoid mass presents a squamous mucosa and a loose fibrous connective tissue core that is lightly infiltrated with lymphocytes and plasma cells.

TUBERCULOSIS OF LARYNX

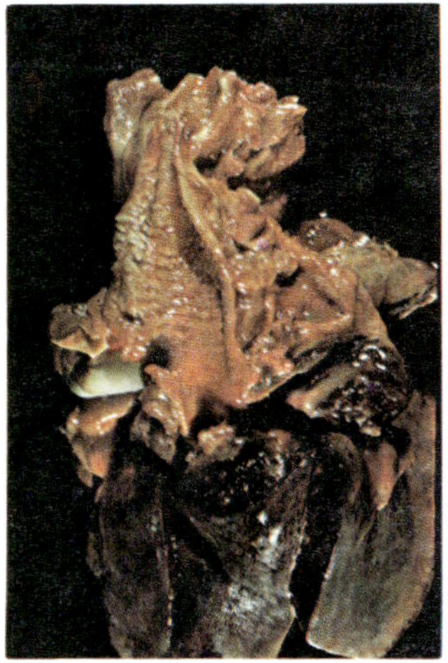

The lungs revealed extensive cavitary tuberculosis. The photograph displays the lung with attached trachea and larynx.

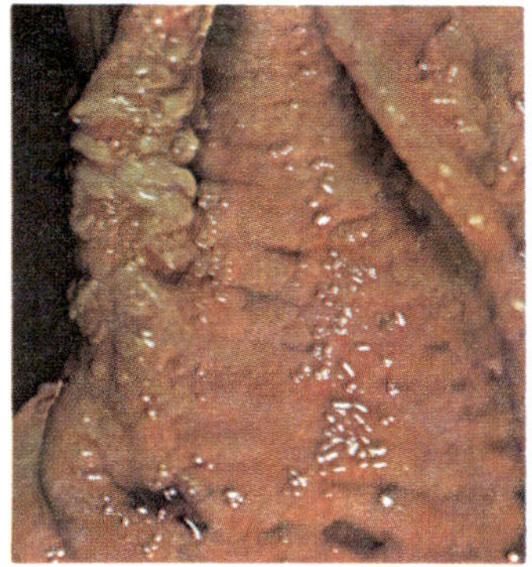

A closer view of the trachea reveals extensive tuberculosis with widespread ulceration. This process extended into the larynx.

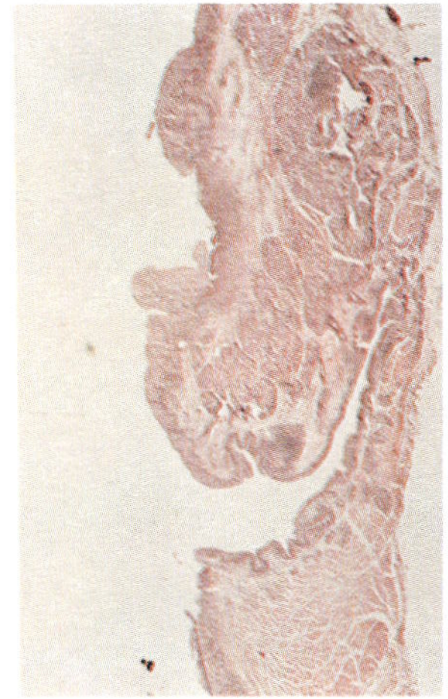

A low power view of the larynx shows the upper vocal cord projecting on the left surface of the section. The mucosa is thickened and focally ulcerated; the subjacent connective tissue is markedly inflamed.

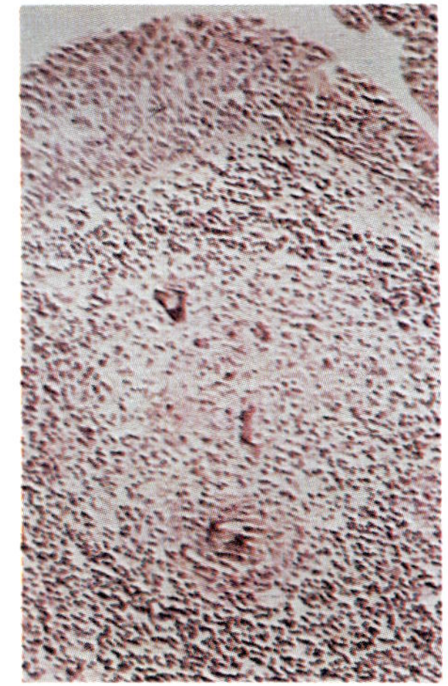

A higher view of the mucosa of the larynx reveals the tuberculous inflammation.

TUBERCULOSIS OF LARYNX

CLINICAL ACCOUNT 443

The patient was a black male twelve years old who was admitted to the hospital because of coughing, hoarseness, and pronounced anemia. Preliminary examination disclosed rhonchi over both lung fields and moderate dependent edema. Before further examination could be completed, the patient collapsed and died. Autopsy examination revealed large tuberculous cavities throughout both lungs and extensive ulcerative tuberculosis of the larynx and trachea. The right and left lungs weighed 680 and 740 Gms. respectively.

THE ENTITY

Tuberculosis of the larynx is now a vanishing lesion because it occurs only as a complication of advanced pulmonary tuberculosis, and such pulmonary disease is diminishing in frequency because of improved hygienic measures and the widespread use of anti-tuberculous chemotherapeutic agents. Nevertheless, the condition does occur and, although uncommon, is occasionally seen where hygienic practices are undeveloped and disease states are allowed to become extreme before medical attention is sought. Tuberculous laryngotracheobronchitis is seen in East Africa. The opened larynx reveals superficial serpiginous ulcers and submucosal granulation tissue that affect especially the arytenoids and vocal cords. These lesions interfere with the function of the larynx so that the clinical consequences are a rough and worsening hoarseness that may progress to complete aphonia (1). The process may extend to the trachea, with the formation of superficial ulcers and thick elevating submucosal granulation tissue. The process may extend into the deeper tissues and cause caseous necrosis and collapse of the cartilaginous structures of the larynx. Ultimately perforation into the esophagus may occur, and the fistula formed may lead to the development of aspiration pneumonia.

1. Smith, L.W., and Gault, E.S. Essentials of Pathology, Second Edition. D. Appleton-Century Co., New York, 1942.

LOBAR PNEUMONIA

CLINICAL ACCOUNT 6141

The patient was a 64-year-old white female who was admitted to the hospital because of dyspnea. She had had emphysema and a cough for the past two years and had smoked a pack of cigarettes daily for many years.

The blood pressure was 260/130 mm. Hg. She was slim, agitated, and short of breath. The chest was hyperresonant, and rhonchi were heard over all lung fields. The urine was normal. The hemoglobin was 14.2 Gm., and the leukocytes numbered 17,100, with a normal differential count. The electrocardiogram disclosed left ventricular strain. X-rays of the chest showed cardiac enlargement to the left, an infiltration of the left lung field, and pleural fluid at the left base. The respiratory difficulty increased. Nasal oxygen was given, a thoracentesis was performed, and a tracheostomy tube was inserted. The temperature rose to 102 degrees F. The bronchi were aspirated and a respirator was applied. Despite these measures, the respiratory difficulty worsened, and the patient died after 41 days in the hospital.

Autopsy examination revealed lobar pneumonia of the right lung, and bronchopneumonia of the left lung. In addition, there was an acute fibrinous pleuritis, recent pulmonary thrombo-emboli, and a recent tracheostomy. Pleural effusions were present; 250 ml. on the right and 350 ml. on the left. The kidneys displayed arteriolar nephrosclerosis with necrotizing arteriolitis; fibrinoid necrosis was also present in the peri-adrenal adipose tissue. A large recent infarct was present in the right adrenal that affected especially the medulla. The right and left lungs weighed 620 and 400 Gm., respectively.

THE ENTITY

Lobar pneumonia is characterized clinically by chills, fever (104 degrees F.), leukocytosis, cough, hemorrhagic or "rusty" sputum, shortness of breath, sometimes cyanosis, pleuritic pain, dullness to percussion, absence of breath sounds, and opacity of lobar distribution on the chest x-ray.

The condition is a diffuse exudative inflammation of pulmonary tissue that affects one or more lobes. It is usually caused by pneumococci, especially types I, II, and III, but may be caused by *Hemophilus klebsiella* or *influenzae*. Any lobe may be affected. The inflammatory process is dynamic and tends to pass through four stages, i.e., congestion, red hepatization, gray hepatization, and resolution. In the first the tissue is soggy and subcrepitant and the alveoli are filled with a serous exudate in which bacteria are numerous and blood vessels are widely dilated. In the second the tissue is red, firm, and dry. The alveoli are filled with fibrin, neutrophils, and large numbers of extravasated erythrocytes which give the tissue its distinctive color. The third stage evolves as the erythrocytes degenerate; the leukocytes and fibrin remain so that the tissue cut surface becomes gray, firm and dry. Throughout these stages, the alveolar walls remain intact. With resolution, the leukocytic enzymes liquefy the exudate which is carried away by macrophages or coughed up and expectorated so that the tissue begins to return to its normal consistency. With antibiotic treatment these stages may be obscured.

Complications include abscess formation, empyema, suppurative pericarditis, and bacteremia with spread to the brain, heart valves, kidneys, or joints. In addition, the stage of resolution may fail so that the exudate organizes and the alveoli become filled with granulation tissue that eventually matures into dense fibrous connective tissue.

LOBAR PNEUMONIA

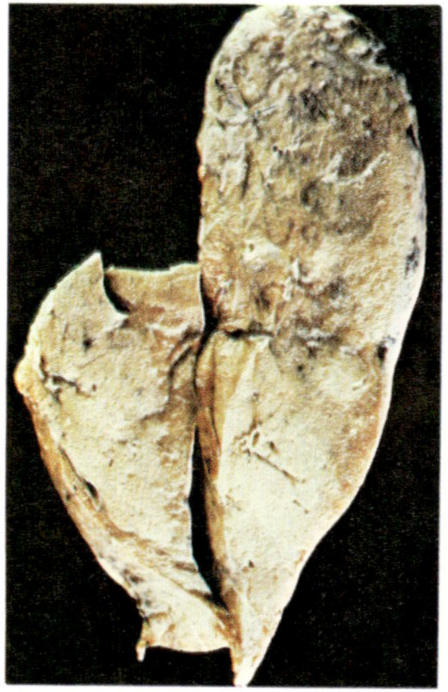

The middle and lower lobes of the right lung display pale brownish gray consolidation. The change in consistency is nearly uniform so that the exudate is lobar in distribution. The pulmonary thrombo-emboli are small, peripheral, and unaccompanied by infarction of tissue.

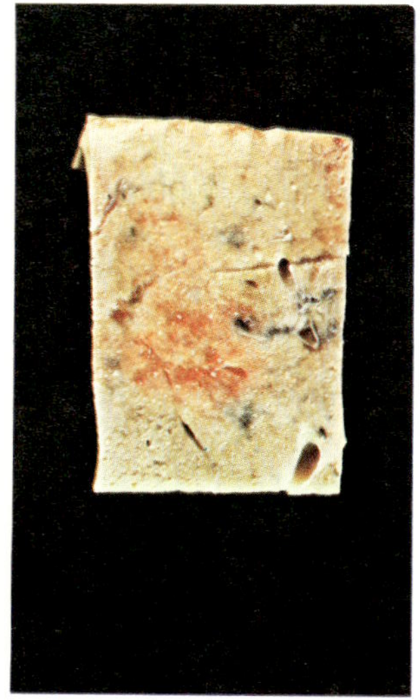

A close-up of the cut surface shows the solid nature of the tissue. The red central region is a zone of poor fixation. The pleural surface at the top is covered with a thin layer of fibrin.

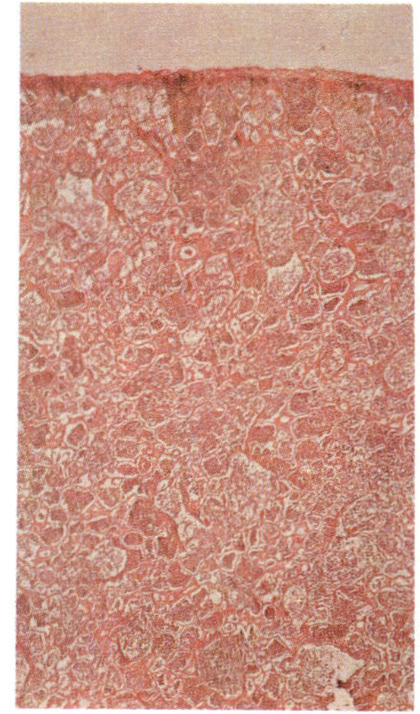

The scanning power reveals the uniform distribution of exudate; it extends evenly throughout all alveoli. This is altogether different from bronchopneumonia in which the exudate is located especially about bronchi and hence forms nodules that are somewhat unevenly dispersed.

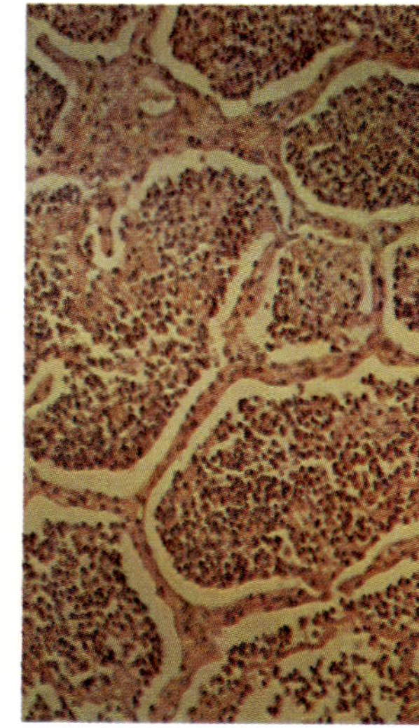

At higher power the exudate is seen to lie within alveoli without necrosis or disruption of the alveolar walls. If the exudate resolves, the alveoli will clear and function will be restored; if the exudate organizes, the alveoli will be filled with fibrous tissue and function will be lost.

ABSCESS OF LUNG

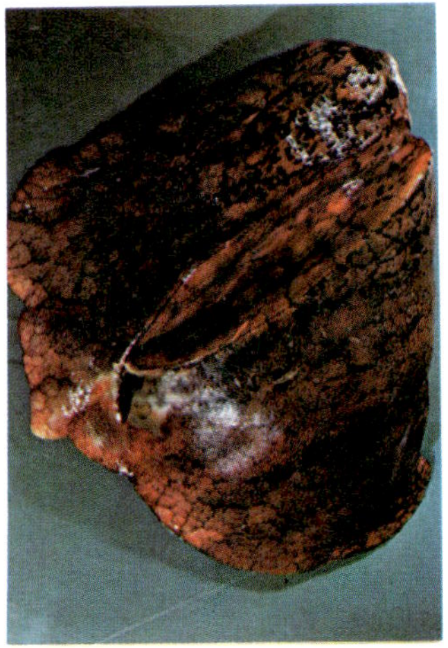

The tissue is firm, hyperemic, and distended. The surface is roughened with fibrinous adhesions.

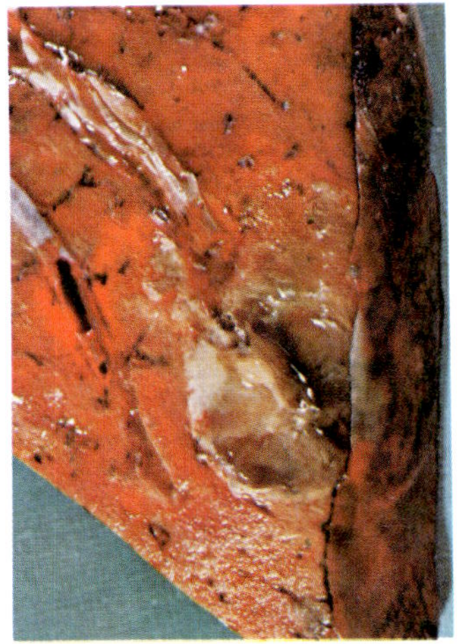

Section reveals the abscess cavity; it is roughly round, immediately adjacent to the pleura, and a dense leukocytic infiltration is present in the marginal tissue.

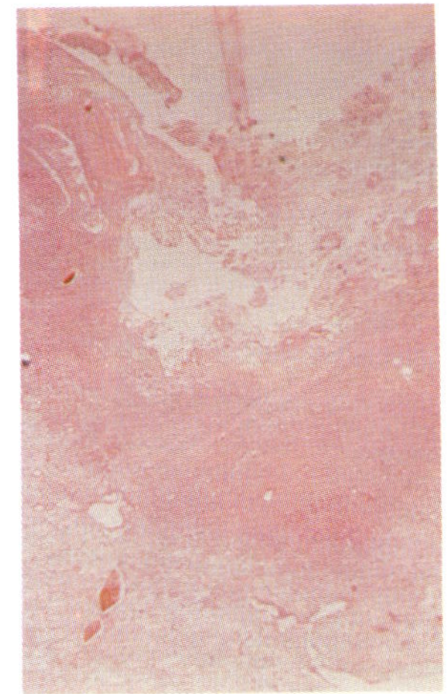

A scanning view shows the abscess cavity above, the wall of the cavity in the middle, and the viable less densely inflamed pulmonary tissue below.

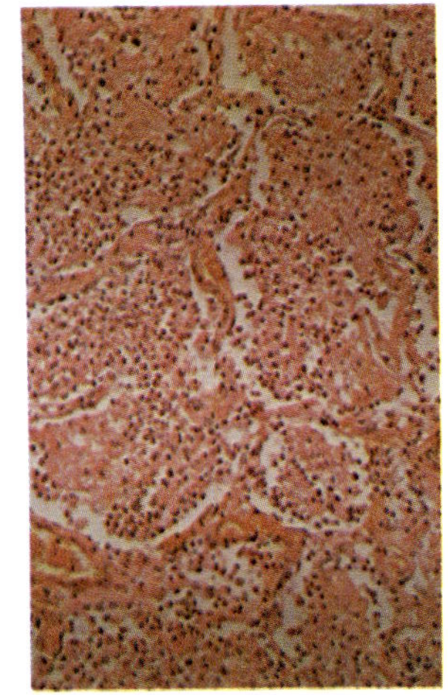

The abscess wall discloses intact alveoli filled with strands of fibrin and masses of segmented granulocytes.

ABSCESS OF LUNG

CLINICAL ACCOUNT 6258

The patient was a white male 67 years old who had a hemiglossectomy and left radical dissection for carcinoma of the tongue 18 months before entering the hospital. His admitting complaints were weakness and dizziness, with a tendency to fall.

The temperature was 98.6 degrees F., pulse 85, respirations 16, and blood pressure 135/95 mm. Hg. The face was swollen, the left half of the tongue was absent, and a draining sinus was present on the left side of the neck. The hematocrit was 40 and the leukocyte count was 13,700, with a slight neutrophilia. A chest x-ray revealed pleural fluid on the left, consolidation at the base of the right lung, enlargement of the heart, and slight displacement of the mediastinum to the right. In the last few days of a 13-week course the temperature rose to 102.2 degrees F., bronchopneumonia was presumed, response to antibiotic therapy was not discernable, and the patient died.

Autopsy examination disclosed recurrent carcinoma of the tongue and metastatic carcinoma of the tissues of the neck. There were also an acute fibrinous pleuritis on both sides, bilateral bronchopneumonia, and an abscess in the lower lobe of the left lung. The right and left lungs each weighed 925 Gms.

THE ENTITY

An abscess is a tissue cavity lined by an inflammatory margin. Abscesses of lung occur at any age and especially in those with a depressed cough reflex such as results from anesthesia, alcoholism, or coma. Common organisms are staphylococci, streptococci, and Friedlander's bacillus. Clinically the lesion is manifested by cough, fever, and copious sputum that is purulent and foul-smelling. X-rays reveal a round focus of translucency that may show a fluid level. The lesion tends to heal by marginal fibrosis and scar formation, although the outlook depends chiefly on the primary cause. Spread to pleura with empyema and to brain with meningitis or cerebral abscess are main complications.

Inhalation abscesses tend to occur in the upper lobes, especially on the right, and are due to inspired pus, teeth, blood clot, or infected tonsil (1). Abscesses also arise from bronchogenic carcinomas that block the tube or discharge necrotic material into it. Pneumonias may fail to resolve so that abscesses form; both lungs are often involved. Septic emboli arising especially from foci of suppuration in the pelvis or lower limbs are an additional cause; the lesions tend to be small, multiple, and subpleural. In the tropics, lung abscess is a consequence of hepatic amebiasis which spreads into the right lower lobe with or without an intervening amebic empyema. In some cases the cause is not apparent.

1. Spencer, H. Pathology of the Lung. Second Edition. Pergamon Press, New York, 1969.

PULMONARY EMPHYSEMA

CLINICAL ACCOUNT 6401

The patient was a 74-year-old white male retired banker who was admitted to the hospital for the eighth time because of gradually progressive dyspnea of ten years' duration. The dyspnea was associated with transient periods of acute bronchitis, peripheral edema, and ascites formation. During the past six months the patient also complained of angina pectoris. His presenting complaints were pronounced dyspnea and extreme weakness. He had smoked one to two packs of cigarettes each day for the past 50 years.

The vital signs were normal except for a respiratory rate of 38 per minute. The chest was elongated, the anterior-posterior diameter was increased, and the intercostal spaces retracted on inspiration. The liver edge was 4 cm. below the right costal margin. The urine was normal. The hemoglobin was 15.3 Gm., the hematocrit was 48, and the leukocyte count was 12,100, with a slight neutrophilia. Chest x-rays revealed lowering of the diaphragm and hyperlucency of the lung fields. The cardiac outline was normal. The electrocardiogram was suggestive of cor pulmonale. The shortness of breath became progressively severe, thick secretions accumulated in his bronchi, and death occurred three weeks after the patient had been hospitalized.

Autopsy examination revealed fibrous adhesions of the pleura, chronic bronchitis, and marked emphysema. Other diagnoses included acute ulcers of the stomach, diverticula of the colon, bilateral inguinal hernias, glandular hyperplasia of the prostate, and hypertrophy of the urinary bladder. The heart weighed 380 Gm.; neither ventricle was hypertrophic.

THE ENTITY

Pulmonary emphysema is a dilatation and destruction of the air sacs of the lung. The condition is extensive and may be centrilobular affecting mainly the upper lobes, or panlobular affecting all of the lobes. The former is more common than the latter and may be an earlier stage of it. The condition is due to a loss of elastic tissue which decreases the recoil of the air sacs and reduces the structural support of them. As a result, forced expiration is required, intra-alveolar pressure is increased, and more dilatation takes place. The condition is thus gradually progressive. As the air sacs dilate and the walls rupture, gaseous exchange is reduced and pulmonary arterial pressure is increased. Air hunger develops and is eventually followed by right heart failure.

Grossly the lungs are large, soft, pale, light, and excessively porous. Microscopically the air sacs are large and the alveolar walls are thin, fibrosed, and often bloodless. The condition is regarded as bullous when the air sacs exceed 1 cm. in diameter. The process may also take place at the site of pulmonary scarring; cicatricial emphysema. The cause is unknown although chronic bronchitis is commonly present and may play a role.

Clinically there are shortness of breath, productive cough, increased anterior-posterior diameter of the chest, and air hunger from difficulty exhaling. Radiographs show elongation of the chest, hyperlucent lung fields, narrowing of the mediastinum, and flattening of the diaphragm. The body is wasted. There are often associated conditions including asthma, chronic bronchitis, pulmonary tuberculosis, and exposure to irritant dusts and gases including cigarette smoke. The course is long. Common terminal events include cor pulmonale with right heart failure, superimposed pulmonary infection, and rupture of a pleural bleb with sudden pneumothorax.

PULMONARY EMPHYSEMA

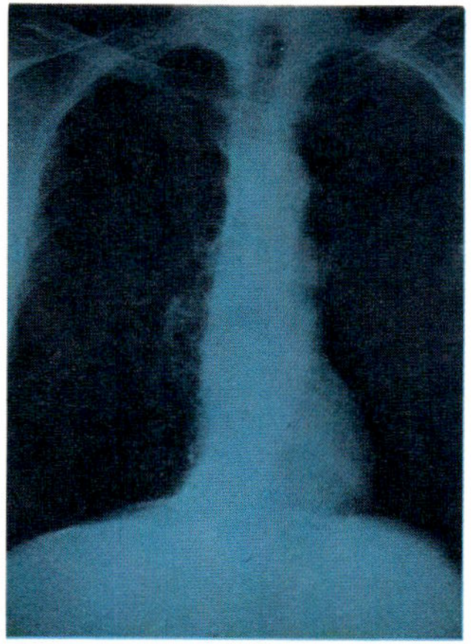

The photograph shows the characteristic findings of advanced pulmonary emphysema, i.e., flat diaphragm, hyperlucent lungs, and elongation of the chest.

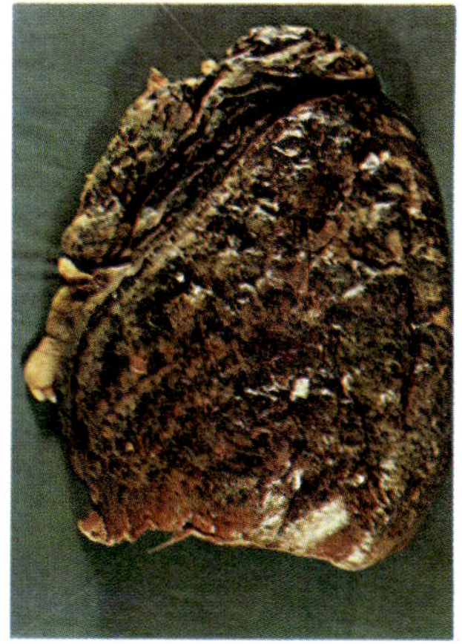

Although partially fixed, the lung readily collapses leaving the pleural surface coarsely wrinkled. There is scant tissue beneath the pleura to support the normal contour.

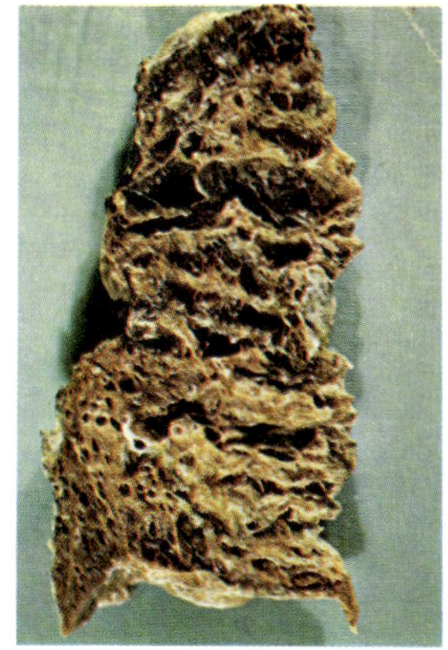

On section the reason for collapse is evident; scarcely any normal tissue remains. The air sacs are vastly dilated and coalesced so that large empty spaces traversed by delicate septae are all that remain.

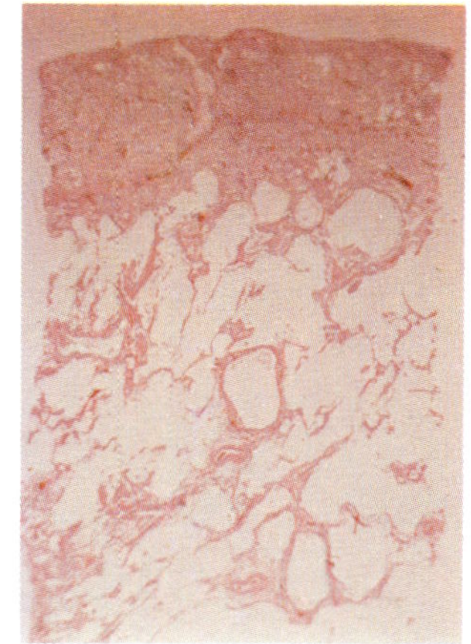

At scanning power the pleura is seen to be thickened with fibrous connective tissue and the subjacent regions reveal coalescence of markedly dilated air sacs.

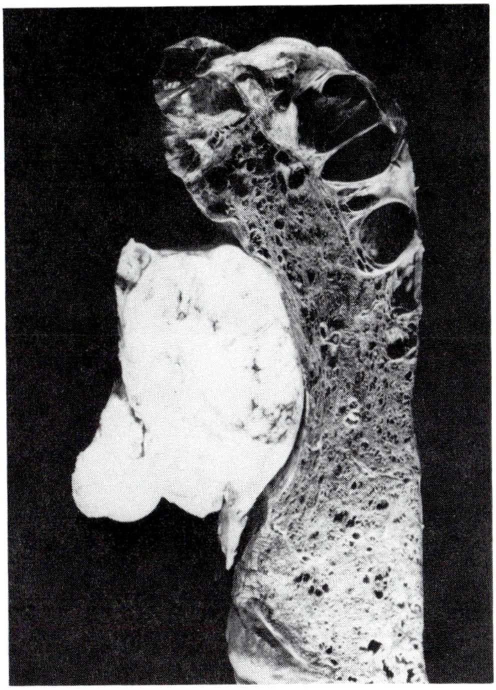

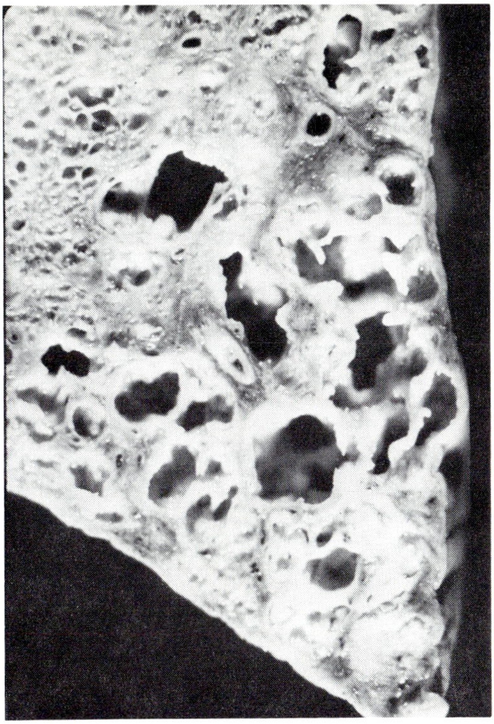

BRONCHIECTASIS

Left: The pale gray solid mass is metastatic tumor in mediastinal lymph nodes. The cut surface of the adjacent left lung shows emphysema with bullae in the upper lobe, bronchopneumonia in the lower lobe, and bronchiectasis in the extreme right lower tip of the cut surface. **Right:** A close-up of the bronchiectasis shows the pronounced surface dilatation of the bronchi extending nearly to the pleural surface. In chambers like these, secretions accumulate, degenerate and cause coughing and expectoration of sputum that is copious in amount and foul in odor.

Left: The unmagnified microsection reveals the dilated bronchi extending nearly to the pleural surface, and the fibrosis of the air sacs between the dilated chambers. Exudate may be seen pooling in the dilated bronchi. **Right:** Higher power reveals a bronchiectatic chamber that contains purulent exudate. Part of the mucosa displays squamous metaplasia. Outside of the mucosa the wall is composed of fibrous connective tissue.

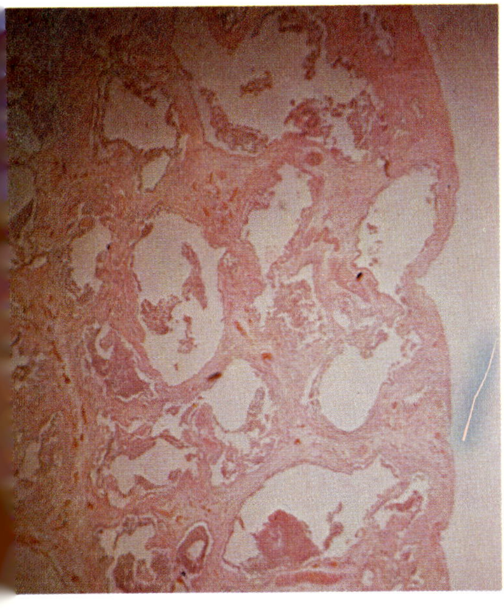

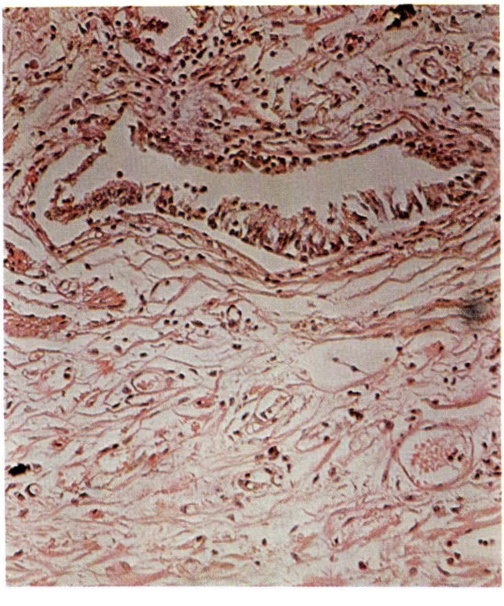

BRONCHIECTASIS

CLINICAL ACCOUNT 6474

The patient was a white male 74 years old who entered the hospital because of dyspnea. He was well until six months previously, when tiredness and anorexia were first noted. These persisted, and there was a slight loss of weight. A chest x-ray revealed "water on the left lung." The dyspnea increased. There had been no hemoptysis, chest pain, orthopnea, cough, or leg edema.

The vital signs were normal except for a respiratory rate of 27. The chest was increased in thickness, the breath sounds were distant, and rales were heard over both bases. The urine was normal except for a trace of albumin. The hemoglobin was 12.1 Gm., hematocrit 36, and leukocytes 30,000, with a slight neutrophilia. A chest x-ray disclosed a large oval mass in the region of the left hilum. Bronchoscopy was normal, and cytologic examination revealed no metastatic tumor. On the eleventh hospital day a thoracotomy was performed, the hilar mass was biopsied, and histologic examination revealed giant cell carcinoma. The patient had a cardiac arrest and died four days later.

Autopsy examination revealed a giant cell carcinoma of the left lung with massive metastasis to the mediastinal lymph nodes. The right and left lungs weighed 1070 and 1000 Gm., respectively. There were also an acute fibrinous pleuritis, bronchopneumonia, and bronchiectasis of both lower lobes. Emphysema was pronounced in both lungs. The heart was hypertrophied and weighed 465 Gm. Incidental diagnoses included a mural thrombus of the pulmonary artery, a mural thrombus of the abdominal aorta, nephrolithiasis of both kidneys, and nodular hyperplasia of the prostate.

THE ENTITY

Bronchiectasis is the combination of dilatation and inflammation of bronchi. The former may be cylindrical or saccular and often extends outward to the subpleura. The latter may be acute or chronic and is associated with necrosis and the pooling of mucous secretions and purulent exudate. The process tends to occur in the lower parts of the lower lobes. Microscopically, columnar cells line the surface, squamous metaplasia is frequent, necrotizing inflammation is prominent, and the dilated tubes fill with exudate, desquamated mucosa, mucinous secretions, and granular debris.

The process occurs in both sexes at all ages and is especially common in those under age 20. The condition is usually secondary to bronchial obstruction which causes secretions to accumulate, become infected, and damage the walls which then dilate. Obstruction is often due to asthma, bronchitis with squamous metaplasia, sinusitis with post-nasal drip, and tumors that compress bronchi. The usual organisms are staphylococci, streptococci, pneumococci, escherichia, and hemophilus. The clinical manifestations are fever, cough, and copious foul-smelling purulent sputum. In advanced cases there may also be dyspnea, orthopnea, cyanosis, and clubbing of the fingers. Complications include pneumonia, lung abscess, broncho-pleural fistula, empyema, and "metastatic" meningitis or cerebral abscess. In addition, bronchial arteries dilate and anastomose with pulmonary arteries so that pulmonary hypertension results; the left ventricle is also strained because its output must exceed that of the right ventricle by the amount that shunts from pulmonary tissue to left atrium, left ventricle, aorta, bronchial arteries, and pulmonary arteries. Thus cor pulmonale or left ventricular failure may result (1).

1. Liebold, A.A., Hales, M.R., and Lindskog, G.E. Enlargement of bronchial arteries, and their anastomoses with the pulmonary arteries in bronchiectasis. Am. J. Path. 25:211, 1949.

INFARCT OF LUNG

CLINICAL ACCOUNT 6200

The patient was a white male 25 years old who was well until six months before admission to the hospital. At that time diarrhea began. The stools were loose, then watery, and finally bloody. During the first two months there were as many as 20 bowel movements per day. The diarrhea then gradually subsided. Ten days before admission, unpleasantness in his home was followed by extreme nervousness and recurrence of the diarrhea. The patient's weight had dropped from 220 to 160 pounds. Two years previously he had seen a psychiatrist for "anxieties."

The patient lived with his parents. He was employed by his father who was described as wealthy, demanding, and intolerant. The patient was hospitalized; the hemoglobin was 5.4 Gm., the hematocrit was 23, and the leukocytes numbered 11,400 with a neutrophilia. A barium enema revealed ulcerative colitis from sigmoid to cecum, transfusions were given. He was discharged to seek psychiatric help.

Two months later he was re-admitted with acute fulminant ulcerative colitis. On the fifth day decompression of the colon was undertaken by cecostomy. Two days later cardiac arrest occurred, and on the following day the patient died.

Autopsy examination revealed acute tracheobronchitis, bronchopneumonia, pulmonary thrombo-emboli, and recent infarcts of both lungs. There were also an acute esophagitis, atrophy of the pancreas, fatty metamorphosis of the liver, and Zahn infarcts of the hepatic tissue. An organizing thrombus was present in the right renal vein.

THE ENTITY

Large emboli to the lung cause sudden death from right heart failure. Small emboli cause only hemorrhage, since the viability of the tissue is preserved by the bronchial circulation. Small emboli cause pulmonary infarcts if passive hyperemia is also present; the essential feature is necrosis of pulmonary tissue. Infarcts tend to occur in the lower lobes and are often multiple. The lesions are firm, hemorrhagic, well defined, peripheral in location and 3 to 4 cm. in diameter; the overlying pleura is bulging, dark red, and covered with fibrin. Microscopically the alveolar walls are necrotic, and the blood is in a state of degeneration. If the emboli are septic, suppuration follows and abscesses form. Otherwise the lesion gradually decolorizes and undergoes cicatrization so that the pleural surface becomes indented and roughened by fibrous adhesions.

Pulmonary infarcts are frequent and serious (1). They occur in older patients, especially those with cancer, heart disease, or recent operation. The emboli arise from the deep leg veins. Clinically there is sudden pain in the chest associated with cough, hemoptysis, tachycardia, pleuritic pain, a friction rub, occasionally fever, and sometimes an opacity on the chest x-ray. Vasoconstriction may cause dyspnea and cyanosis. Anticoagulation, early ambulation and ligation of the inferior vena cava tend to prevent recurrence of the problem.

1. Hodgson, C.H., and Good, C.A. Pulmonary embolism and infarction. Med. Clin. N. Am. 48:977, 1964.

INFARCT OF LUNG

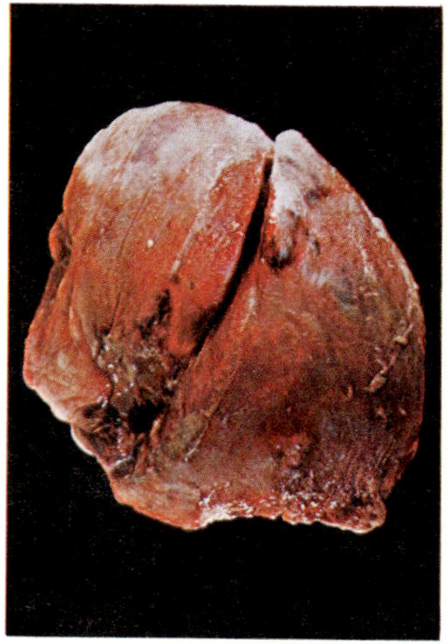

The pleura of the left lung is roughened by friable pale yellow fibrinous adhesions. In the lower part of the upper lobe there is a bulging focus of dark red discoloration. A similar appearance is seen in the lower part of the lower lobe. These are the external appearances of recent infarcts.

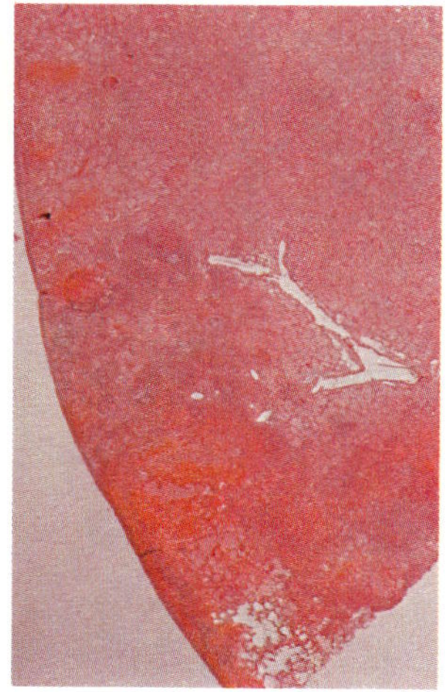

The scanning power reveals an infarct; it is pyramidal in shape with the base toward the pleura, the pleura bulges and is covered with fibrin, and the infarct is hemorrhagic.

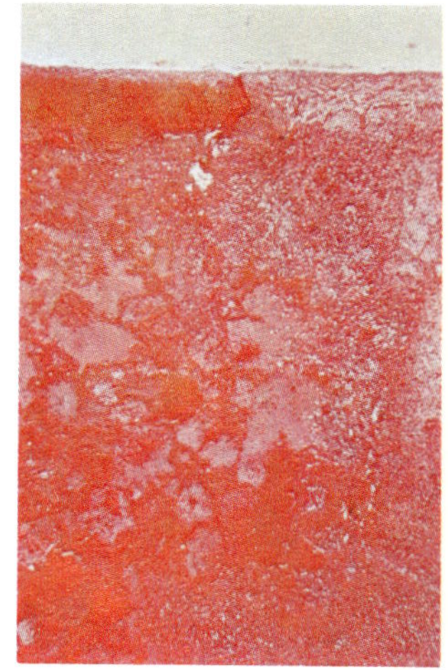

At low power, the hemorrhagic necrosis of recent infarction is present on the left while the inflamed, viable, and noninfarcted tissue is present on the right.

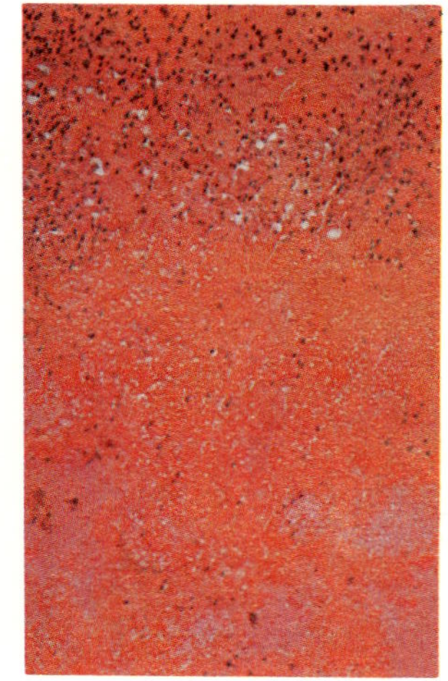

At higher power the extensive hemorrhagic necrosis of recent infarction can be seen.

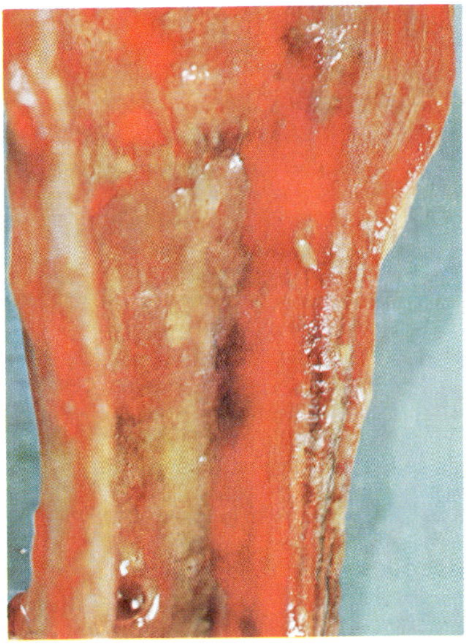

The microsection of trachea reveals necrotic mucosa and a thick exudate overlying the surface. This richly cellular exudate is attributed to secondary bacterial infection.

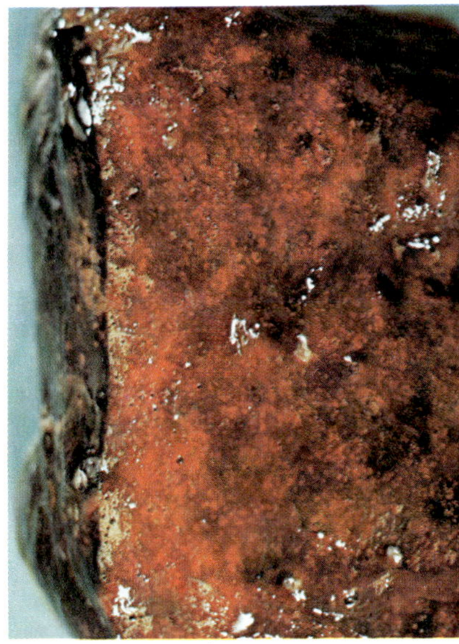

The cut surfaces of both lungs are wet, dark brownish red, and of uniformly increased firmness. The pleural surfaces are mottled with black as the result of anthracotic pigmentation.

PRIMARY ATYPICAL PNEUMONIA

At low magnification the pulmonary tissue reveals small foci of recent hemorrhage, widespread infiltration with macrophages, enlargement and desquamation of alveolar lining cells, and proteinaceous fluid within the air sacs.

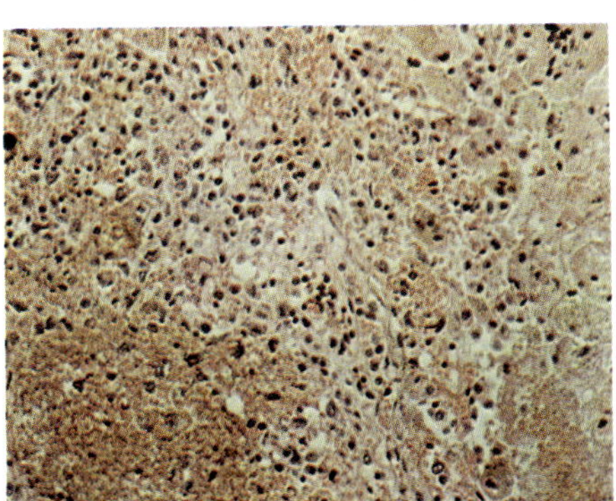

At higher magnification macrophages, lymphocytes, and desquamated alveolar lining cells may be seen. The alveolar walls are thickened, and the air sacs contain proteinaceous fluid. Although hyaline membranes usually line the air sacs in this condition, they are not present in this instance. This reaction is altogether different from bacterial pneumonia in which the alveoli remain intact and the air sacs become filled with solid masses of polymorphonuclear leukocytes.

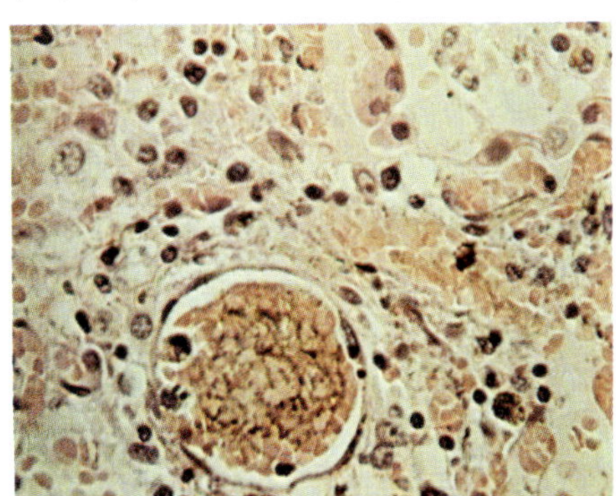

PRIMARY ATYPICAL PNEUMONIA

CLINICAL ACCOUNT 6013

The patient was a white male 57 years old who had been well until eight days before admission, when he developed malaise, weakness, muscle aches, a slight cough, and a low-grade fever. There were also dizziness and slight shortness of breath on exertion. On the morning of admission he was acutely dyspneic and entered the hospital for this reason. For the past several months he had had slight dyspnea on walking two blocks or climbing one flight of stairs. He smoked one pack of cigarettes daily and was taking antihypertensive medication.

The temperature was 97.4 degrees F., pulse 96, respirations 22, and blood pressure 130/90. The skin was pale. Coarse rales were audible over both bases. The physical examination was not otherwise remarkable. The urine was normal except for a few leukocytes in the sediment. The hemoglobin was 5.7 Gm., the hematocrit was 17 per cent, and the leukocytes numbered 5,000 with 14 segmented granulocytes, 12 band cells, 2 myelocytes, 62 lymphocytes, 7 monocytes, and 3 eosinophiles. Bone marrow examination revealed no maturation arrest. A chest x-ray disclosed "diffuse interstitial fibrosis."

During the hospital course the temperature ranged from 98 degrees to 104 degrees F. Digitalis, antibiotics, and transfusions were given. The anemia and leukopenia persisted. The dyspnea gradually increased. On the sixth day the chest x-ray revealed increased interstitial infiltration and enlargement of the cardiac outline. On the eleventh day a tracheostomy was performed and a respirator was applied. On the fourteenth day the temperature rose to 104 degrees F., the blood pressure fell, and the patient died.

Autopsy examination revealed interstitial pneumonitis; the right and left lungs weighed 1360 and 1425 Gm., respectively. There were also an acute ulcerative tracheobronchitis, a recent infarct of the right lung, acute fibrinous pericarditis, passive hyperemia of the liver with centrilobular necrosis, and recent infarcts of the spleen and prostate.

THE ENTITY

The condition called "flu" is known in morphologic terms as primary atypical pneumonia (1), and more recently, as usual interstitial pneumonia (2). The conditions are identical and are caused by various viruses as well as the Eaton agent, *Mycoplasma pneumoniae*. The clinical manifestations range from mild upper respiratory congestion to an acute toxic febrile illness with a fulminant course in which respiratory failure is progressive and death occurs in a few days. Bacterial infection often complicates the terminal period.

The lungs are wet and heavy. The pleural surfaces are usually smooth and glistening. The tissue is somewhat soft; there is no consolidation. The characteristic histologic feature is a cellular exudate within the interstitial tissue, i.e., within the alveolar walls which are uniformly thickened. The alveoli contain proteinaceous fluid, hyaline membranes, and cellular exudate. The cells are monocytes, macrophages, and desquamated septal or alveolar cells. Neutrophils and plasma cells may be seen in small numbers. Most cases undergo resolution.

1. Parker, F., Jr., Jolliffe, L.S., and Finland, M. Primary atypical pneumonia. Arch. Path. 44:581, 1947.
2. Liebow, A.A., and Smith, D. The Lung. The Williams and Wilkins Co., Baltimore, 1968.

ALVEOLAR PROTEINOSIS

CLINICAL ACCOUNT 5915

The patient was a Negro woman 28 years old who took a steroid medication for two weeks because of swelling and tenderness of the thyroid. The symptoms subsided; the medication was continued. One week before admission her morning cough became worse, malaise was noted, and the temperature rose to 99.6 degrees F. On the day of admission she had a sharp pain in the right chest that was accentuated by deep breathing. She then became short of breath, the cough worsened, and abundant "dirty" sputum was raised.

The temperature was 102 degrees F., pulse 120, respirations 32, and blood pressure 120/70. Breath sounds were decreased, and coarse rales were heard. The urine disclosed 3 plus protein. The hemoglobin was 15.0 Gm., hematocrit 47, and leukocytes 11,000, with 66 neutrophils and 18 band cells. The serum glutamic transaminase and lactic dehydrogenase were elevated. During the hospital course an anemia developed. The leukocytes rose to 24,000, with 59 neutrophils, and 22 band cells. A right thoracentesis yielded 300 ml. of bloody fluid. Dyspnea increased. A chest x-ray disclosed a widespread infiltration in both lung fields. Oliguria developed, and peritoneal dialysis was performed. Respiratory distress increased, coma supervened, and death occurred on the fifteenth hospital day.

Autopsy examination revealed alveolar proteinosis, focal acute interstitial pancreatitis, and passive hyperemia of the liver. Other diagnoses were incidental. The heart weighed 325 Gm., the right and left lungs, 950 and 775 Gms., respectively.

THE ENTITY

Alveolar proteinosis is a noninflammatory diffuse accumulation of lipid-rich, PAS positive, proteinaceous material within alveolar sacs (1). The lungs are heavy and sink in water, the cut surfaces are uniformly firm, and the pleural surfaces are usually smooth. Alveolar macrophages increase in number, accumulate within the lumens, and disintegrate there. The intra-alveolar PAS positive material may also be present within bronchopulmonary lymph nodes.

The condition occurs in adults, more often in males. The onset is gradual, with dyspnea and cough productive of yellow gelatinous sputum. There are rales, diminished breath sounds, and occasionally clubbing of the fingers. X-rays reveal a fine diffuse mottling suggestive of edema. Leukocytosis and a high serum lactic dehydrogenase are expected. The course is one of either spontaneous improvement, or, more often, steady progression. Pulmonary lavage is useful therapy (2). Death is due to respiratory failure.

The cause is uncertain, but the findings suggest impairment of the pulmonary clearing process; i.e., the material is abnormal and the alveolar lining cells cannot remove it, or the alveolar lining cells are abnormal and the material consists of accumulated normal secretions and debris.

1. Rosen, S.H., Castleman, B., and Liebow, A.A. Pulmonary alveolar proteinosis. N. Eng. J. Med. 258:1123, 1958.
2. Ramirez-R, J. Pulmonary alveolar proteinosis. Treatment by massive broncho-pulmonary lavage. Arch. Int. Med. 119:147, 1967.

ALVEOLAR PROTEINOSIS

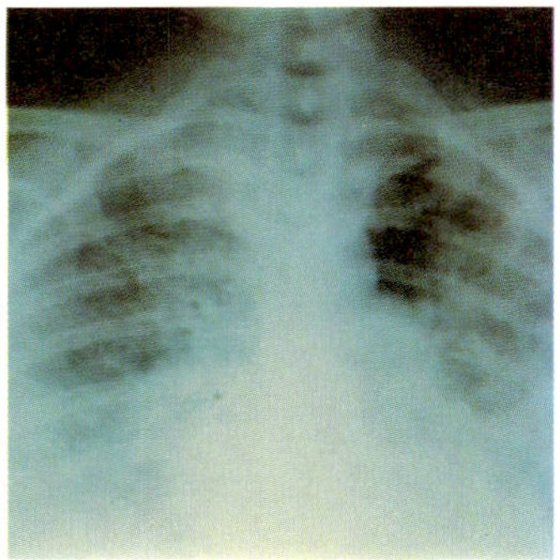

The chest x-ray discloses an extensive infiltration throughout both lung fields.

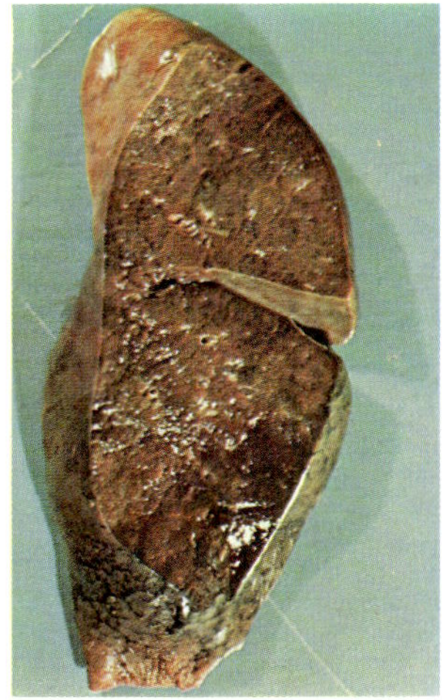

The cut surfaces are brownish red mottled with dark red. All cut surfaces are uniformly increased in firmness; pleural surfaces smooth and glistening.

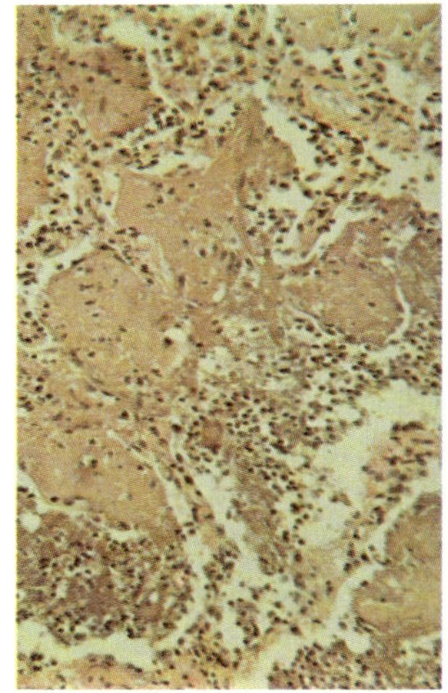

A characteristic of alveolar proteinosis is a positive reaction of the alveolar semifluid to the Schiff-periodic acid stain (PAS). The photograph shows the pink positive reaction.

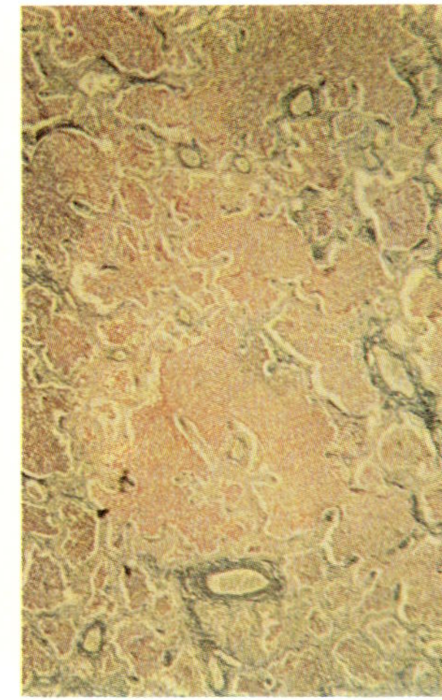

Histologic sections reveal alveoli to be filled with a protein-rich semifluid in which cells are sparse. Most of these are macrophages; only a few segmented granulocytes are present.

METASTATIC CALCIFICATION

The chest x-ray reveals oval masses of radio-opaque tissue in the patient's right upper lung field. These bear a similarity to metastatic neoplasm.

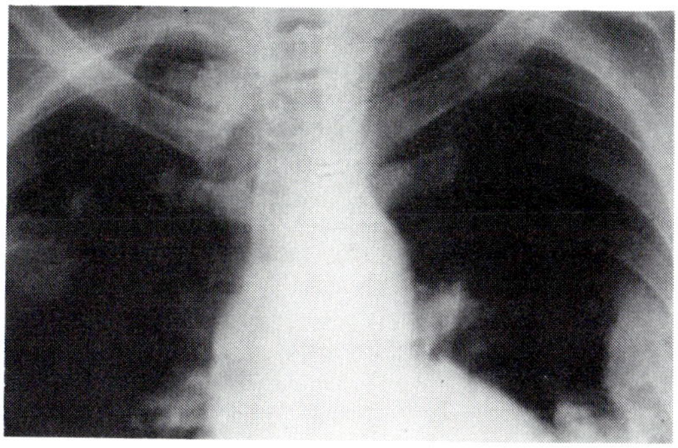

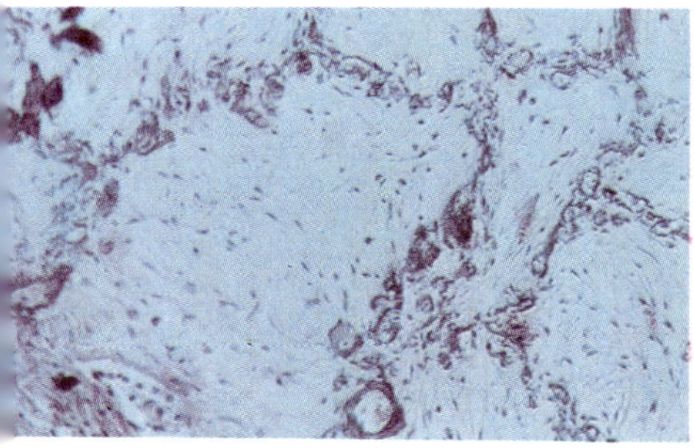

A portion of fixed lung reveals discrete pallid foci of increased firmness that cut with a gritty sensation.

Microsections disclose a reticulated pattern of calcium deposition that lies within alveolar walls. In this section the alveoli are occupied by loosely constructed fibrous connective tissue. Elsewhere the air sacs were empty and the alveolar walls were equally the seat of calcium deposition.

At higher power the coarse nature of the calcium deposition is evident. While connective tissue is abundant, a leukocytic infiltration is conspicuously absent.

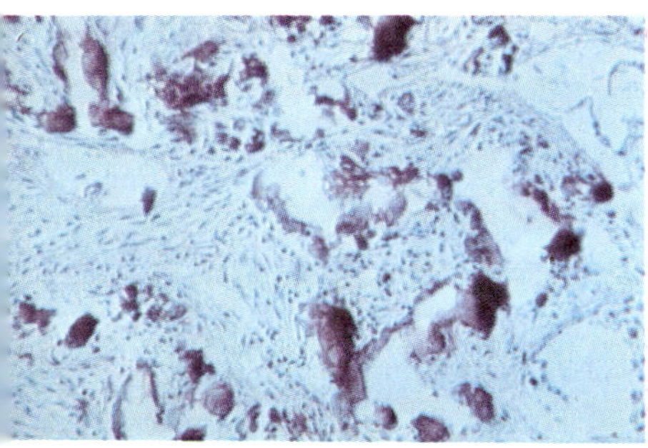

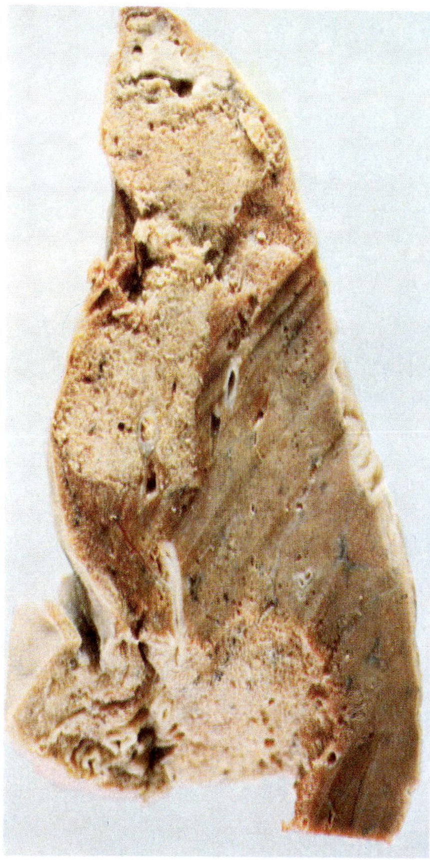

METASTATIC CALCIFICATION OF LUNG

CLINICAL ACCOUNT 5722

The patient was a white male 43 years old who complained of weakness, lethargy, and stupor. At age 32 bilateral polycystic renal disease was discovered. At age 39, hypertension developed. Uremia was noted at age 40. Since then peritoneal dialysis had been performed repeatedly. Chest x-rays fourteen months before admission were normal; two months later patchy densities were attributed to pneumonia, and one month before admission discrete oval densities were found on biopsy to be foci of metastatic calcification. The blood pressure was 140/95. Physical examination revealed pallor, widespread subcutaneous edema, and large masses in both flanks. The urine contained protein, and the blood revealed anemia. The blood urea nitrogen was 138 mgs. per 100 ml., and the serum calcium and phosphorus were 6.9 and 12.0 mgs. per 100 ml. respectively. The patient died of uremia after fifteen days in the hospital.

The principal autopsy diagnoses were congenital polycystic renal disease, ascites (450 ml.), hypertrophy of the heart (650 Gm.), metastatic calcification of lungs and metastatic calcification of old pulmonary thrombo-emboli. The right and left lungs weighed 750 and 700 Gms., respectively.

THE ENTITY

Deposition of calcium in injured or abnormal tissue is common and is called dystrophic calcification. Deposition of calcium in normal tissue is uncommon and is called metastatic calcification. The sites of predilection are especially the stomach, kidneys, and lungs. The gastric deposition is usually mucosal and consists of scattered flecks that do not affect function and are usually discernible only on microscopic examination of the tissue. Metastatic calcification of the kidneys also tends to be slight but may occasionally be sufficient to impair function and become recognizable on the abdominal x-ray. Calcification of the lung is often widespread and pronounced. The calcium deposits in the alveolar walls, the structures become fixed, and granulation tissue may fill the air sacs. The gross and microscopic features are shown on the photographs.

Metastatic pulmonary calcification is associated with five conditions, i.e., chronic renal failure, parathyroid adenoma, excessive ingestion of calcium salts, excessive intake of Vitamin D, and destructive lesions of bone including leukemia, myelomatosis, and widespread metastatic carcinoma (1). In renal disease phosphate is retained, the serum calcium falls, and hypertrophy of the parathyroids produces excessive parathormone. In parathyroid adenoma, the parathormone liberates calcium, nephrocalcinosis with renal failure follows, and phosphate is secondarily retained. In both instances the calcium-phosphate product exceeds the solubility level of the blood which is 75 mg. per cent. Over that figure, calcium deposition in normal tissues begins. Bone decalcification in children causes dwarfism and renal rickets; in adults it causes osteitis fibrosa cystica generalisata.

1. Smith, J.C., Stanton, L.W., Kramer, N.C., and Parrish, A.E. Nodular pulmonary calcification in renal failure, report of a case. Am. Rev. Resp. Dis. 100:723, 1969.

RADIATION PNEUMONITIS

CLINICAL ACCOUNT 1860

The patient was a white girl four years old who complained of cough and dyspnea of two weeks' duration. The lymph nodes of the left axilla were enlarged, and biopsy of them revealed lymphosarcoma. A chest x-ray disclosed a mass in the right lung field that merged with the mediastinum. The mediastinum was irradiated on 49 days over the following four months. The central tissue dose was 2915r. During the last month of treatment, respiratory distress markedly increased. Amethopterin, nitrogen mustard, prednisone, penicillin, and oxygen were given. Two weeks before death, an x-ray of the chest revealed an infiltration especially on the right that suggested radiation pneumonitis or metastatic tumor. The patient died of respiratory failure five months after the onset of her illness and four months after the beginning of her treatment.

Autopsy examination revealed the right and left lungs to weigh 220 and 270 Gm., respectively. Both had the consistency of liver. No tumor was found in either lung. Tumor was found, however, in both ovaries, one kidney, the uterine cervix, the vaginal mucosa, the bone marrow, and the abdominal lymph nodes. Focal fibrosis was extensive in the thoracic bone marrow.

THE ENTITY

Although the lung is relatively resistant to radiation, pulmonary tissue does reveal early and late reactions to the ionizing energy. The early stage, or acute radiation pneumonitis, which is common, begins one to four months after treatment and consists of slight dyspnea and a dry, hacking, nonproductive cough. During this time the chest x-ray reveals scattered fluffy densities throughout all lung fields. Morphologic examination shows desquamation of alveolar lining cells, filaments of fibrin within alveolar spaces, and accumulation of macrophages in the interstitial tissue. Neutrophils are scarce and necrosis is not seen. The reaction subsides gradually and spontaneously.

The pathogenesis of the lesion is uncertain but has been attributed to a proliferative response of macrophages to the ionizing injury, and a lymph blockage in which outflow obstruction causes macrophages to accumulate in a system normally balanced between cell renewal and cell depletion (1). The possibility also exists that viruses are liberated by the radiation; this explanation is especially attractive when the reaction develops in tissue shielded from the ionizing rays.

The late reaction is rare and arises two to eight years after treatment. It is also characterized by cough and dyspnea but in this instance the symptoms are relentessly progressive. The tissue shows dense adhesions and massive fibrosis with attachment to adjacent structures, eventually leading to gross deformity of the lungs, thorax, and spine. The pulmonary fibrosis causes respiratory insufficiency, and the kyphoscoliosis of the chest distorts the structure of the mediastinum with eventual vessel blockage, cor pulmonale, and right heart failure.

1. Smith, J.C. Radiation pneumonitis; a review. Am. J. Resp.Dis. 87:647, 1963.

RADIATION PNEUMONITIS

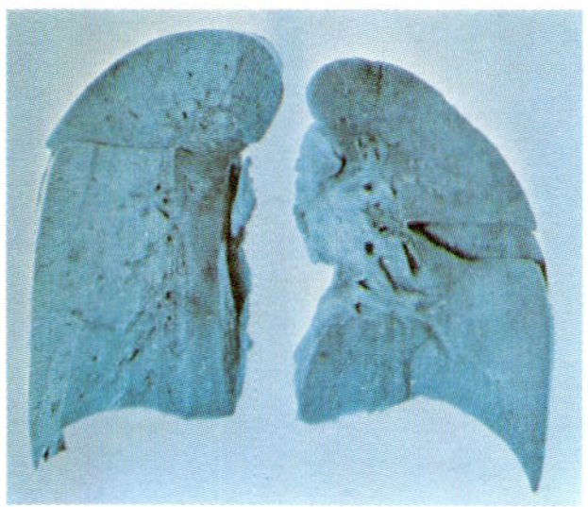

The lungs were similar and the cut surfaces before fixation were firm, subcrepitant, and pale brownish gray. In the photograph the tissue is fixed and the color is artefactual.

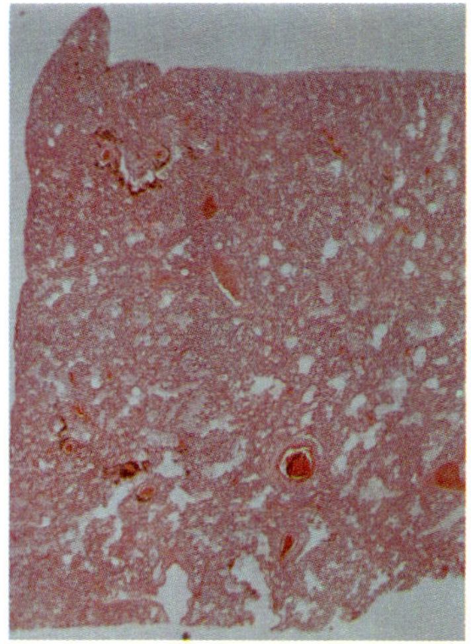

An unmagnified histologic section reveals diffuse filling of alveoli so that few open air sacs remain. All sections of both lungs were similar. A leukocytic infiltration is sparse.

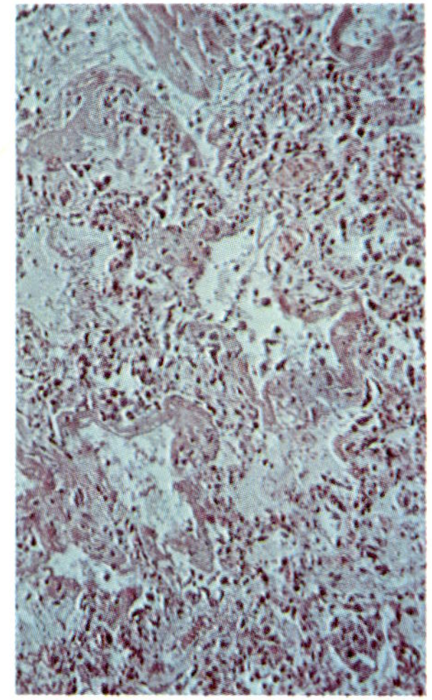

At low magnification, hyaline membranes lining the alveoli are evident and the lumens contain occasional lymphocytes and moderate numbers of large macrophages.

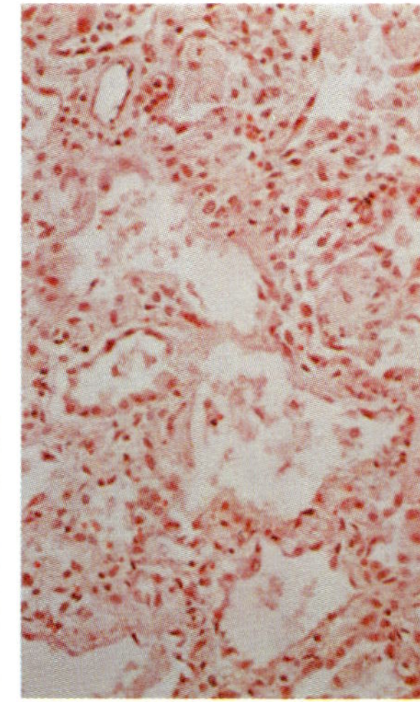

At higher magnification, thickening of the alveolar walls is conspicuous. Large macrophages are present within the alveolar walls and at the margins of the patent air sacs.

INTERSTITIAL PULMONARY FIBROSIS

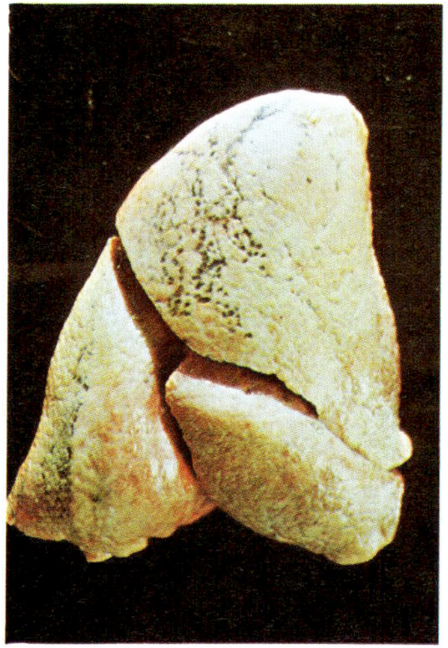

The right lung presents a glistening, pinkish gray, finely nodular pleural surface. The tissue is firm and retains its shape without need for fixation or inflation.

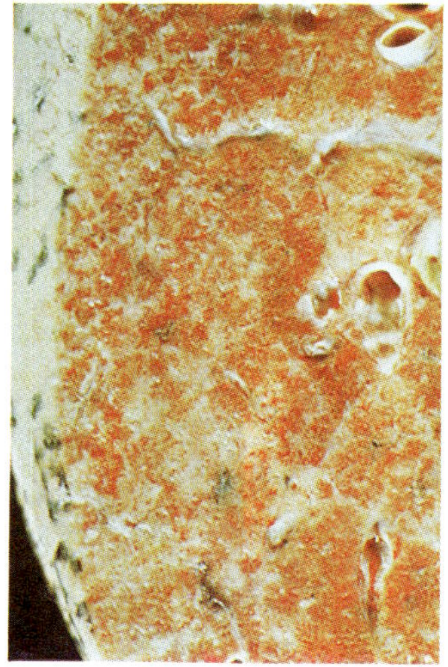

The cut surfaces are uniformly firm and pale mottled with light red. Neither fluid nor exudate can be expressed. The firmness and discoloration are uniform.

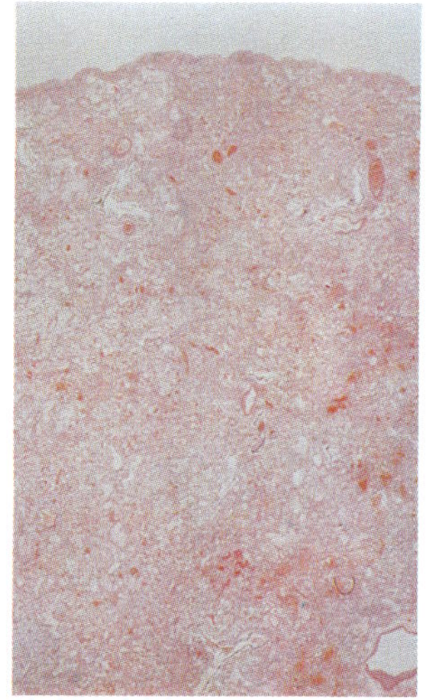

The unmagnified section shows extensive fibrosis that obliterates most of the air sacs.

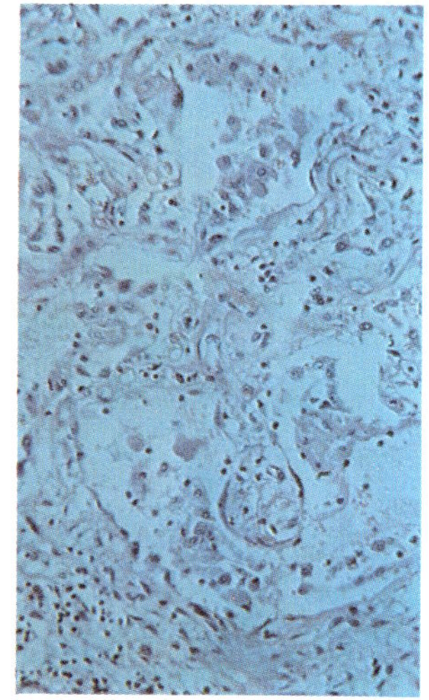

The magnified section discloses abundant interstitial connective tissue, conspicuous macrophages in the alveolar sacs and within the alveolar walls, and the presence of only occasional lymphocytes.

INTERSTITIAL PULMONARY FIBROSIS

CLINICAL ACCOUNT 5813

The patient was a white female 92 years old who was admitted to the hospital because of dyspnea. Shortness of breath had been pronounced on several occasions over the past three years. The patient had never been in congestive heart failure, she had never taken digitalis, and she had never been hypertensive. She had been diabetic for the past eight years, had had a right radical mastectomy for cancer of the breast 20 years previously. She was thin, undernourished, confused, and extremely dyspneic. Rales and rhonchi were present over both lung fields. A chest x-ray was interpreted as showing pulmonary edema. The heart was not enlarged, the rhythm was regular, and no murmurs were heard. She was treated with penicillin, aminophylline, digitalis, and a diuretic. Her condition steadily worsened, and she died after three days in the hospital.

The right and left lungs weighed 650 and 550 Gm., respectively. The heart weighed 375 Gm. and disclosed a pronounced calcification of the mitral valve annulus. Other diagnoses included effusions (600 ml. each side), and marked arteriolar nephrosclerosis.

THE ENTITY

Widespread fibrosis of pulmonary tissue is caused by many diseases including organizing pneumonia, silicosis, tuberculosis, sarcoidosis, berylliosis, asbestosis, scleroderma, rheumatoid disease, and systemic lupus erythematosus. When these conditions are excluded, there remain cases of primary interstitial fibrosis for which the cause is obscure. For such cases, four mechanisms of injury are suggested, i.e., organization of exudate with incorporation of fibrin into the alveolar walls, particulate damage to alveolar cells with accumulation of macrophages in air sacs and interstitial tissues, capillary damage from altered immune response, and chronic lymphedema with stimulation of collagen production (1). While the cause of the interstitial fibrosis in the present case is not clear, calcification of the mitral annulus was pronounced, annulus calcification may cause mitral insufficiency, and mitral insufficiency is associated with increased venous pressure and pulmonary lymphedema (2). It is thus possible that the persistent lymphedema stimulated the formation of reticulin and collagen fibers which eventually led to the diffuse interstitial fibrosis.

In interstitial fibrosis the lungs are firm and heavy with more or less solid cut surfaces. The pleura is often glistening and nodular with coarse indentations representing interstitial bands of fibrous tissue. Microscopically the alveoli show fibrin membranes and plump alveolar cells. The interstitial tissue is edematous, reticulin and collagen bands are laid down, and fibrous tissue gradually replaces the air sacs. Inflammation is slight and bacteria are absent. The process is bilateral and diffuse. The clinical features are dyspnea, cough, late cyanosis, and eventually weight loss. Tachypnea and fever are indications of superimposed infection. Death is due to respiratory insufficiency.

1. Spencer, H., in Liebow, A., and Smith, D.E. The Lung. The Williams and Wilkins Co., Baltimore, 1968.
2. Simon, M.A., and Liu, S.F. Calcification of the mitral valve annulus and its relation to functional valve disturbance. Am. Heart J. 48:497, 1954.

METASTATIC CALCIFICATION

CLINICAL ACCOUNT 5907

The patient was a white female 43 years old who was admitted to the hospital because of subcutaneous edema and shortness of breath. Nine months previously swelling of the right leg was noted; this was followed by widespread edema. Oliguria developed, and proteinuria and hypoproteinemia were discovered. One month before admission dyspnea began, and swelling of the abdomen was noted. The latter progressed, and during the three days preceding admission the dyspnea became severe.

The patient had had pulmonary tuberculosis for the past 20 years. There had been no complaints referable to the urinary tract before the onset of the present illness. The lungs revealed rales, the abdomen was distended with fluid, and edema of the extremities was pronounced. The urine disclosed 4 plus protein and the blood revealed anemia. There was no leukocytosis, and the blood urea nitrogen was normal. The total serum protein was 4.3 Gm. with 1.8 Gm. albumin and 2.5 Gm. globulin. A renal biopsy revealed amyloidosis.

Over the ensuing nine months renal failure progressed, acid-fast bacilli were identified in the sputum, and peritoneal dialysis became necessary because of oliguria and azotemia. During this time the blood calcium ranged from 6.4 to 10.2 mg. and the serum phosphorus from 6.9 to 12.6 mg. The two maximum values occurred together six weeks before death. The patient died of renal failure.

Autopsy examination revealed cavitary tuberculosis of the upper lobes of the right and left lungs, amyloidosis of the right and left kidneys, and anasarca. Additional diagnoses were incidental.

THE ENTITY

Calcification occurs in normal tissue when the product of the serum calcium and serum phosphorus expressed in milligrams per cent exceeds the solubility concentration of the blood, which is 75 mg. per 100 ml. (1). This is called metastatic calcification; when calcium is deposited in abnormal tissue the solubility product does not hold, and the process is called dystrophic calcification. The latter is, of course, much more common than the former.

Metastatic calcification is usually due to primary parathyroid hyperfunction due to adenoma formation, or secondary parathyroid hyperfunction due to renal failure. In the former instance, the high blood calcium causes nephrocalcinosis and eventually renal failure. In the latter instance, the tubules fail to excrete phosphorus, the blood level rises, and the serum calcium falls in response to this. As a result, the parathyroids undergo hypertrophy, and the serum calcium rises so that the product of the two ions eventually exceeds the critical solubility level.

Often the clinical problem is to decide whether the process is primarily renal with secondary hyperparathyroidism or primarily parathyroid disease with secondary renal failure. A helpful feature is that the excretion of calcium in the urine tends to be high with primary parathyroid disease and tends not to be raised with primary renal failure (1).

1. Smith, J.C., Stanton, L.W., Kramer, N.C., and Parrish, A.E. Nodular pulmonary calcification in renal failure, report of a case. Am. Rev. Resp. Dis. 100:723, 1969.

METASTATIC CALCIFICATION

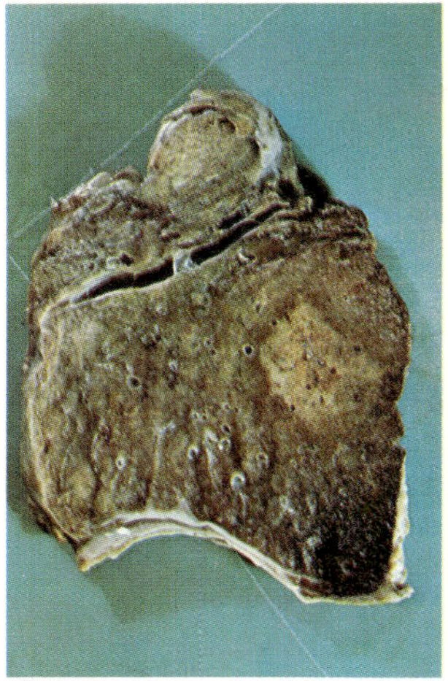

The cut surface of the right lung reveals a nearly collapsed upper lobe, and a pale brownish gray oval focus in the lower lobe that cuts with a gritty sensation. The latter is a focus of metastatic calcification.

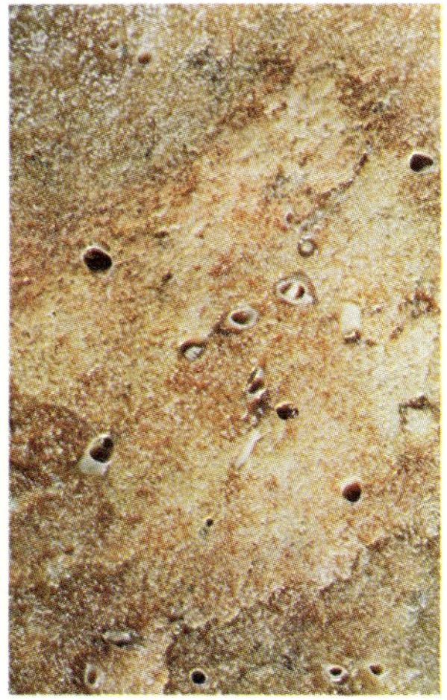

A closer view shows the pallid tissue that is firm, porous, and gritty. Elsewhere the tissue is soft and compressible.

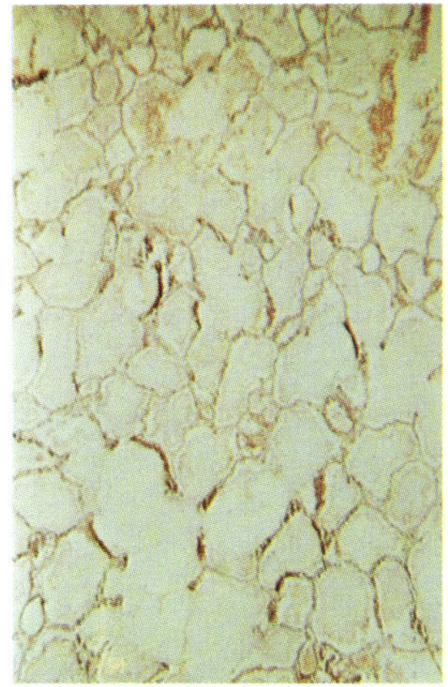

In the microsection, scattered alveolar walls reveal dark calcium deposits.

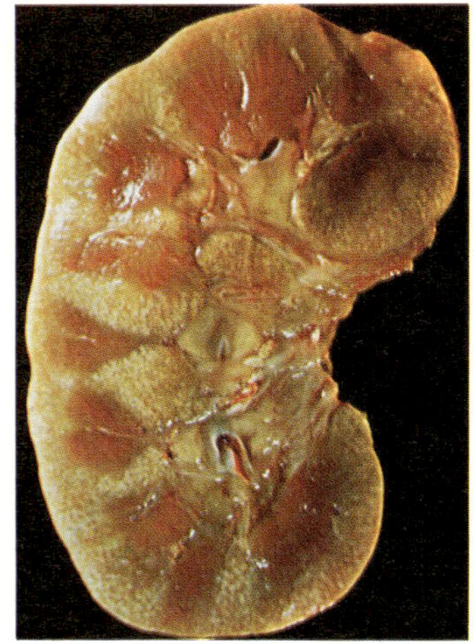

A cut surface of kidney shows a fine pale yellow speckling that is due to widespread macrophage infiltration. The glomeruli were large, avascular, and laden with amyloid.

HAMMAN-RICH SYNDROME

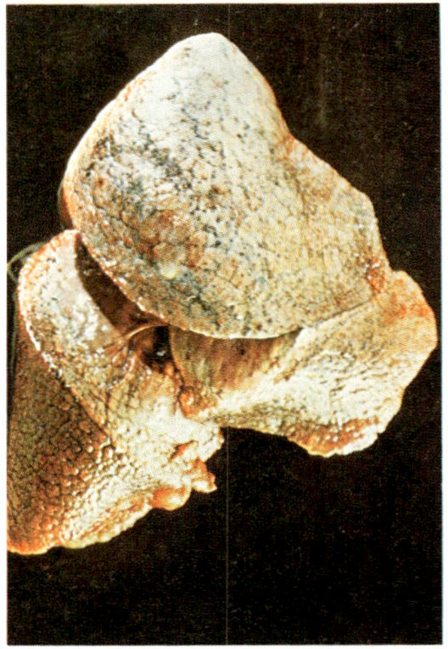

The right lung weighs 825 Gm. The pleural surface is finely nodular and glistening. The tissue is firm; it retains its shape without inflation with fixative. The left lung was similar and weighed 700 Gm.

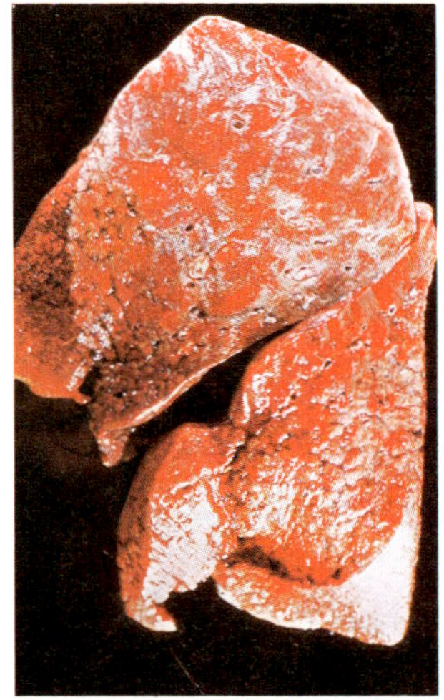

The cut surface is red, firm, more or less dry, and mottled with pale gray.

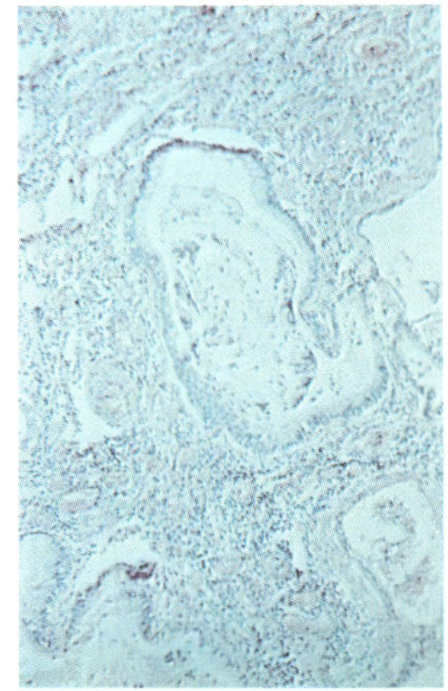

Microsections reveal dilated bronchi filled with mucin, squamous metaplasia of the lining cells, fibrosis of the intervening parenchyma, and a liberal infiltration with lymphocytes.

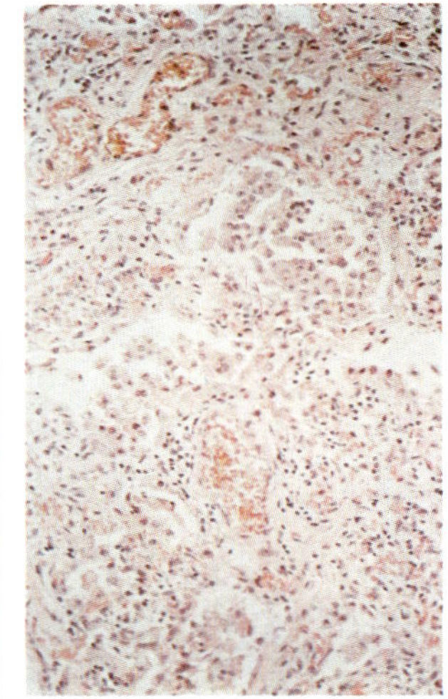

At higher magnification the alveoli disclose clusters of desquamated lining cells, and fibrosis of the alveolar walls. The latter process contributes especially to the increased firmness of the tissue.

HAMMAN-RICH SYNDROME

CLINICAL ACCOUNT 6018

The patient was a white male 51 years old who was known by biopsy to have diffuse interstitial fibrosis of both lungs. This caused dyspnea that had been gradually progressive for four years and rapidly progressive for the past year. At home the patient required 2.5 liters of nasal oxygen per minute to aid respiration. A few days before admission, sinusitis developed. A post-nasal drip followed, and the dyspnea increased. Six liters of oxygen per minute were then required. The patient did not smoke. There was no history of tuberculosis, respiratory infections, or occupational exposure to respiratory disease. The pulse rate was 120, respiratory rate 50, and blood pressure 120/70. Rales were present over both lungs. The fingers were clubbed. The hemoglobin was 16.2 Gm., the hematocrit was 47 per cent, and the leukocytes numbered 26,300, with a neutrophilia. Digoxin, aminophylline, and corticosteroids were given. Tachypnea increased, cyanosis developed, and the patient died on the fourth hospital day. The clinical diagnosis was Hamman-Rich Syndrome with cor pulmonale.

Autopsy examination revealed marked interstitial fibrosis of the lungs, cor pulmonale, and chronic passive hyperemia of the liver. The heart weighed 650 Gm., and the right ventricle measured 0.7 cm. in thickness. The liver weighed 2100 Gm.

THE ENTITY

After an earlier report, Hamman and Rich in 1944 described four cases of a pulmonary condition that was clinically and pathologically unusual (1). The clinical features were progressively worsening dyspnea, often with cyanosis, and death from relentless pulmonary insufficiency or cor pulmonale with intractable right heart failure. X-ray changes are often inconspicuous, and neither fever nor leukocytosis is common. The illness ordinarily lasts about two years, although fulminant cases occur; i.e., death in one to six months after onset (2). All ages are affected, especially adults of 30 to 50 years. The condition is slightly more common in males.

Of the eight pathologic features given by the original authors, three are particularly characteristic: enlargement (and detachment) of alveolar lining cells, edema and fibrin deposition within alveolar walls, and diffuse proliferation of fibrous tissue throughout all lobes of both lungs (1). Exudative inflammation is scant, and bacteria are not demonstrable. The cause is unknown, although infection, hypersensitivity, and collagen disease have been suggested (2). Death follows progressive respiratory insufficiency with or without right heart failure.

1. Hamman, L., and Rich, A.R. Acute diffuse interstitial fibrosis of the lungs. Bull. John Hopkins Hospital. 74:177, 1944.
2. Muschenheim, C. Some observations on the Hamman-Rich disease. Am. J. Med. Sci. 241: 279, 1961.

SCLERODERMA LUNG

CLINICAL ACCOUNT 5948

The patient was a Negro female 46 years old who was admitted to the hospital because of severe shortness of breath. She had been treated for the past four years for disseminated scleroderma with pulmonary involvement. There had been a persistent cough, occasionally productive of blood-tinged sputum. Dyspnea had been present for the past six months and had become severe over the past two days. The temperature was 98.6 degrees F., respirations 30, pulse 120, and blood pressure 100/80 mm. Hg. Physical examination revealed moderate obesity and rales and wheezes over all lung fields.

The hemoglobin was 14.6 Gm., the hematocrit was 45 per cent, and the leukocytes numbered 11,900 with a slight neutrophilia. Radiographs were interpreted as showing diffuse interstitial fibrosis. The patient suffered a cardiac arrest and was revived. She was placed on a respirator. The blood pressure fell, vasopressor agents were ineffective, and death occurred on the day after hospital admission.

Autopsy examination revealed scleroderma of the skin, interstitial fibrosis of the lungs, fibrous adhesions of the pleura, and marked passive hyperemia of the liver. Additional diagnoses were incidental. The right and left lungs weighed 560 and 500 Gms., respectively.

THE ENTITY

Scleroderma is most common in young adult and middle-aged women, in whom it is frequently associated with Reynaud's phenomenon. Atrophy and fibrosis occur especially in the skin, esophagus, and lungs. For this reason the condition is also known as progressive systemic sclerosis. Atrophy and fibrosis, especially the latter, are the principal changes. The condition is slowly progressive. The clinical manifestation is relentlessly progressive dyspnea.

The pleura tends to be smooth, since the condition is regressive rather than inflammatory. The visceral pleura may thus be thick without adhesions or attachment to the parietal pleura. The gross cut surface is firm and flecked with gray. As the fibrosis proceeds, especially in the outer parts of the lower lobes, distension of air sacs and small bronchi produces a honeycomb appearance. Micro-sections reveal pronounced and more or less even thickening of the alveolar walls, with collagen that may become hyalinized. A small number of macrophages, lymphocytes, and desquamated alveolar cells occupy the air sacs. Hyperplasia of alveolar lining cells is frequent. The interstitial fibrosis obstructs capillaries and causes an alveolar capillary diffusion block and an increased pressure in the pulmonary blood vessels. Exudative inflammation is not seen unless secondary bacterial infection occurs. Death is due to respiratory insufficiency, often with right heart failure.

SCLERODERMA LUNG

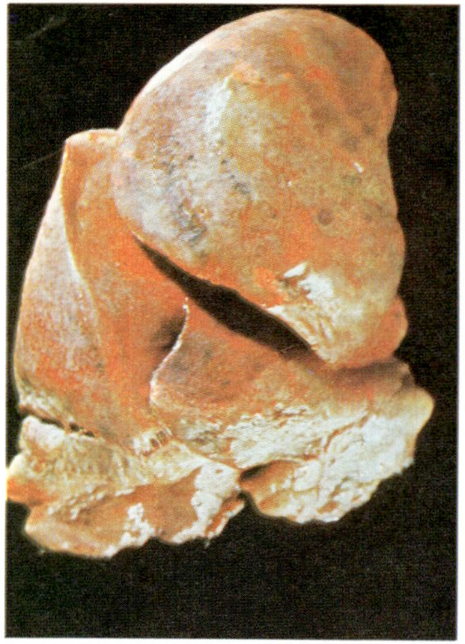

The pulmonary tissue is firm and rubbery. Much of the pleura is smooth, glistening, and red. At some sites, especially within lobar fissures, the tissue is pale pinkish gray and dense fibrous adhesions are evident.

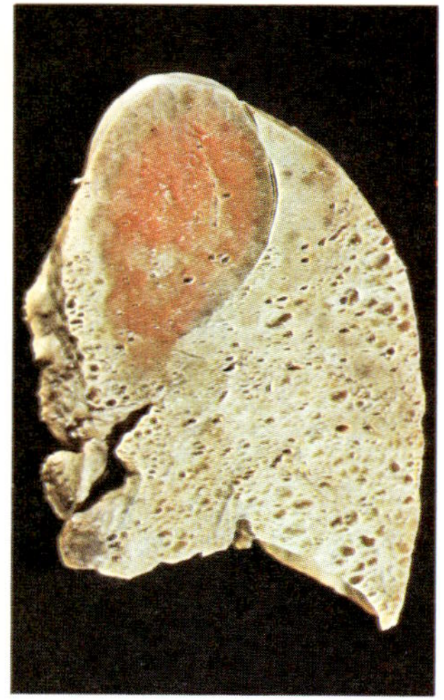

The cut surfaces, semifixed in formalin, are extensively fibrosed with pronounced intervening emphysema and bronchiectasis. The red portion of the upper lobe is unfixed and is a nearly solid mass of fibrous connective tissue.

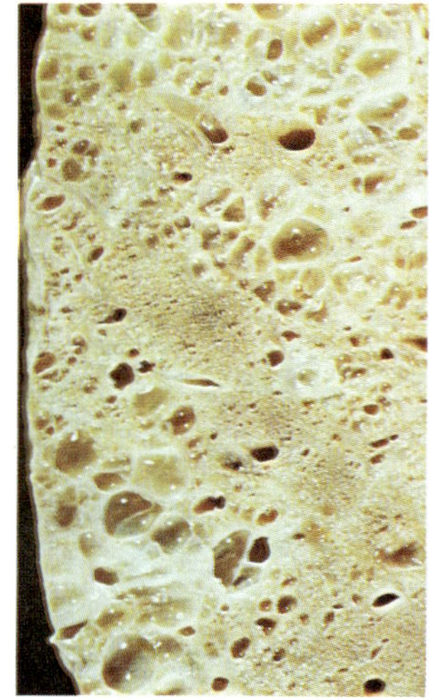

Between the dilated air sacs (emphysema) and dilated bronchi (bronchiectasis), the tissue is solid, pale gray, and fibrosed. The essentially noninflammatory nature of the process is indicated by the lack of adhesions on much of the pleural surface.

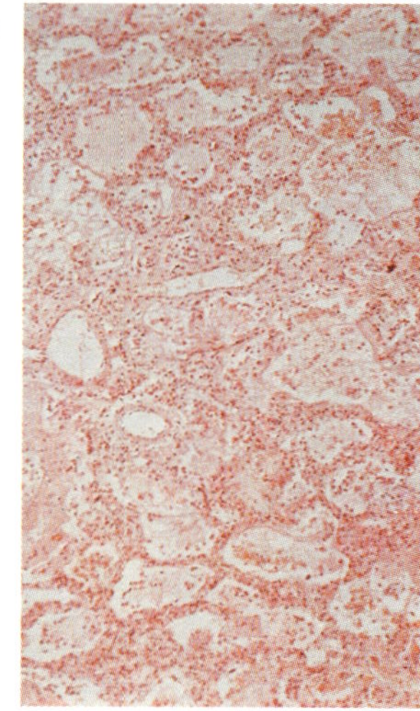

The photomicrograph reveals connective tissue thickening of the alveolar walls, lymphocytic infiltration of the interstitial and subpleural tissue, and accumulation of macrophages in the air sacs.

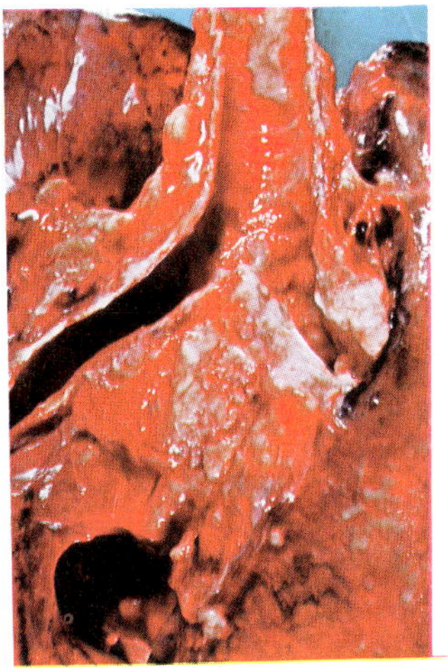

The tissue is opened from the posterior surface; it shows a carcinoma of the right main bronchus that causes stenosis of the lumen, fixes the carinal structures, and metastasizes to both lungs and to regional lymph nodes.

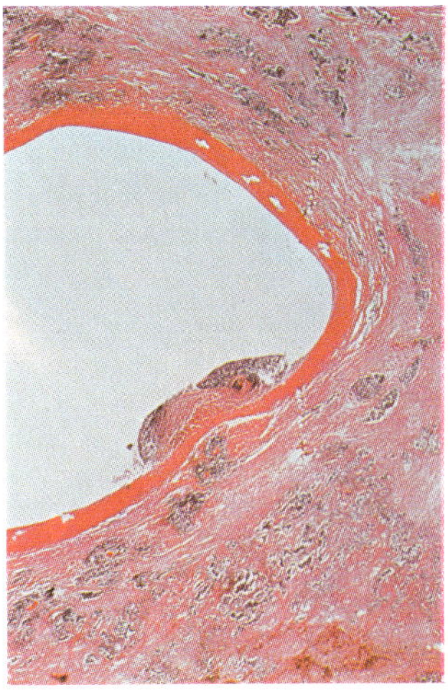

The tumor is an undifferentiated small cell carcinoma. In the photograph, penetration of tumor into a large pulmonary vein is shown. In this way tumor cells gain access to the systemic circulation.

CARCINOMA OF LUNG

Left: At scanning power, tumor cells can be seen to lie mainly within lymphatics around vessels and bronchi. This distribution is attributable to retrograde lymphatic flow that courses outward from the hilum toward the pleura. **Right:** At higher magnification, undifferentiated tumor cells lie in perivascular lymphatics. The vessels are occupied by canalized thrombi. Tumor cells in perivascular lymphatics, especially about arterioles, tend to cause thrombosis of them. This may be widespread and the effect so pronounced that cor pulmonale and right heart failure may ensue.

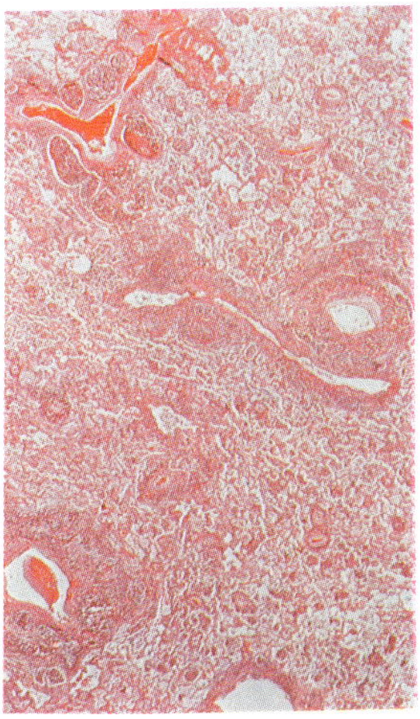

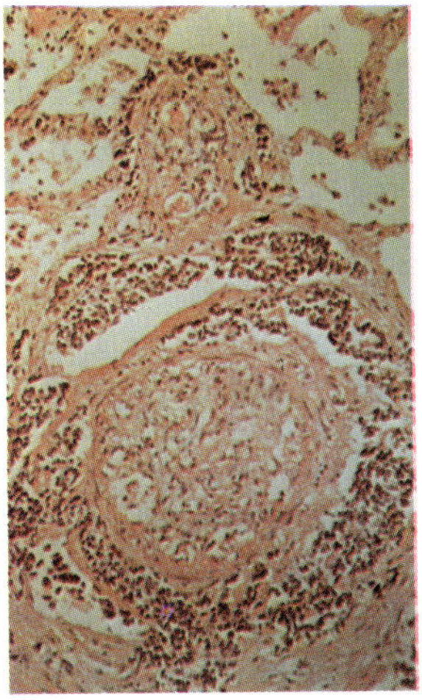

CARCINOMA OF LUNG

CLINICAL ACCOUNT 6142

The patient was a Negro male 58 years old who was admitted to the hospital because of shortness of breath. He had felt well until three months previously, when anorexia began and nausea occurred. Over the past two months there had been a weight loss of 20 pounds. During the past month, night sweats were pronounced, and dyspnea began. The latter was progressive and for the past three weeks was accompanied by coughing that produced yellowish gray mucus occasionally streaked with bright red blood. The patient smoked one pack of cigarettes daily.

The temperature was 99.8 degrees F., pulse 96, respirations 32, and blood pressure 110/70. The patient was thin and dyspneic. All lung fields revealed coarse rhonchi. The heart, abdomen, and extremities were not remarkable.

The urine and blood were normal. The serum glutamic transaminase was 70 units per 100 ml., and the lactic dehydrogenase was 465 units per 100 ml. An x-ray of the chest revealed consolidation of the right lower lobe. Biopsy of the bronchus disclosed an oat cell carcinoma with scalene node metastasis. The patient's condition rapidly worsened, his shortness of breath increased, and his neck veins became distended. He died of respiratory failure on the sixth hospital day.

A carcinoma of the right main bronchus was found. There were also bronchopneumonia, a healed gastric ulcer, and widespread metastases that included both adrenals. Additional diagnoses were incidental. Permission for examination of the brain was not granted.

THE ENTITY

Cancer of the lung is increasing in incidence; it occurs in middle age and more frequently in men. The time, age, and sex factors correlate directly with the practice of smoking cigarettes.

Carcinoma is the commonest primary tumor of the lung. There are five main kinds: squamous, adenocarcinoma, oat cell, undifferentiated, and alveolar cell. About half are squamous, and about one-fourth are adenocarcinomas. Only squamous, undifferentiated, and oat cell cancers are associated with smoking (1).

Squamous carcinomas arise in the hilum, obstruct bronchi, and lead to atelectasis, focal pneumonia, abscess formation, and pleural extension with empyema. They may compress and obstruct the superior vena cava. Adenocarcinomas occur more often in women, arise in the periphery of the lung tissue, and spread to the surface to cause pleural and pericardial effusions. Invasion of the brachial plexus causes pain and muscle wasting of the hand as described by Pancoast (2). Oat cell carcinomas arise between the periphery and hilum; they infiltrate lymphatics early and spread widely. Alveolar carcinomas line the air sacs with a single layer of columnar cells that secrete abundant mucin. They grow slowly, consolidate large areas, and metastasize late.

Metastasis is most frequent to the opposite lung. Thereafter, spread is common to the liver, adrenals, brain, bone, and kidneys in that order. Metastasis may be the first clinical manifestation, especially in brain.

1. Doll, R., Hill, A.B., and Kreyberg, L. The significance of cell type in relation to the etiology of lung cancer. Brit. J. Cancer 11:43, 1957.
2. Pancoast, H.K. Superior pulmonary sulcus tumor; tumor characterized by pain, Horner's syndrome, destruction of bone and atrophy of hand muscles. JAMA 99:1391, 1932.

BRONCHOGENIC CARCINOMA

CLINICAL ACCOUNT 6205

The patient was a white male 89 years old who had been treated for obstructive uropathy, transient episodes of cerebral ischemia, and gall bladder disease. He had had hepatosplenomegaly which recently increased in size and was associated with ascites formation and fever of 100° F.

Although the vital signs were normal, the patient was incontinent of urine and stool. The chest was clear to auscultation. The heart was not remarkable. The abdomen was soft and the liver edge was firm, nontender, and 15 cm. below the right costal margin. The spleen was palpable.

The hemoglobin was 11.9 Gm., hematocrit 35, and leukocytes 15,200 with a normal distribution. The urine was normal. A chest x-ray revealed a dense infiltration in the upper lobe of the left lung that was suggestive of neoplastic disease. The patient died after nine days in the hospital.

Autopsy examination revealed a carcinoma of the upper lobe of the left lung with metastases in the liver, spine, and lymph nodes (bronchopulmonary and para-aortic). The metastatic disease in the liver was especially pronounced, and that organ weighed 3050 Gm. The heart weighed 350 Gm. and disclosed calcification of the mitral annulus. Arteriosclerosis of the aorta was pronounced, especially in the abdominal portion. The right and left lungs weighed 585 and 475 Gm., respectively. Both displayed pulmonary emphysema, and there were 250 ml. of clear pale yellow fluid in the pleural space on the left. Incidental diagnoses included an adenoma of the transverse colon, diverticula of the colon, and ascites (180 ml.).

THE ENTITY

Cancer of the lung occurs most frequently between 50 and 70 years of age, and arises approximately six times more often in men than women. Slightly less than half of all lung cancers arise in the central region of the lung, slightly more than half at the periphery (1). About 50 per cent are squamous (epidermoid) cancers, 30 per cent are undifferentiated or oat cell carcinomas, and 15 per cent are adenocarcinomas. Giant cell and alveolar cell carcinomas also occur. Squamous, undifferentiated, and oat cell carcinomas are associated with smoking.

Squamous cancers arise from the mucosa of large bronchi near the hilus. They invade and encircle the bronchus so that obstructive pneumonitis develops. The tumor is bulky and often undergoes central necrosis with cavity formation. It grows somewhat slowly, metastasizes to hilar lymph nodes, and has the longest life expectancy without treatment. Clinical signs arise from the bronchial block and are due to obstructive pneumonitis, suppurative pneumonia, abscess formation, bronchiectasis, and extension to the pleura with empyema formation. The tumor is radioresistant and cure requires lobectomy or pneumonectomy.

Undifferentiated or oat cell carcinoma arises in the center or periphery of the lung from germinal (deep) cells of the bronchial mucosa. The primary lesion is often minute, the cells deploy in solid clusters, and the tumor is extremely malignant with widespread metastasis usually preceding clinical diagnosis. The cells display large hyperchromatic nuclei and may resemble lymphocytes. Patients seldom live more than six months after the diagnosis is established. The tumor is radiosensitive and may exhibit endocrine effects including Cushing's syndrome, carcinoid syndrome, and hyponatremia from the inappropriate excretion of antidiuretic hormone.

1. Spencer, H. Pathology of the Lung. Second Edition, Pergamon Press, New York, 1968.

BRONCHOGENIC CARCINOMA

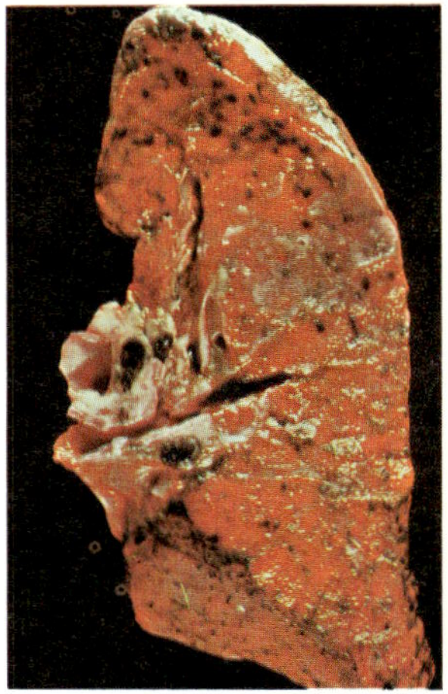

The cut surface of the left lung reveals a carcinoma in the hilar region; it is especially conspicuous in the vertically oriented bronchus. The pale gray peripheral discoloration in the upper middle portion is secondary neoplastic disease,

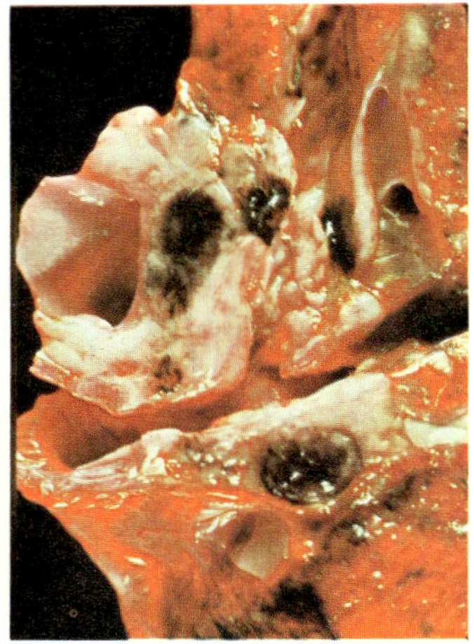

A close-up of the bronchus reveals the pale gray corrugated surface of the primary tumor. As the lesion obstructs the lumen, atelectasis, infection, and abscess formation are prone to develop in the distal airless tissue. The hilar lymph nodes are discolored pale gray with tumor, and black with anthracotic pigment.

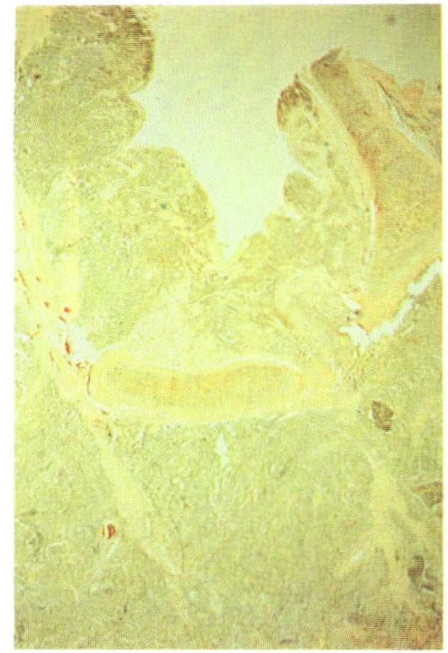

A scanning section shows tumor masses elevating the mucosa of the bronchus and extending between cartilaginous plates to the peribronchial tissue.

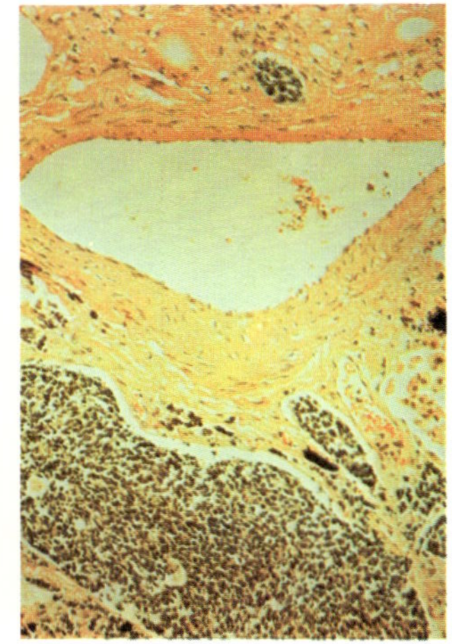

At higher power, the small cell undifferentiated nature of the cancer is evident. Such tumors spread widely and early. Clusters of tumor cells show in perivascular lymphatic spaces.

ALVEOLAR CELL CARCINOMA

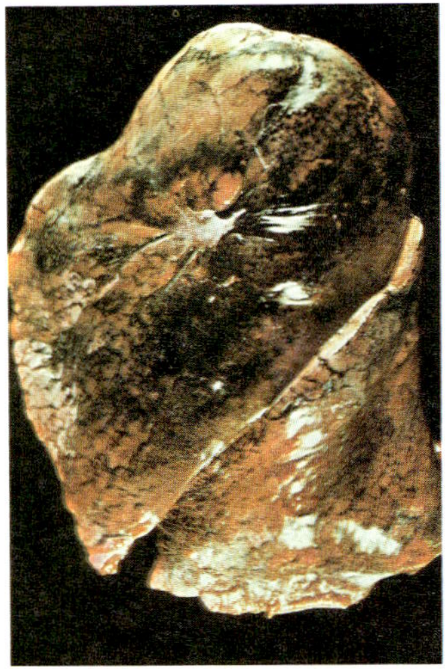

The pleural surface of the left lung presents a firm pale gray indentation of the upper lobe about which fibrous adhesions roughen the surface.

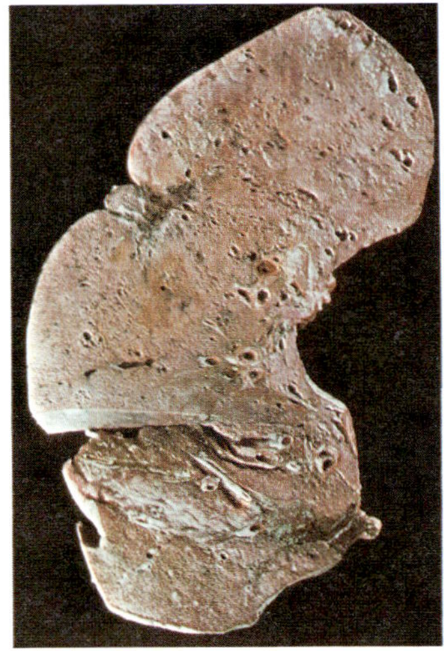

Section reveals an indented subpleural scar in which the cancer is not grossly visible. Pneumonia of nearly lobar distribution is present elsewhere in the upper lobe which is solid, airless, and firm. In contrast, the lower lobe is soft, crepitant, and finely porous.

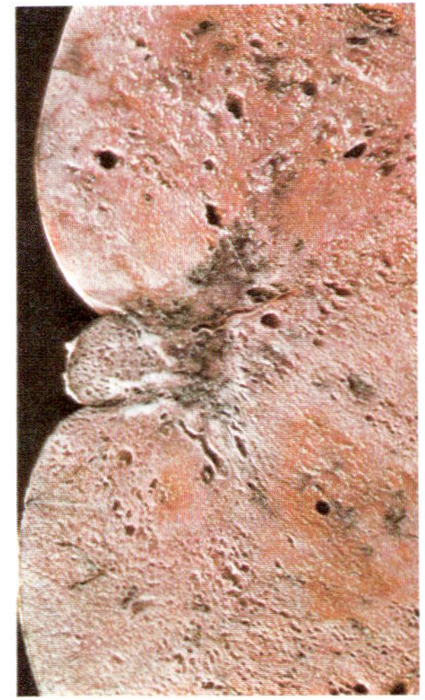

Even a close-up gross examination fails to reveal more than pneumonic consolidation, anthracosis, and cicatrization.

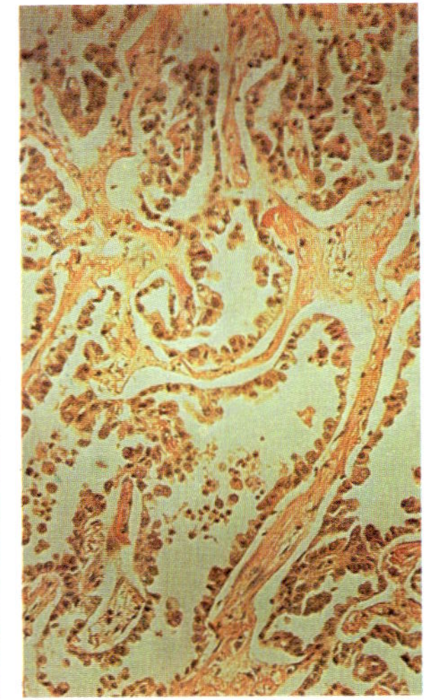

The alveoli at the base of the scar are lined by a single layer of columnar epithelial cells that leaves the wall intact. There is very little anaplasia, and only an occasional mitotic figure is found. This well differentiated pattern of a single layer of tall columnar cells lining air sacs without destroying them is characteristic of alveolar cell carcinoma.

ALVEOLAR CELL CARCINOMA

CLINICAL ACCOUNT 6176

The patient was a white male 62 years old who was admitted to the hospital because of crampy abdominal pain, diarrhea, and black stools. He was previously well except for chronic alcoholism and six months of treatment for pulmonary tuberculosis two years before the present admission.

The temperature was 103 degrees F. Coarse rales were present over the right posterior lung field. The heart was not enlarged, the rhythm was regular, and no murmurs were heard. The abdomen was soft, no organs were felt, and rectal examination was not remarkable. The hemoglobin was 11.6 Gm., hematocrit 32, and leukocytes 8,200 with a normal distribution. An x-ray of the chest disclosed an infiltration in the right lower lung field consistent with pneumonitis. Bronchoscopy revealed only mucus accumulation. The pneumonic infiltration spread to the right and left upper lung fields, the patient became cyanotic, and death occurred after the patient had been in the hospital for fourteen days.

The lungs displayed bronchopneumonia and acute fibrinous pleuritis. The left lung also disclosed a small alveolar cell carcinoma. The heart was hypertrophic and weighed 560 Gm. Additional diagnoses included acute ulcers of the duodenum, a polypoid adenoma of the rectum, acute suppurative prostatitis with abscess formation, and a double right renal artery.

THE ENTITY

Alveolar cell carcinoma constitutes only 3 to 4 per cent of primary malignant tumors of the lung. It arises in the periphery of the pulmonary tissue and slowly spreads through the pores of Kohn to line the alveoli with a single layer of tall columnar mucus secreting epithelial cells that often show slender papillary projections. The alveolar walls tend to remain intact, necrosis is not conspicuous, and anaplasia is extremely slight. The tumor arises from terminal bronchioles or from alveolar lining cells. The gross cut surface displays single or coalescing multiple nodules that are poorly defined and glairy because of mucus production. Spread to regional lymph nodes occurs late, and widespread metastasis is uncommon.

The tumor occurs approximately equally in the sexes, is not related to smoking, and may arise adjacent to pulmonary scars (1). Histologically it resembles jaagsiekte, an infectious lung disease of sheep. It occurs over a broad age span beginning with the second decade. In contrast to bronchogenic carcinomas that are characterized by cough, pain, and hemoptysis, alveolar carcinoma is more likely to be manifested by dyspnea, cyanosis, and copious mucin production. Although spread is late, recognition also tends to be delayed so that survival is low.

1. Beaver, D.L., and Shapiro, J.L. A consideration of chronic pulmonary parenchymal inflammation and alveolar cell carcinoma with regard to a possible etiologic relationship. Am. J. Med. 21:879, 1956.

LYMPHANGITIC PULMONARY METASTASES

CLINICAL ACCOUNT 6248

The patient was a white female 55 years old who developed an inflammatory carcinoma of the left breast. Biopsy disclosed abundant lymphatic invasion. Mastectomy was not recommended; oophorectomy was performed. Approximately two years later metastatic carcinoma appeared in the skin, lungs, mediastinum, and left axilla. Hypophysectomy was performed. Thereafter, metastases appeared in the bones of the pelvis. X-rays of the chest revealed the fine shadows of lymphangitic metastases. Shortness of breath developed and became progressive. Ankle edema appeared, the patient became obtunded, and dyspnea became pronounced. Cyanosis developed in the terminal period; the patient died six years after the onset of the breast cancer.

Autopsy examination revealed carcinoma of the left breast with metastatic tumor of the lungs, liver, lymph nodes, bone marrow, brain, dura mater, pleura, right and left ureters, skeletal muscle, and spine. Other diagnoses included absence of the pituitary, radiation dermatitis of the skin, hydronephrosis on the right, and a submucosal leiomyoma of the ascending colon. The right and left lungs weighed 600 and 480 Gms., respectively.

THE ENTITY

Metastatic carcinoma of the lungs is ordinarily in the form of multiple discrete nodules. Uncommonly metastases are lymphangitic so that no gross nodules are evident. In this form the pleural surfaces show fine white lines of tumor in subpleural lymphatics. The cut surfaces feel gritty, as vessels and bronchioles, surrounded by tumor, stand above the soft adjacent tissue. The perivascular tumor stimulates thrombosis of arterioles, the thrombi organize, and as a result pulmonary hypertension, right ventricular strain, and eventually cor pulmonale with right heart failure all develop.

Primary tumor sites from which lymphangitic spread arises include especially the breast, lung, stomach, and pancreas. The hilar nodes are regularly involved, and it is not clear whether the tumor cells move from the nodes to the pulmonary lymphatics in a retrograde direction or gain the lymphatics after direct hematogenous spread.

The primary tumor is often silent, and the main clinical feature is breathlessness that may be paroxysmal and mistaken for asthma. Moreover, the dyspnea, while clinically unexpected, is relentlessly progressive and becomes severe. X-rays characteristically show fine string-like shadows, apart from bronchovascular markings, that stretch from hila to the periphery of all lobes. Once dyspnea begins, death ordinarily follows within a few months (1).

1. Harold, J.T. Lymphangitis carcinomatosa of the lungs. Quart. J. Med. 21:353, 1952.

LYMPHANGITIC PULMONARY METASTASES

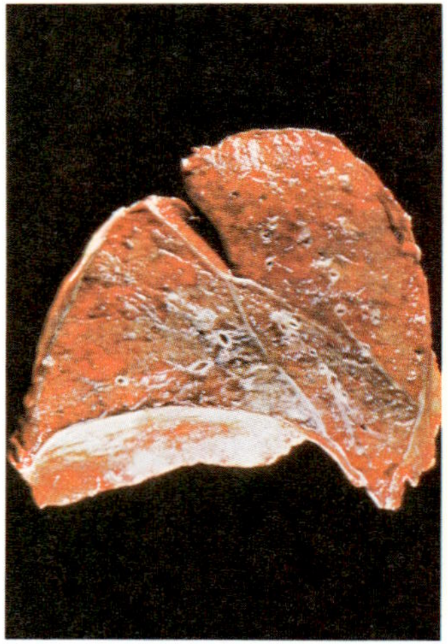

While the cut surface reveals no nodular masses of metastatic tumor, there are thickened septae, bronchi encased in thin collars of pale gray tissue, and thickening of the pleura with pale gray discoloration. All of these changes are due to metastatic disease.

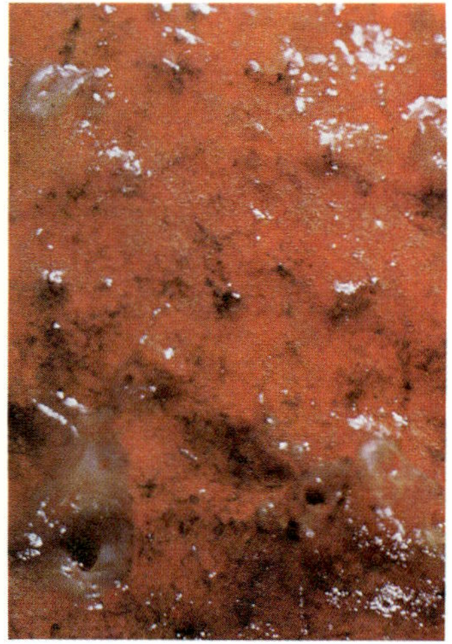

A close-up of the cut surface displays pale gray tumor that surrounds medium sized bronchi.

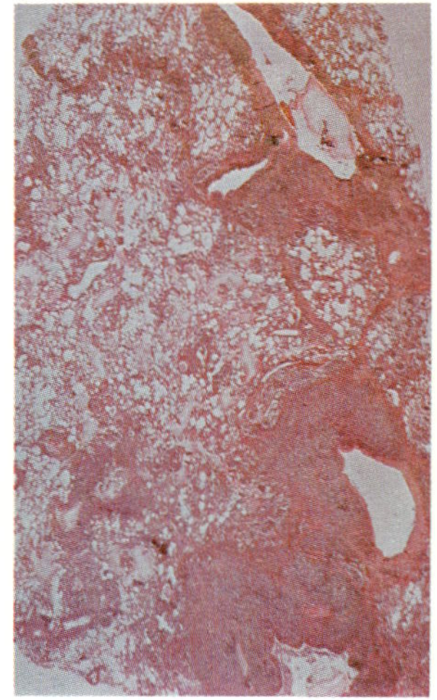

The low power microsection reveals the distribution of tumor that is principally in peribronchial and perivascular sites.

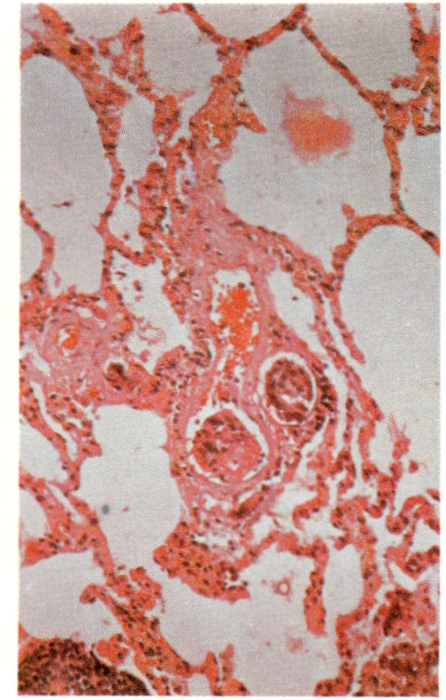

At higher power the tumor cells are seen within minute vascular spaces. The effect of such tumor, especially that in perivascular lymph spaces, is to cause thrombosis of the adjacent blood vessels which are for the most part arterioles and small arteries.

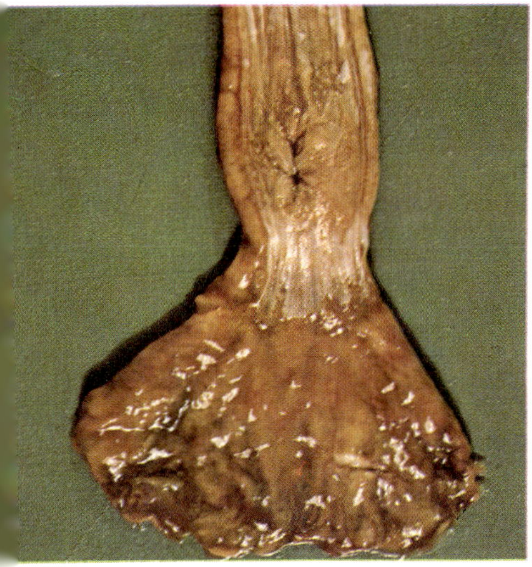

The opened esophagus is shown with a portion of attached stomach below. The "dimple" of the diverticulum is present just above the gastric junction.

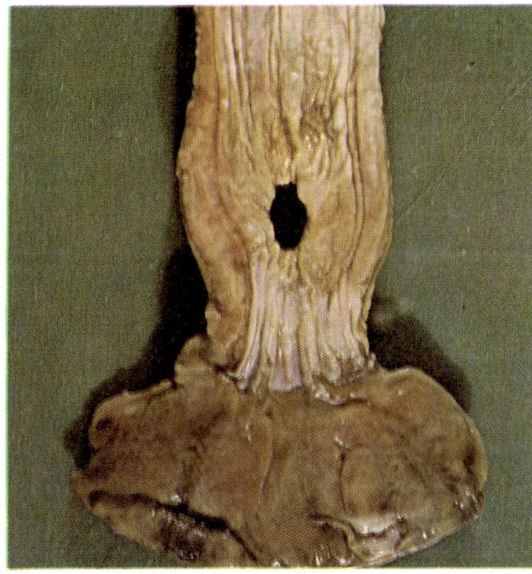

The specimen has been fixed in formalin with a wad of cotton in the diverticulum. On account of this the mouth of the diverticulum is more apparent.

Below: The cut surface of the fixed tissue shows the diverticulum extending to the right. The wall is thin and squamous mucosa lines most of the surface. The mouth of the diverticulum is large.

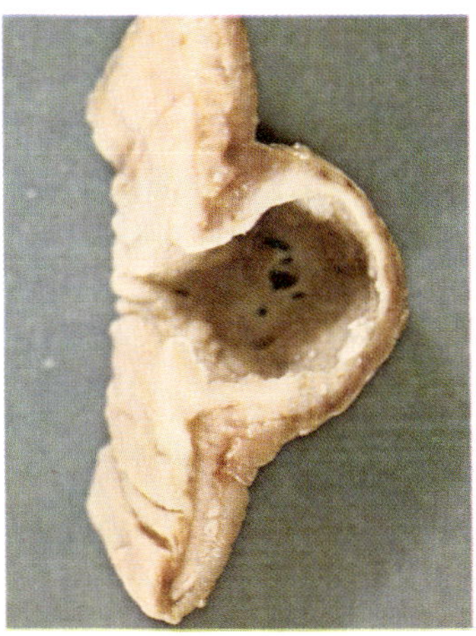

Right: An unmagnified histologic section shows the contour of the lesion. It is a true diverticulum although the external muscle layers are thin. Exudate covers a portion of the lining surface.

DIVERTICULUM OF ESOPHAGUS

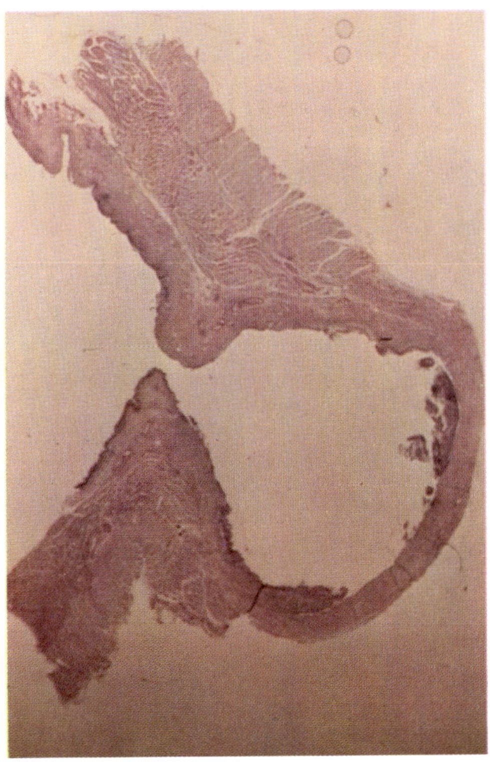

DIVERTICULUM OF ESOPHAGUS

CLINICAL ACCOUNT 6849

The patient was a white male 76 years old who was admitted to the hospital because of shortness of breath, nocturnal dyspnea, and cervical recurrence of a mucoepidermoid carcinoma of the sublingual salivary glands on the left. There were no complaints referable to the esophagus. At a previous admission a traction diverticulum of the mid-esophagus had been identified by barium studies. The patient had been a diabetic for many years. He was found dead in bed the morning after admission.

Autopsy examination revealed pronounced emphysema of the right and left lungs and metastatic carcinoma of the lungs, liver, spleen, adrenals, pericardium, and mediastinal lymph nodes. There was a fusiform aneurysm of the abdominal aorta and a saccular diverticulum of the mid-esophagus. Additional diagnoses were incidental. No tuberculosis was found in the lungs or bronchopulmonary lymph nodes.

THE ENTITY

Diverticula of the esophagus occur principally at two sites, the upper end of the posterior surface and the midportion on the anterior or right anterolateral surface. The former are attributed to an excess of pressure within the esophagus or to a weakness of the esophageal wall, or both. They are accordingly regarded as pulsion diverticula. They become large, retain food, cause symptoms, and require treatment.

The latter are single and small, usually not exceeding 2 cm. in diameter. They arise opposite the tracheal bifurcation and are attributed to the tug of infected hilar lymph nodes that have become attached to the wall of the esophagus and contract with the healing process. The nodal infection is usually tuberculous (1). The mouth of the diverticulum is large, the sac remains at or above the level of the mouth, and all layers of the wall participate in the sacculation. Food is accordingly not retained, and the condition is rarely symptomatic. The radiographic appearance with a barium swallow is characteristic. The condition is unassociated with other diseases of the esophagus. Treatment is ordinarily not required. Inflammation may cause rupture with the formation of an esophagobronchial fistula or an acute suppurative mediastinitis.

1. Bockus, H.L. Gastroenterology, Vol. I, W.B. Saunders Company, Philadelphia, 1963.

VARICES OF ESOPHAGUS

CLINICAL ACCOUNT 5867

The patient was a white male 50 years old who developed ankle edema, ascites, and muscle wasting nine years before the last hospital admission. Biopsy of the liver at that time revealed cirrhosis. Varices of the esophagus were detected by radiographic studies four years after the onset of this illness. One year before admission a cerebrovascular accident caused a right hemiparesis. Four months before the onset of symptoms, the patient was exposed to a hydrocarbon insecticide (malathion); there had been no jaundice or alcoholism prior to that time.

The patient was emaciated. The temperature was 98.6 degrees F., pulse 100, respirations 20, and blood pressure 120/80 mm. Hg. The heart and lungs were normal. Veins were prominently dilated over the lower chest, the abdomen was markedly dilated, and a fluid wave was elicited. The right arm and leg were spastic.

The urine revealed a trace of albumin, an occasional hyaline cast, and a few bacteria. The hemoglobin was 13.8 Gm., the hematocrit was 43 per cent, and the leukocytes numbered 12,100 with a moderate neutrophilia. The total serum bilirubin was 2.4 mg. with 1.2 mg. conjugated. The condition of the patient gradually worsened. He was found unresponsive, and he died on the eleventh hospital day.

Autopsy examination revealed Laennec cirrhosis of the liver with esophageal varices and massive recent gastro-intestinal hemorrhage. There were also cholelithiasis, hyperemia of the spleen, atrophy of the testes, gynecomastia, and wasting of skeletal muscle. An old infarct was found in the internal capsule of the brain. Additional diagnoses were incidental.

THE ENTITY

Varices of the esophagus are caused by prolonged obstruction to the flow of portal blood through the liver. Causes include cirrhosis, organizing pylephlebitis, veno-occlusive disease, and thrombosis of the hepatic vein. Of these causes, cirrhosis is the most common. The most frequent kind of cirrhosis is that of Laennec, which is also known as portal or nutritional cirrhosis. Portal vein obstruction occurs in about two thirds of such cases. It is less common in postnecrotic and pigmentary cirrhosis and is decidedly uncommon in biliary and cardiac cirrhosis.

The varices are especially frequent at the lower end of the esophagus. Dilatation is due to the weak supporting tissue of the submucosa and the proximity of the lumen, into which the bulging may take place. The actual perforation may be due to increased venous pressure during coughing or vomiting, mucosal abrasion from swallowing coarse particulate matter, or inflammation from reflux of gastric acid. The hemorrhage is often massive and sudden with the attendant features of shock and collapse. If the patient survives, recurrence is nearly certain. Approximately half the patients die from recurrence within twelve months of the first hemorrhage.

It may be pointed out that the most common cause of the vomiting of blood is peptic ulceration of the stomach. The most common cause of hematemesis in patients with cirrhosis is rupture of an esophageal varix. Although patients with cirrhosis may also have ulcers of the stomach, the presence of jaundice, spider angiomas of the skin, enlargement of the liver, and gynecomastia help make this distinction and indicate that the esophagus is the site of the bleeding.

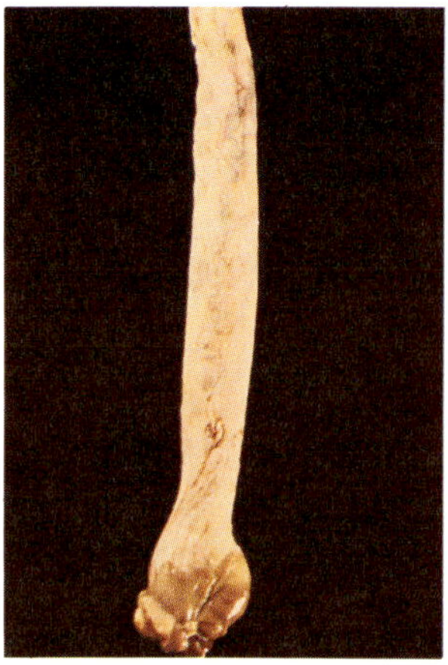

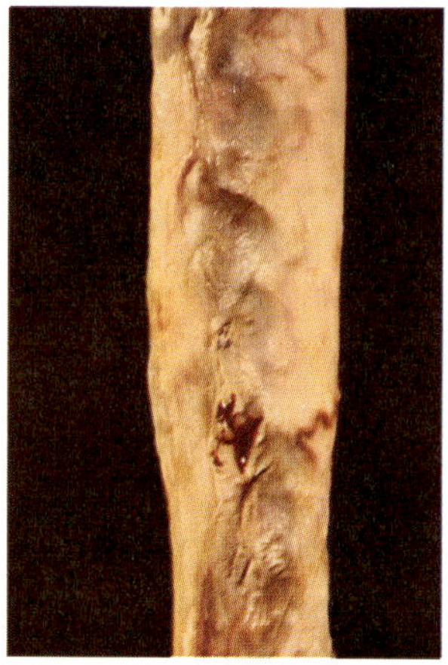

Left: The esophagus, turned inside-out, reveals prominent dilatation of submucosal veins. The junction with gastric mucosa is at the lower part of the picture; just above this a rent in the mucosa may be seen. The hemorrhage occured at this site. **Right:** Applying gentle pressure to both ends of the inverted esophagus causes the veins to dilate and a trickle of blood to emerge from the mucosal rent at the site of rupture.

Left: Cross section of the esophagus, now restored to its normal orientation with the mucosa on the inside, shows the dilated veins of the submucosa, one of which projects into the lumen. Increased pressure within the vein or ulceration of the overlying mucosa causes rupture with hemorrhage that is often massive and not infrequently fatal. **Right:** When cirrhosis blocks the flow of portal blood through the liver, channels open up that allow the portal blood to enter the systemic veins and thus by-pass the liver. These collateral channels are indicated in the diagram. Chief among them is the coronary-esophageal-azygous vein route.

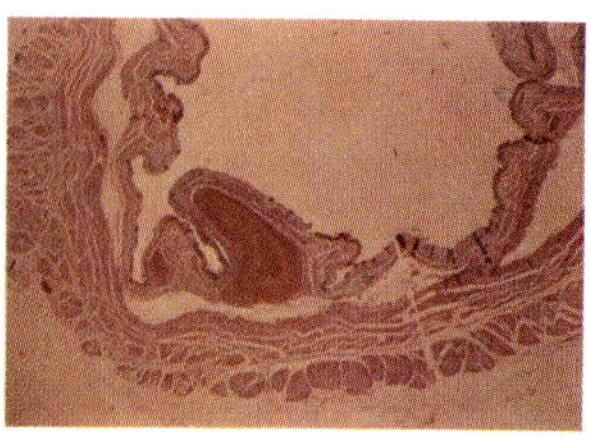

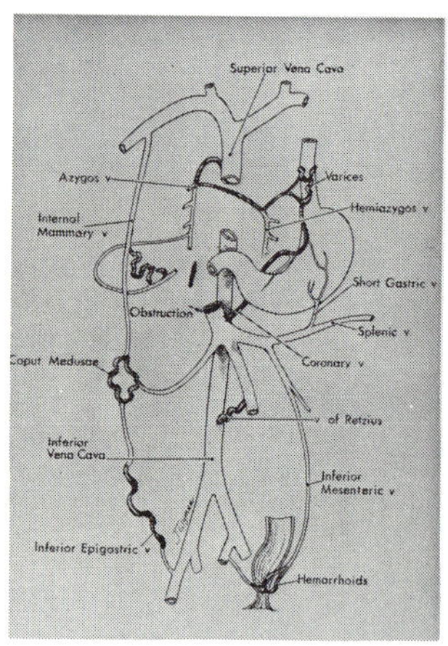

MALLORY-WEISS LESION

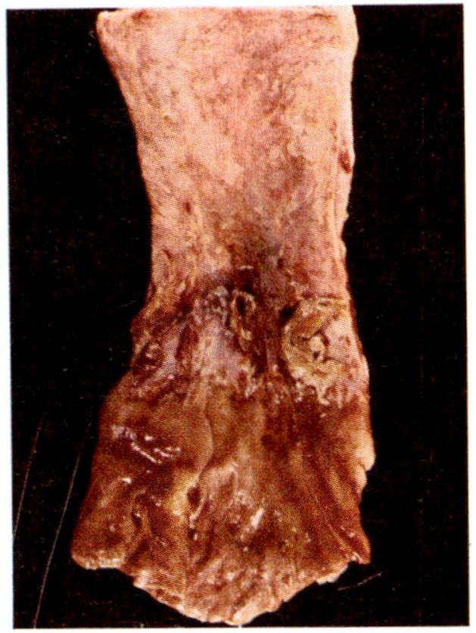

The photograph reveals the gastroesophageal junction. Linear ulcers are apparent in the distal esophagus, and the surfaces are covered by projecting irregular thrombi. The gastric mucosa is hyperemic and the esophageal mucosa displays slight leukoplakia above the ulcers.

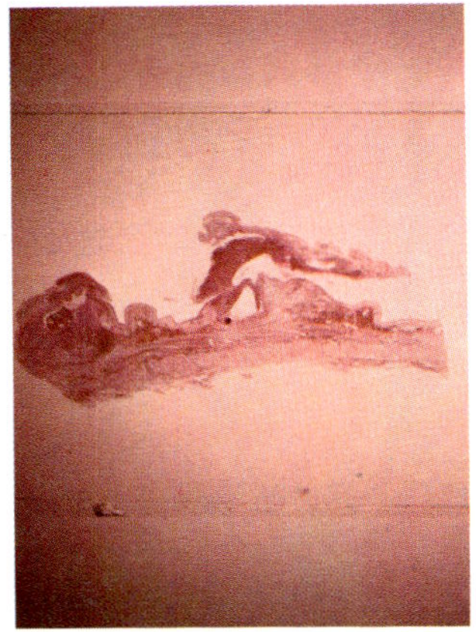

An unmagnified cross section of the lesion reveals large vascular spaces filled with blood over which there are projections of fibrin that extend into the esophageal lumen.

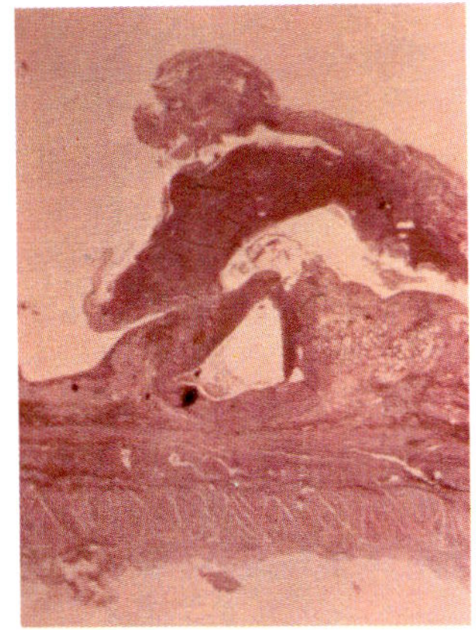

At scanning power a small varix, a rent in the vessel wall, and an overlying fibrin mass are apparent.

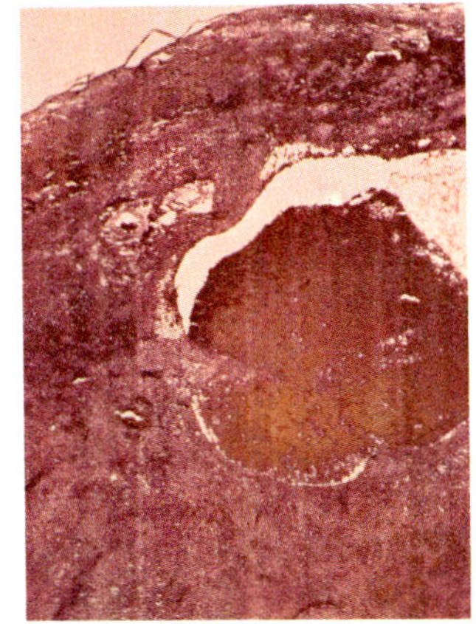

At low power another varix is revealed. It is partially filled with a recent thrombus and the overlying portion of esophageal wall is denuded of mucosa and richly infiltrated with leukocytes. Hemorrhagic necrosis is also focally present and a fibrin mass clinging to the surface is seen in the right upper portion of the picture.

MALLORY-WEISS LESION

CLINICAL ACCOUNT 6365

The patient was a Negro male 53 years old who was a chronic alcoholic. He experienced nausea and vomiting six times on the day of admission, the last time vomiting "2 quarts of blood." He stated that he had had a gastrointestinal hemorrhage 12 years before, that he had a "nervous stomach," and that he had lost 15 pounds over the past three months. His blood pressure was 90/60 mm. Hg., and his pulse was 90. Physical examination revealed the liver margin to be 4 cm. below the right costal margin. The abdomen was soft. Rectal examination was not remarkable. Transfusions of whole blood were started. The hemoglobin was 12.9 Gm., hematocrit 41, and leukocyte count 18,600 with a neutrophilia. The patient had a cardiac arrest and died on the second hospital day.

Autopsy examination revealed linear ulcers of the esophagus at the gastroesophageal junction. There was a massive recent gastro-intestinal hemorrhage. The liver weighed 2500 Gm. and disclosed marked fatty metamorphosis. Cirrhosis was not present. The pancreas revealed pronounced chronic inflammation with atrophy and fibrosis. Incidental diagnoses included hypertrophy of the heart (400 Gm.), atelectasis of the lower lobes of both lungs, and pleural effusion (200 ml., right, 100 ml., left).

THE ENTITY

In 1929 Mallory and Weiss described a syndrome of massive gastro-intestinal hemorrhage that occurs after vomiting, usually in alcoholics, and is associated with linear tears of the mucosa of the cardio-esophageal junction (1). The vomiting is often prolonged and vigorous. The cause of the vomiting is usually alcoholism. The hemorrhage is frequently massive and is occasionally fatal. The mucosal tears extend into the wall but do not perforate the esophagus. The tears are arranged around the circumference of the cardia parallel to the long axis of the esophagus. They measure 0.5 to 3.0 cm. in length and up to 0.7 cm. in width. Cure may be achieved by gastrotomy and ligature (2). The diagnosis rests on the observation that the patient does not have gastric or duodenal ulcers, cirrhosis of the liver, varices of the esophagus, or carcinoma of the stomach, and does have vigorous vomiting, usually associated with alcoholism, and massive hemorrhage, often with hematemesis, that comes on at the end of the vomiting.

1. Mallory, G.K., and Weiss, S. Hemorrhages from lacerations of cardiac orifice of stomach due to vomiting. Am. J. Med. Sci. 178:506, 1929.
2. Baue, A.E. Bleeding from lacerations of the cardia: The Mallory-Weiss syndrome. JAMA 184:325, 1963.

CARCINOMA OF ESOPHAGUS

CLINICAL ACCOUNT 6815

The patient was a black male 64 years old who came to the hospital because of dysphagia, vomiting, anorexia, and weight loss. He had felt well until ten months previously, when anorexia began. Soon weight loss was noted. At seven months before admission retrosternal pain developed; this was gnawing in character and occurred during meals. Somewhat later, difficulty in swallowing developed, and the patient remarked that "food seems to stick in my throat." At four months before admission vomiting occurred when the patient attempted to swallow solid foods. The vomitus lacked blood or bile and consisted of recently chewed food particles. The dysphagia worsened and the vomiting came to be occasioned also by the swallowing of liquids. The body weight loss was 35 pounds by the time of admission. The patient had smoked one pack of cigarettes daily for the past ten years, and had drunk one pint of whiskey daily for the past 20 years.

The physical examination was not remarkable. The urine was essentially normal. The hemoglobin was 14.1 Gm., the hematocrit was 43 per cent, and the leukocytes numbered 4,700 per cmm. with a normal differential count. An x-ray of the chest revealed clear lung fields. An electrocardiogram was normal. A barium swallow disclosed a filling defect of the esophagus 7 cm. in length that was consistent with carcinoma. A laparotomy revealed metastatic epidermoid carcinoma in the retroperitoneal lymph nodes. The patient was treated with 4000 rads of x-radiation. Symptomatic improvement was temporary, and his condition gradually regressed. Death occurred eight months after the diagnosis was established and 18 months after the onset of the illness.

THE ENTITY

Carcinoma of the esophagus occurs after the age of 50 years, and seven times more often in males than females (1). Most arise in the middle third at the level of the tracheal bifurcation, some occur at the lower end, and a few arise at the upper end. The tumor may fungate into the lumen and cause obstruction, it may diffusely infiltrate the wall, which becomes thick and stiff, or it may perforate the wall with excavation into the mediastinum, pericardium, or airway. In the last event, broncho-esophageal or tracheo-esophageal fistulae form. Almost all are squamous carcinomas; the few adenocarcinomas, which are especially frequent at the cardia, presumably arise from mucous glands of the submucosa or ectopic gastric glands. All metastasize to regional lymph nodes, although those of the lower third often spread below the diaphragm, while those of the upper and middle thirds are usually confined to the thorax.

The cardinal symptom is progressive dysphagia which develops gradually. There may also be indigestion, substernal distress, and epigastric pain. Loss of weight follows and debilitation may become extreme. The diagnosis is established by contrast x-rays and endoscopy with biopsy. Treatment is usually unsuccessful because of deep spread of the tumor. Most die within one year of the onset of symptoms.

While the cause is unknown, the incidence of cigarette smoking, alcoholism, and lye burns of the esophagus with prolonged stricture is high. In addition, the lesion is inordinately frequent in parts of the Middle East and South Africa; environmental factors are suspect.

1. Spiro, H.M. Clinical Gastroenterology. The MacMillan Company, London, 1970.

CARCINOMA OF ESOPHAGUS

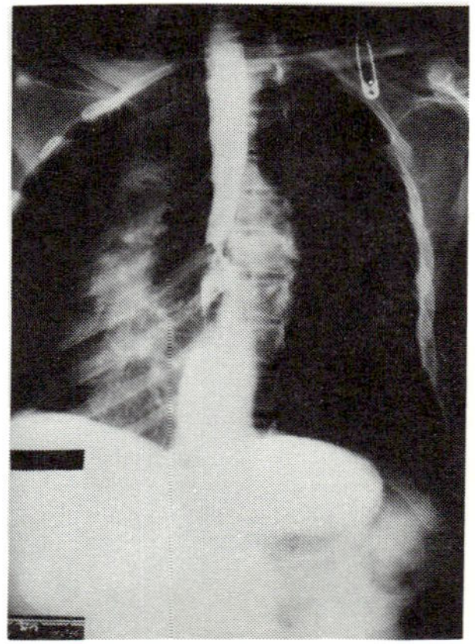

The chest x-ray with barium swallow reveals the disfiguration of the mid-esophagus caused by the cancer.

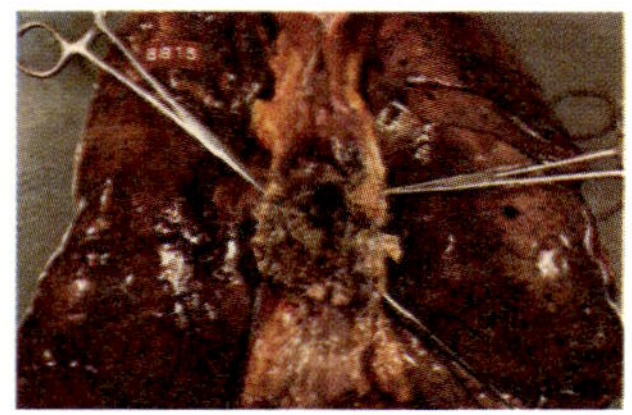

The opened esophagus discloses the carcinoma. It can be foreseen that extension into a bronchus is a frequent consequence of the lesion.

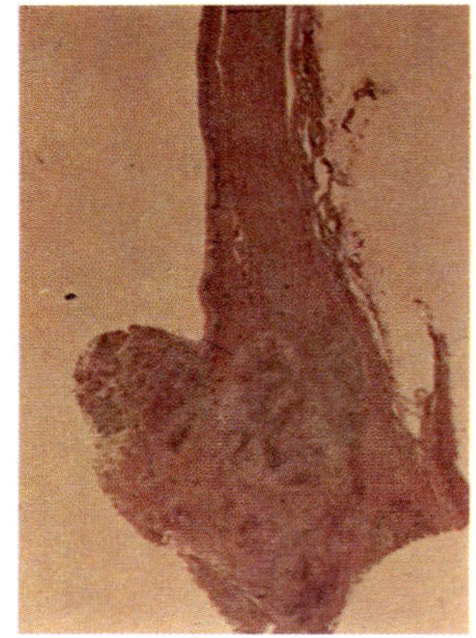

The unmagnified histologic section shows normal esophageal wall above with mucosa on the left. The cancer in the lower portion extends into the lumen on the left, and into the wall on the right.

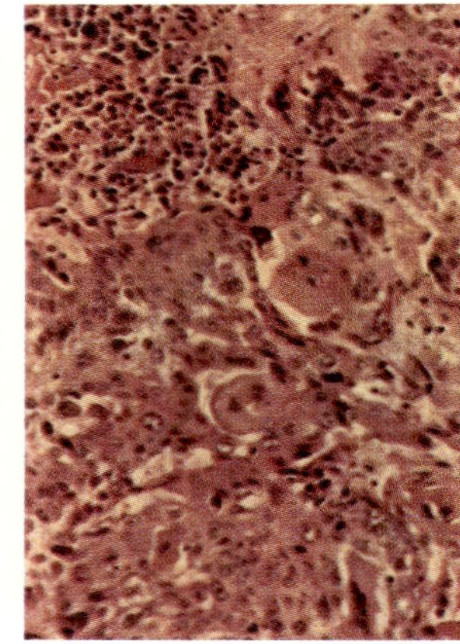

The cancer is composed of epithelial cells in which cytoplasmic keratinization is frequently evident. The lesion is thus a poorly differentiated squamous cell carcinoma.

CHRONIC ULCER OF STOMACH

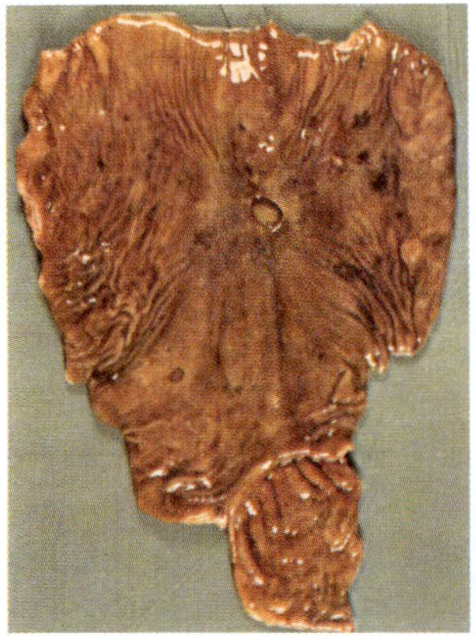

The ulcer is seen in the center of the stomach. It is on the lesser curvature in the upper part of the pyloric antrum. The pylorus with attached segment of duodenum is present at the lower part of the picture.

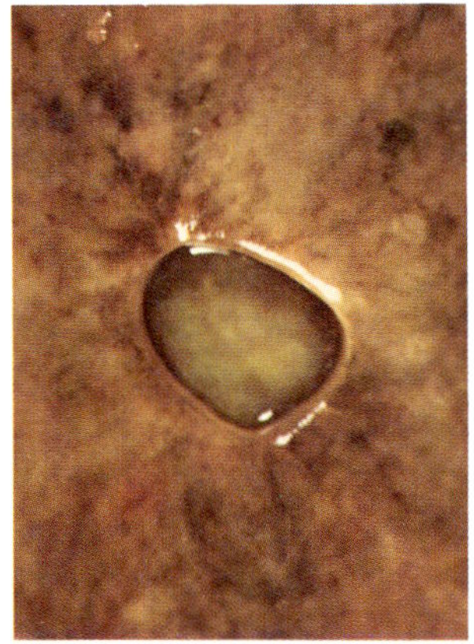

A close-up reveals the oval outline, sharp margins, steep walls, and clean base of the ulcer.

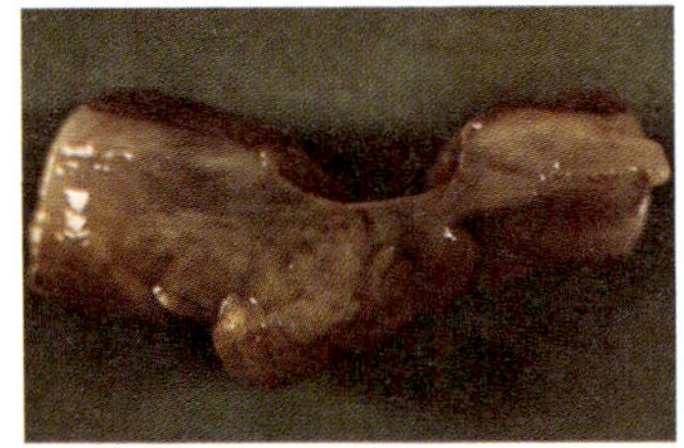

At cross section, the extension of the defect through the muscle layers is evident. The excavation has extended to the fibroadipose tissue of the mesentery along the lesser curvature of the stomach.

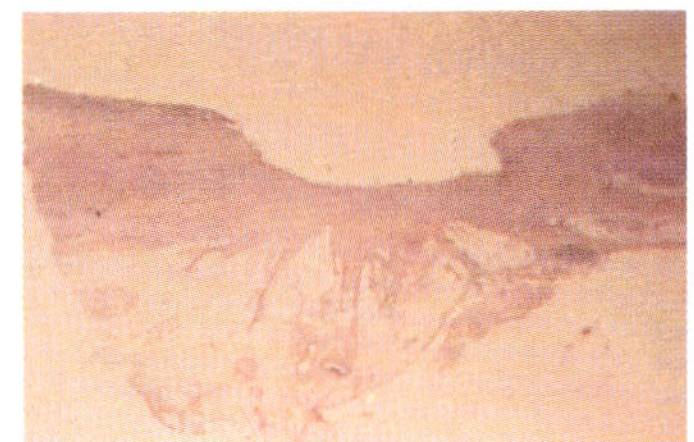

Without magnification the histologic section discloses the tissue pattern of the previous picture. Exudate lies on the surface of the ulcer base, granulation tissue lies beneath this, and atherosclerotic arteries and small nerves are present in the deeper fibrous connective tissue.

CHRONIC ULCER OF STOMACH

CLINICAL ACCOUNT 7376

The patient was a black female 52 years old who was admitted to the hospital because of back pain and shortness of breath. Seven years previously a radical mastectomy had been performed for cancer of the left breast. Three years later metastatic disease was first noted; tumor deposits were found in the spine, ribs, and calvarium. A bilateral oophorectomy was performed, cytotoxic drugs were given, and prednisone was administered. The latter was discontinued because of an episode of gastro-intestinal bleeding. Enlargement of the liver developed, hypercalcemia was noted, and her condition steadily deteriorated.

The temperature was 37.2 degrees C., pulse 108, respirations 24, and blood pressure 100/60 mm. Hg. Physical examination revealed emaciation, enlargement of the liver and spleen, a fluid wave in the abdomen, and marked subcutaneous edema of the lower legs.

The hemoglobin was 9.0 Gms., hematocrit 28, and leukocyte count of 9,300 with a normal cell distribution. The total serum protein was 6.0 Gms. with 2.0 Gms. albumin, the serum bilirubin was 4.7 mgs., and the blood calcium was 10.9 mgs./100 ml. The serum alkaline phosphatase was 1700 mU/ml., lactic dehydrogenase 349 mU/ml., and glutamic transaminase 256 mU/ml. Symptomatic treatment was given and the patient died on the second hospital day.

Autopsy examination revealed massive metastatic carcinoma of the liver, abdominal lymph nodes, and spine. There were also ascites (2,000 ml.) pleural effusions (200 ml. on each side), and extensive subcutaneous edema. Additional findings were incidental.

THE ENTITY

Peptic ulcers occur principally in the stomach and duodenum. In the stomach they tend to arise in the pyloric antrum and on the lesser curvature. In the duodenum, most occur within 2 cm. of the pyloric ring. At both sites they tend to be round, measure 1 to 2 cm. in diameter, and are deep, with steep walls and a clean base. Those that do not heal or perforate become chronic. Chronic ulcers reveal four histologic layers, i.e., leukocytes on the ulcerated surface, an underlying layer of necrotic debris, a subjacent layer of granulation tissue, and a deep zone of fibrous connective tissue that forms a dense scar. Nerves are bound in the scar tissue, and vessels at the ulcer base reveal pronounced arteriosclerosis.

Gastric ulcers are associated with normal or hypoacidity, are twice as common in males as females, and often occur in the elderly. Duodenal ulcers are associated with hyperacidity, are four times more frequent in males, and occur more often in young adults. Duodenal ulcers are five to ten times more common than gastric ulcers.

Clinical features include a gnawing midabdominal pain that is relieved by food, an x-ray defect visible after barium swallow, and occult blood in the stool. Most heal with bland diet, frequent feedings, and antacids. Healed ulcers leave a stellate mucosal scar that occasionally progresses to an hourglass constriction. Without healing there are four complications. The most common is perforation with acute suppurative peritonitis. Less common are pyloric stenosis with gastric retention, and duodenal penetration with massive hemorrhage. Least common is malignant transformation of a gastric ulcer. Other peptic ulcer sites are the lower esophagus, the stoma of a gastro-intestinal anastomosis, the jejunum, and the tip of a Meckel's diverticulum.

CARCINOMA OF STOMACH

CLINICAL ACCOUNT 6643

The patient was a white male 65 years old who was well until four weeks before coming to the hospital. At that time he noted anorexia, malaise, epigastric discomfort, and back pain. All gradually progressed. There had been a weight loss of 20 pounds.

The vital signs were normal. A firm lymph node was present in the left supraclavicular fossa. The lungs, heart, and abdomen were not remarkable. Rectal examination revealed prostatic enlargement.

The hemoglobin was 8.9 Gms., the hematocrit was 28 per cent, and the leukocytes numbered 19,500 with a pronounced neutrophilia. The blood urea nitrogen was 104 mgs. A barium enema revealed diverticula of the colon. An upper gastro-intestinal study was normal. Biopsy of the left supraclavicular lymph node revealed carcinoma. The patient was discharged after eleven days in the hospital; he died at home two weeks later.

Autopsy examination revealed a superficial spreading carcinoma of the gastric fundus, widespread metastatic disease, glandular and stromal hyperplasia of the prostate, and an adenoma of the mucosa of the ascending colon.

THE ENTITY

Carcinoma of the stomach arises twice as often in men as women, three times as often in the impoverished as the affluent, and most frequently between the ages of 50 and 69 years. Common complaints are epigastric distress, anorexia, and loss of weight. Usual signs are anemia, achlorhydria, and occult blood in the stool. X-rays of the stomach with contrast material usually reveal a defect in the gastric wall.

The tumors are predisposed to the lesser curvature, and more than half arise in the pyloric antrum. Most are flat, ulcerated, and spreading, although some are papillary with the bulk of the lesion projecting into the lumen. Least common is a diffuse spread throughout the wall that reduces the stomach to a thick rigid structure through which peristaltic waves cannot pass. This is due to a desmoplastic effect of the tumor cells so that the cut surface resembles "glistening threads of woven linen" and is hence named linitis plastica. Most are adenocarcinomas, usually of poor differentiation, and some, including linitis plastica, are undifferentiated. In the latter the tumor cells produce mucin, the nuclei are pushed to the periphery, and "signet ring" forms take the mucicarmine stain.

The tumor spreads to the lymph nodes of the lesser curvature, cardia, and mediastinum, to the liver and lungs, and to the left supraclavicular fossa (Virchow's or sentinel node) via the thoracic duct. It also spreads via the peritoneum to both ovaries, which become large firm discrete masses, and to the pouch of Douglas to form a hard "shelf" that can be palpated per rectum. The bilateral ovarian metastases, originally thought to be primary cancers, are still known as "Krukenberg tumors". Surgical excision produces five-year survivals of under 10 per cent.

While the cause is unknown, the cancers are often preceded by atrophic gastritis, and the patients frequently have pernicious anemia and are of blood group A. In addition, the incidence is especially high in Japan, Chile, and Finland, whereas in America it is rapidly declining, i.e., from 28 per 100,000 in 1930 to 9.7 in 1967 (1). Environmental factors are suspect.

1. Lilienfeld, A. Epidemiology of gastric cancer. New Eng. J. Med. 286:316-317, 1972.

CARCINOMA OF STOMACH

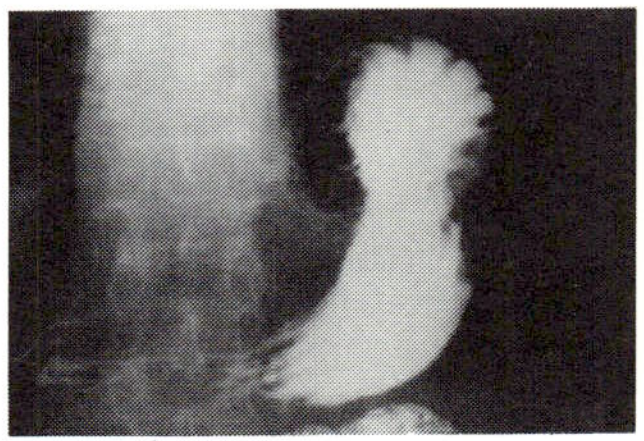

An x-ray study of the stomach after a swallow of barium fails to reveal an abnormality. The tumor is located in a portion of the stomach that is "blind" to radiographic examinations.

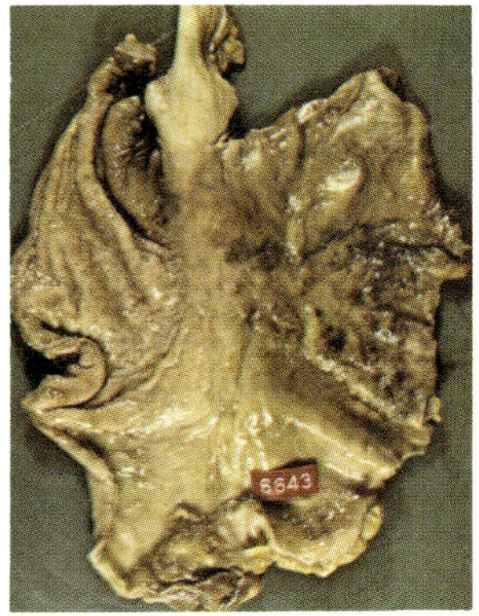

The tumor is flat and infiltrating and lies in the fundus along the greater curvature on the right.

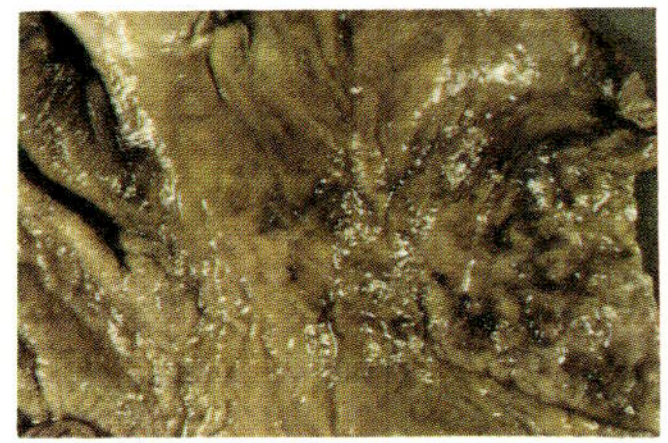

A closer view shows the flat nature of the cancer and the slight disfiguration of the mucosal pattern.

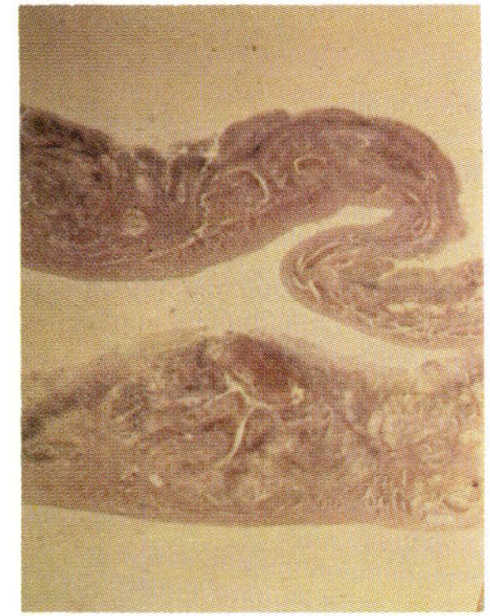

Two cross sections reveal thickening of the gastric wall and extension of tumor glands into the submucosa and external muscle layers. The tumor is a well differentiated adenocarcinoma.

ACUTE NECROTIZING PANCREATITIS

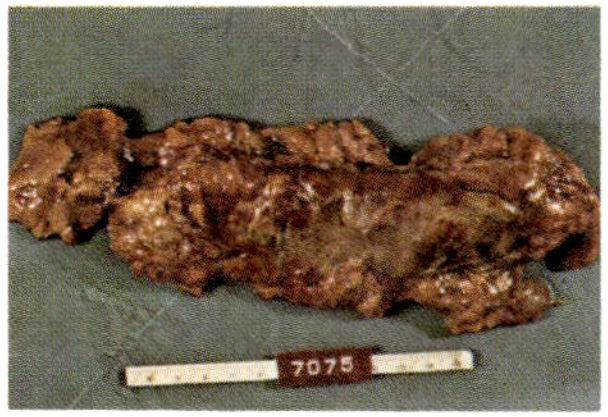

The pancreas is swollen and focally hemorrhagic and large central portions reveal much fat necrosis.

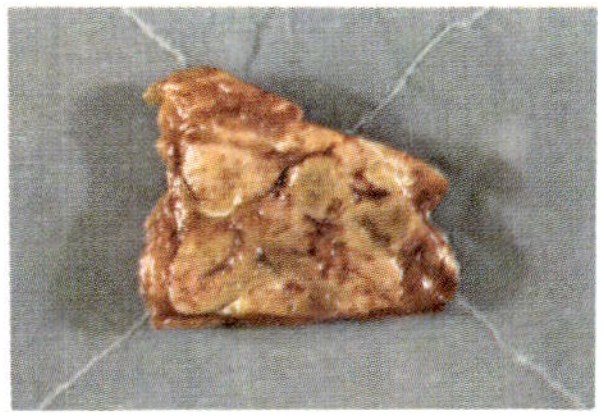

The cut surface discloses large confluent foci of necrosis that extend throughout the cross section of the gland.

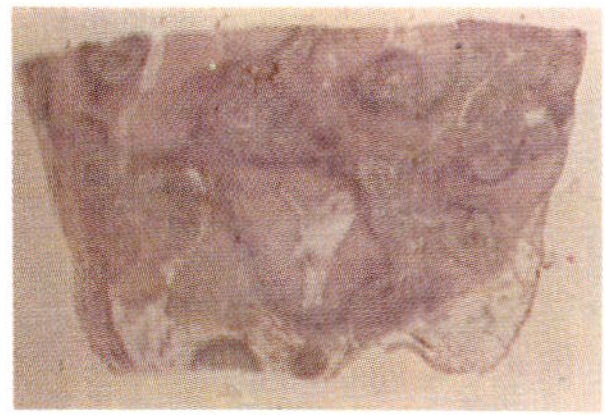

The unmagnified histologic section reveals massive necrosis with the blue marginal discoloration (basophilia) of pronounced leukocytic infiltration.

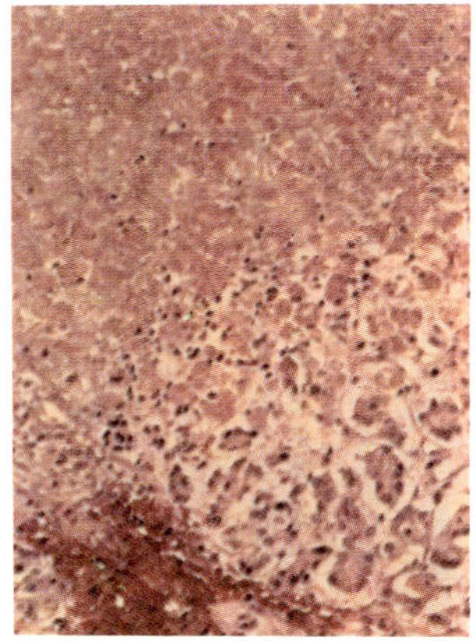

At higher power focal hemorrhage, intact parenchyma, and massive necrosis may be made out. Only slight marginal leukocytic infiltration is present in this field.

CARCINOMA, HEAD OF PANCREAS

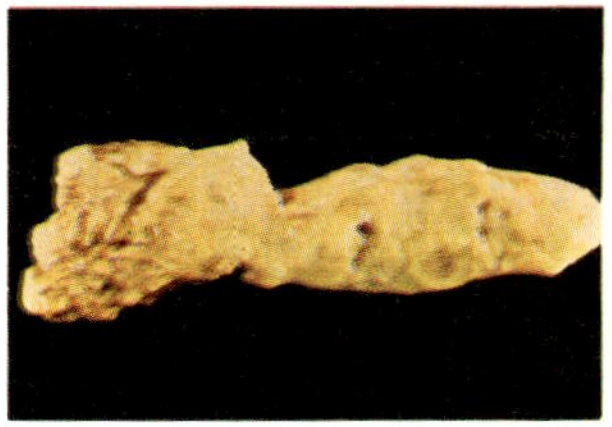

The photograph is orientated with the head at the bottom and the tail at the top. The light brownish gray lobulated appearance of normal pancreas is evident about the head. In the midportion, at the site of the tumor, the cut surface is gray, the lobules are obscure, and the tissue is firm.

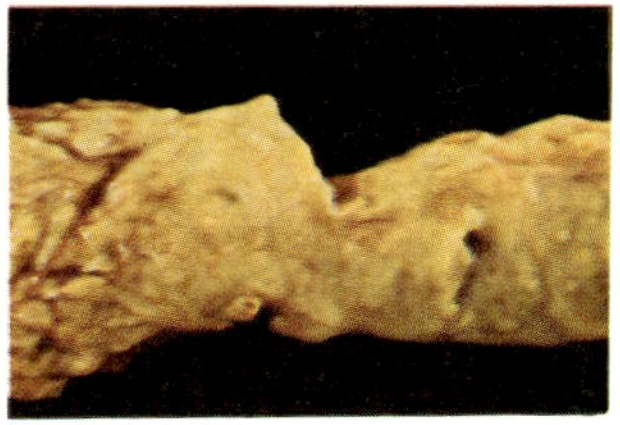

A closer view reveals the tumor. It obstructed the pancreatic duct and the secretory pressure backed up into the tributaries of the ductal system. As a result, dilated ducts are present in the tail, and the parenchyma of this region has undergone pronounced pressure atrophy.

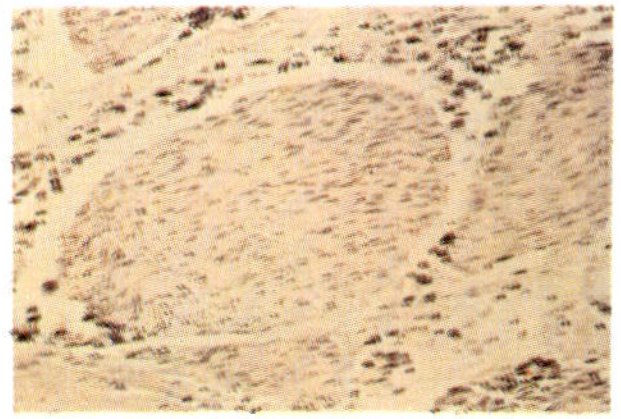

Nerves are present in the para-pancreatic tissue about the head. Sections reveal clusters of tumor cells in the perineural lymph sheaths. Elsewhere the tumor was seen to be a well differentiated adenocarcinoma.

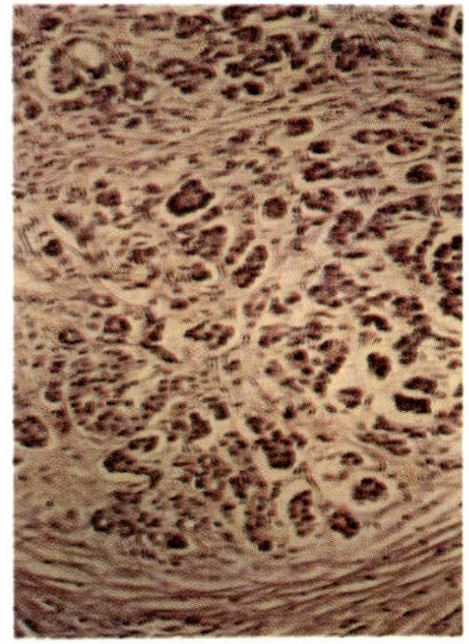

Microsections of the tail region disclose atrophy of the pancreatic lobules with marked perilobular fibrosis evident.

CARCINOMA, BODY-TAIL OF PANCREAS

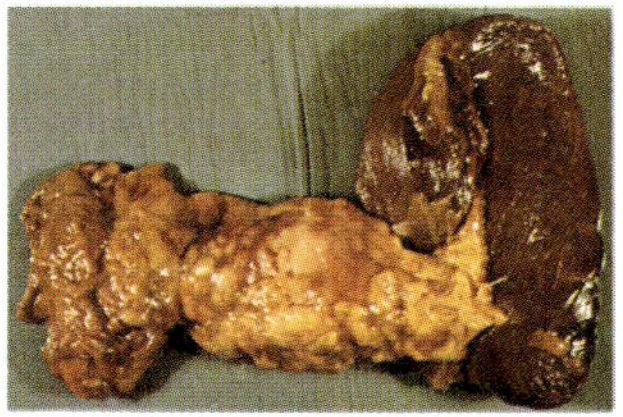

The uncut pancreas reveals the head at the left and the tail at the right with attached spleen. A firm gray mass in the body and tail of the pancreas may be seen.

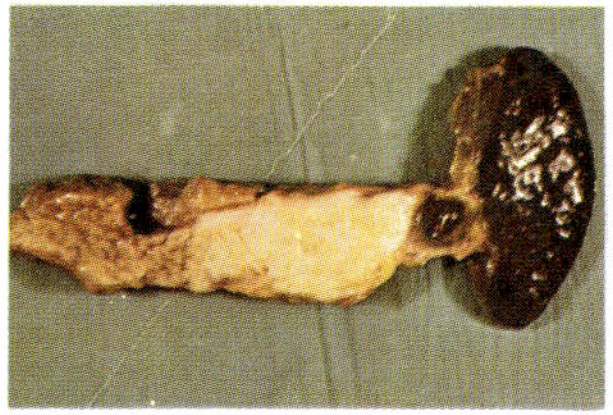

Coronal sections disclose the cut surfaces; the gray firm mass in the body and tail of the pancreas is scirrhous adenocarcinoma. An accessory spleen is evident.

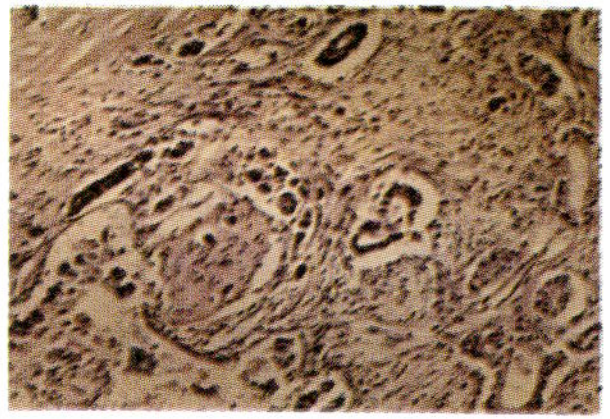

A microsection reveals dense connective tissue with irregularly dispersed small glandular masses of tumor.

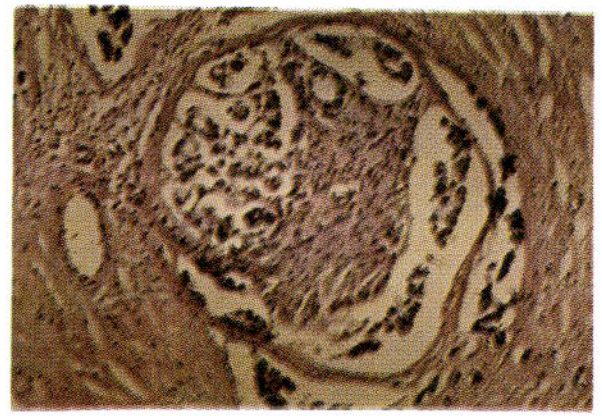

At higher power, gland-forming clusters of tumor cells are present within a perineural lymphatic space.

CARCINOMA, BODY-TAIL OF PANCREAS

CLINICAL ACCOUNT 6825

The patient was a white male 53 years old who was well until two weeks before hospital admission. At that time he developed persistent and generalized abdominal discomfort. On the day of admission, nausea and vomiting began. There had been no change in bowel habit. He had previously had a cholecystectomy for calculi, and a partial colectomy for diverticulitis.

The patient was well nourished and the vital signs were normal. Physical examination revealed a mass in the left upper quadrant of the abdomen, distension of the abdomen, and hypoactive bowel sounds.

The urine was normal. The hemoglobin was 15.6 Gm., and the leukocyte count was 16,800 with a slight neutrophilia. X-rays of the abdomen disclosed dilated loops of bowel with air-fluid levels consistent with intestinal obstruction. Laparotomy revealed massive replacement of the omentum with metastatic tumor. The obstruction was relieved and histologic examination of the omentum revealed mucinous adenocarcinoma. The patient was discharged to his home after fourteen days in the hospital.

He returned two weeks later because of recurrent intestinal obstruction. His condition progressively worsened, and he died after 23 days in the hospital. The total duration of his illness was approximately two and one-half months.

Autopsy examination revealed carcinoma of the body of the pancreas, metastatic carcinoma of the liver and peritoneum, fibrous adhesions of the peritoneum with intestinal obstruction, acute suppurative peritonitis, bronchopneumonia, and cachexia.

THE ENTITY

Carcinoma of the pancreas affects men twice as often as women and occurs predominantly in persons 50 to 70 years of age. The tumors arise in the ducts and are adenocarcinomas. The patients suffer loss of weight, pain in the abdomen, anorexia, nausea, vomiting, weakness, and malaise. The cancers are hard to diagnose, the spread of tumor tends to be rapid, and five-year survivals are seldom achieved with any form of treatment.

Carcinoma of the head is about three times as frequent as carcinoma of the body and tail (1). Because of its location, carcinoma of the head often ulcerates the duodenum, blocks the common bile duct, and is limited in its spread to the regional lymph nodes. As a consequence, blood is often detectable in the stool, and jaundice is frequent, early, and pronounced. The bile ducts are dilated, the gall bladder may be markedly distended and palpable, and biliary cirrhosis may affect the liver. Since the common bile duct is affected early, biliary obstruction dominates the illness, pain tends to be localized in the epigastrium and right upper quadrant, and early demise precludes widespread metastatic disease.

This is in noticeable contrast to carcinoma of the body and tail. Because of its location, jaundice is absent, the gall bladder is not distended, and blood is less frequent in the stool. The epigastric pain penetrates to the back and radiates to the left upper quadrant. In addition, the tumor borders on a peritoneal surface and lies adjacent to the splenic vein so that early invasion causes widespread metastatic disease of both liver and peritoneum.

1. Gullick, H.D. Carcinoma of the pancreas. A review and critical study of 100 cases. Medicine 38: 47, 1959.

CARCINOMA, AMPULLA OF VATER

CLINICAL ACCOUNT 476

The patient was a Ugandan male 72 years old who was well until two months before coming to the hospital. At that time he developed icterus, abdominal pain, dark urine, and swelling of the feet. Shortly thereafter the abdomen became swollen, anorexia developed, and the patient was aware of a loss of weight. Cough and itching of the skin developed one week before hospital admission. The principal physical finding was an abdomen distended with fluid, and a liver border palpated eight fingerbreadths below the right costal margin. The urine was positive for bile, negative for urobilinogen. The hemoglobin was 8.4 Gms., hematocrit 24 per cent, and leukocyte count 9,200 per cmm. The total serum protein was 7.4 Gms. with 1.5 Gms. albumin. The serum bilirubin was 8.1 mgs. with 5.7 direct reacting. The serum alkaline phosphatase was 350 international units (20-90*), and the serum alpha fetoprotein was negative. On the sixth day a liver biopsy revealed bile stasis. On the next day the abdomen became tender, and on the following day the patient died.

Autopsy examination revealed a carcinoma of the ampulla of Vater, bile stasis of the liver, acute fibrinopurulent peritonitis, and pronounced dilatation of the gall bladder and common bile duct. The duct was patent through the tumor at the ampulla. No metastases were found.

THE ENTITY

Carcinoma of the ampulla of Vater is uncommon; the average age of persons affected is 55 years, and the condition occurs three to four times more often in men than women. The tumor is usually flat, ulcerated, and invasive, but may be bulky and sessile without ulceration. Most are adenocarcinomas. Invasion of the duodenal mucosa, common bile duct, and head of the pancreas occurs early. Clinical detection usually precedes widespread metastasis. Metastases extend to the lymph nodes of the porta hepatis, and later to the para-aortic and mediastinal lymph nodes. While the cause is not known, chronic inflammation and aberrant metabolism of bile acids, which resemble the carcinogen methylcholanthrene, have been suggested (1).

Clinically jaundice is early and constant. The urine turns dark and the stool becomes acholic. Vague pain may be present in the hypochondrium. The abdomen reveals hepatomegaly and a palpably dilated gall bladder. Liver function tests decline, the prothrombin time is prolonged, and the serum alkaline phosphatase rises. Diagnosis is aided by contrast radiographs of the duodenum. Without treatment the patient lives six to eight months before succumbing to hepatic failure and ascending cholangitis.

Differential diagnosis includes hepatitis and stone in the common duct. The latter is characterized by fever, lancinating pain, and intermittent course rather than constant jaundice and vague upper abdominal discomfort. With hepatitis the patient experiences a distinct constitutional illness that precedes the onset of jaundice. It is to be recalled that a tumor blocking the common bile duct distal to the cystic duct causes a normal gall bladder to dilate several times its original size. Stone in the common duct, however, is usually preceded by cholecystitis with fibrosis of the wall so that dilatation is prevented. Hence Courvoisier's Law: a palpably distended gall bladder in the presence of obstructive jaundice is more likely due to tumor than to stone.

1. Smith, R. The Surgery of Pancreatic Neoplasms. E. & S. Livingstone, London, 1953.

*Normal range.

CARCINOMA, AMPULLA OF VATER

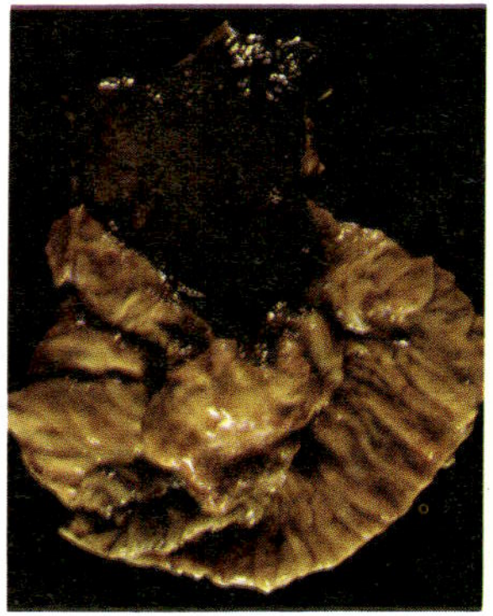

The tumor lies in the middle of the picture under the extremely dilated common bile duct above, and inside the U-shaped curl of the duodenum at the bottom of the picture. The tumor is covered by intact mucosa, and the open ampulla of Vater can be seen on the upper margin of the lesion.

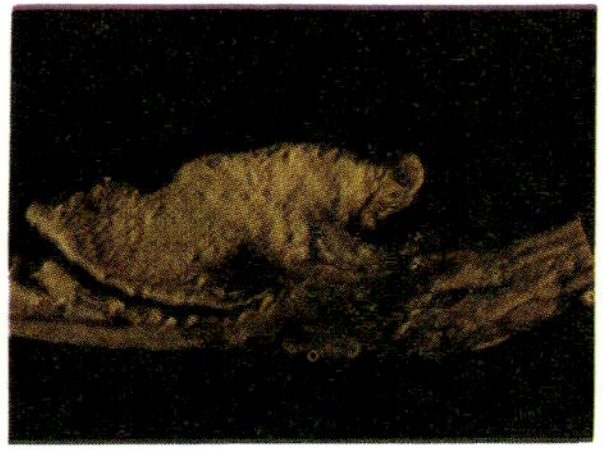

The section reveals a pale gray cut surface bulging into the duodenum. Pancreatic tissue can be seen underneath the duodenal mucosa.

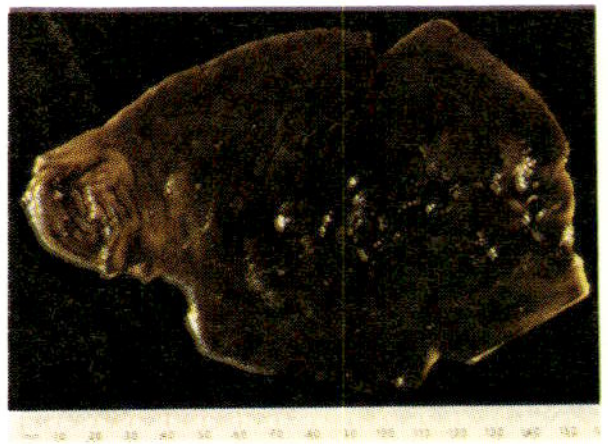

The gall bladder is enormously dilated, measuring about 15 cm. in length and 10 cm. in circumference.

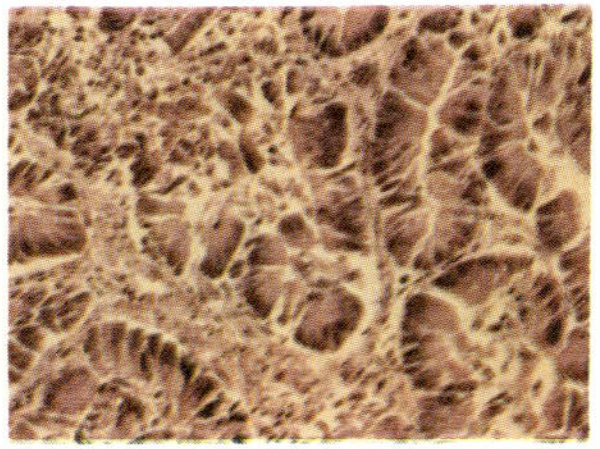

A microsection of the tumor reveals the glandular configuration of an adenocarcinoma.

NORMAL LIVER

The right lobe is somewhat elongated and there is a focus of roughening of Glisson's capsule by a fibrous adhesion. The external surface is not otherwise remarkable except for two grooves on the upper surface. These are an insignificant anomaly; the subjacent tissue is not affected. Despite the history which indicates the probability of passive hyperemia, none was found.

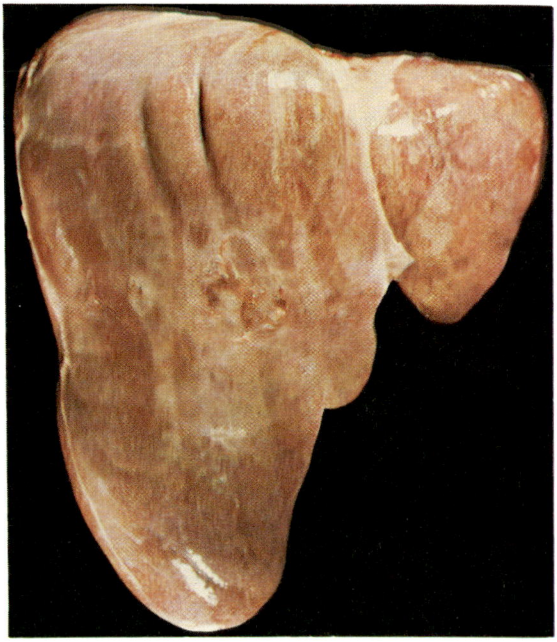

Below, left: The cut surface between the vessels is uniformly light brownish red. **Below, center:** The close-up view shows a finely reticulated pattern in which the pallid parts are clusters of parenchymal cells (hepatocytes), and the light red regions are accumulations of blood that lie principally within the centers of the hepatic lobules. **Below, right:** At scanning power the portal triads, central veins, and intervening sinusoids are evident. The basophilia about the portal triads is due to clusters of lymphocytes which are normally present. All portal zones contain one portal venule, one hepatic arteriole, and one bile ductule. Blood enters the lobule at the portal triad, progresses through the sinusoids, and leaves the lobule through the central vein.

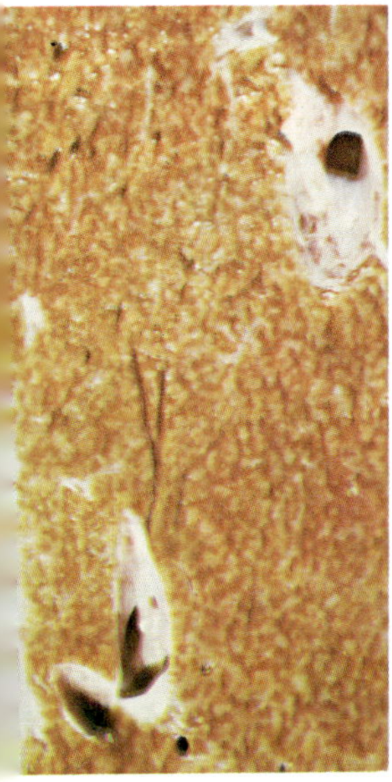

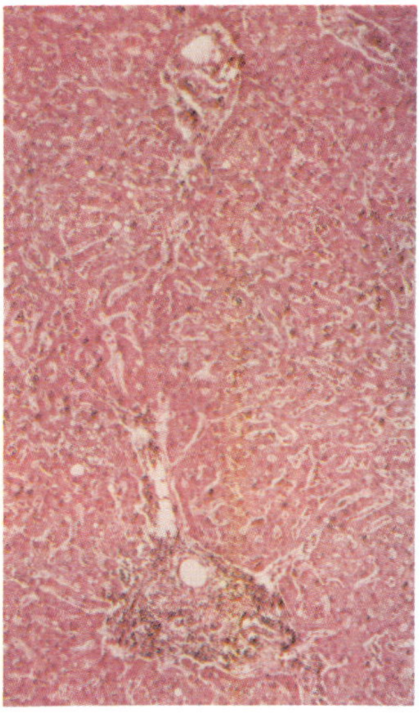

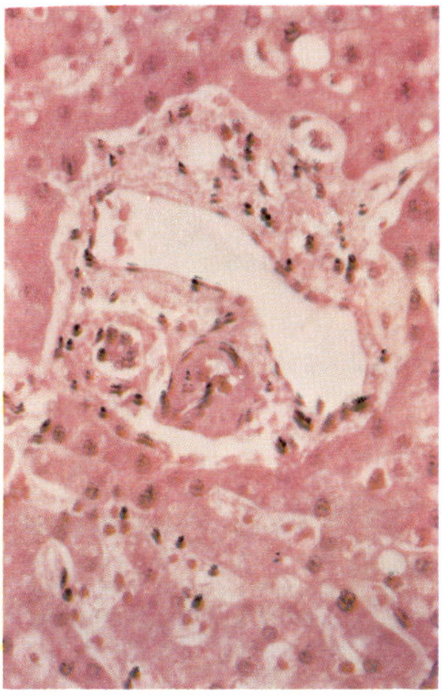

NORMAL LIVER

CLINICAL ACCOUNT 6196

The patient was a white female 75 years old who had experienced angina pectoris for the past five years. For some months she had also had shortness of breath, dyspnea on exertion, two-pillow orthopnea, nocturia, and ankle edema which disappeared in the morning. On the night before admission she had had a severe pain in the left anterior chest that radiated to both shoulders and was not relieved by nitroglycerine.

The temperature was 98.6° F., pulse 150, respirations 32, and blood pressure 92/60 mm. Hg. Rales were audible over the lower posterior lung fields. The heart was enlarged to the left, the rhythm was regular, and no murmurs were heard. The abdomen was protruberant; no masses were palpated. There was no fluid wave. There was no ankle edema.

The hemoglobin was 12.9 Gm., hematocrit 41, and leukocytes 9,000 with a normal differential count. An electrocardiogram disclosed atrial fibrillation. The patient was digitalized, the heart rate decreased, and a harsh systolic murmur radiating to the neck and axilla was then heard. A chest x-ray indicated pulmonary hyperemia, pleural effusions, and cardiac enlargement. On the fourteenth hospital day dyspnea became pronounced and the patient died.

Autopsy examination revealed hypertrophy of the heart (475 Gm.), rheumatic disease of the aortic valve with stenosis, hyperemia of the lungs, carcinoma of the thyroid, and carcinoma of the right breast. There was no metastatic disease from either primary tumor. The liver weighed 1200 Gm.

THE ENTITY

The liver consists of four main components, hepatocytes, biliary channels, Kupffer cells, and blood vessels. The hepatocytes constitute 90 per cent of the liver cell mass. Blood enters the liver in the amount of 1500 ml. per minute at the hilum (porta hepatis) through the portal vein and the hepatic artery. The former carries 80 per cent of this total at a pressure of 8-12 mm. Hg.; the latter carries the remainder at a pressure of 120 mm. Hg. (1). Slightly more than half of the total oxygen supply is delivered by the portal vein, and either vessel is able to maintain the viability of the tissue without the other. At the portal triads (portal vein, hepatic artery, and bile duct) the venous and arterial bloods join in the hepatic sinusoids to flow past the columns of liver cells. The mixed blood then enters the hepatic veins which constitute the beginning of the venous outflow tract. Kupffer cells, which are phagocytic, attach to the sinusoidal surfaces of the hepatocytes, and a finely porous membrane separates the liver cells from the blood flow within the sinusoids. The space created by this membrane between sinusoid and surface of hepatocyte is the space of Disse. Two rows of liver cells ordinarily abut each other; a groove between the cells on the adjoining surfaces forms the beginning of the biliary tract. These convey bile to the preductules (canals of Hering) and thence to the smallest bile ducts of the portal triads. Thus the columns of liver cells sit between sinusoids on the outside moving blood from the portal triads to the central veins and minute bile channels on the inside moving bile in the opposite direction toward the portal triads. The bile proceeds to the common duct, diverts to the gall bladder, and then enters the duodenum, while the blood continues from the central veins to the main hepatic vein which joins the inferior vena cava, perforates the diaphragm, and enters the right atrium of the heart.

1. Wright, G.P., and Symmers, W. St.C. Systemic Pathology, American Elsevier Publishing Company, Inc., New York, 1966.

PASSIVE HYPEREMIA OF LIVER

CLINICAL ACCOUNT 5915

The patient was a Negro woman 28 years old who had taken a steroid medication for two weeks because of swelling and tenderness of the thyroid. The symptoms subsided; the medication was continued. One week before admission her morning cough became worse, malaise was noted, and the temperature rose to 99.6 degrees F. On the day of admission she had a sharp pain in the right chest that was accentuated by deep breathing. She then became short of breath, the cough worsened, and abundant "dirty" sputum was raised.

The temperature was 102 degrees F., pulse 120, respirations 32, and blood pressure 120/70. Breath sounds were decreased and coarse rales were heard. The urine disclosed 3 plus protein. The hemoglobin was 15.0 Gm., hematocrit 47, and leukocytes 11,000 with 66 neutrophils and 18 band cells. The serum glutamic transaminase and lactic dehydrogenase were elevated. During the hospital course an anemia developed. The leukocytes rose to 24,000 with 59 neutrophils, and 22 band cells. A right thoracentesis yielded 300 ml. of bloody fluid. Dyspnea increased. A chest x-ray disclosed a widespread infiltration in both lung fields. Oliguria developed and peritoneal dialysis was performed. Respiratory distress increased, coma supervened, and death occurred on the fifteenth hospital day.

Autopsy examination revealed alveolar proteinosis of the lungs which weighed 950 and 775 Gms., respectively. Other diagnoses included focal interstitial pancreatitis and passive hyperemia of the liver. The liver weighed 1450 Gm.

THE ENTITY

Blood enters the liver at the hilum through the portal vein and hepatic artery. After passing through the vascular subdivisions, the venous and arterial components join at the periphery of the lobules, mix in transit through the sinusoids, and enter the central veins. Thereafter, egress is provided by even larger tributaries that merge to form the hepatic vein, which conveys the blood to the superior surface of the liver and into the inferior vena cava. It then passes through the diaphragm and enters the right atrium of the heart.

When this flow of blood is obstructed, the hydrostatic pressure rises in the venous channels, and when this increased back-pressure reaches the liver, the central portions of the lobules are affected first. If the pressure rise is sudden and marked and pronounced, as with myocardial infarction and acute heart failure, the liver cells lining the sinusoids in the central portions undergo frank necrosis. More often, however, the rise in pressure is slight and gradual and prolonged, as with arteriosclerotic heart disease with congestive failure. In this event, the centrilobular sinusoids widen, and the hepatic cells become thin and disappear. With this central atrophy and the Kupffer cell pigmentation due to blood stagnation and hemosiderin deposition, the cut surface of the organ comes to have a reddish brown mottled with pinkish gray cut surface. That is the hallmark of chronic passive hyperemia of the liver. The viable cells about the portal triads are ordinarily sufficient to maintain normal hepatic function.

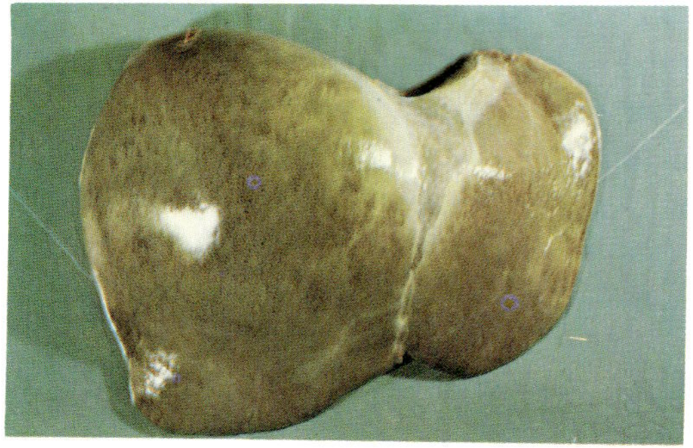

The serosa is smooth, glistening, and light pinkish brown.

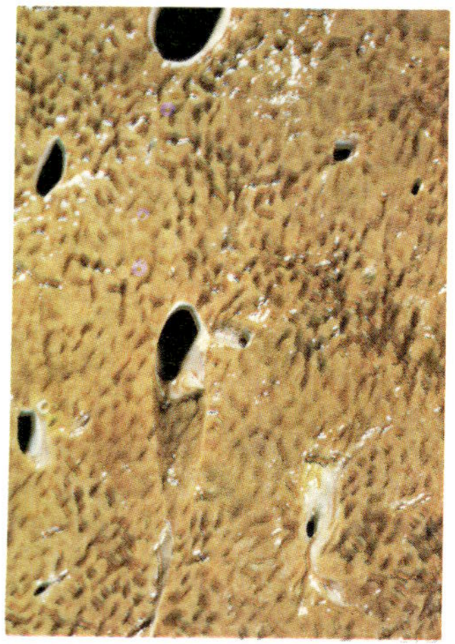

A close-up photograph reveals the reticulated pattern of dark brown discoloration. The light portions are portal regions; the dark brown zones are central regions in which the dilated vessels are packed with blood and hemosiderin. The mottling produced by this irregular distribution of pigment resembles the cut surface of a nutmeg.

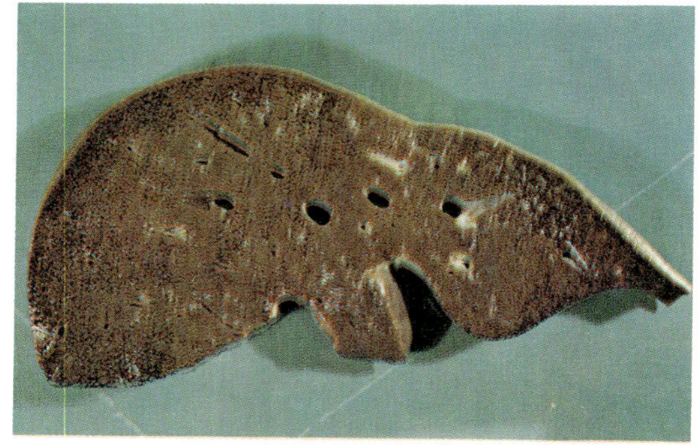

The cut surface is brown, evenly flecked with dark brown.

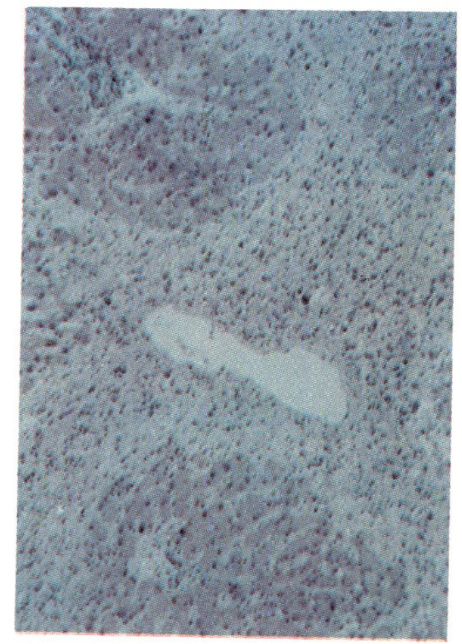

Higher power reveals intact hepatocytes about portal triads. Elsewhere fibrous tissue replaces the parenchyma. Obstruction of outflow of blood in the liver causes the sinusoids to dilate, then atrophy, and finally to be replaced with connective tissue. This begins first in the pericentral regions of the lobules. When the fibrosis is pronounced and widespread, the condition is called cardiac cirrhosis.

FATTY METAMORPHOSIS OF LIVER

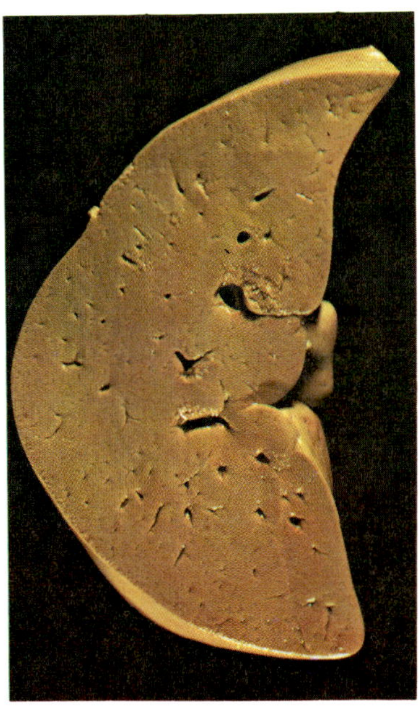

The cut surface of the liver is pale and distinctly yellow. Also, the liver is often enormously enlarged.

An unmagnified section shows extreme pallor because the cytoplasm of every hepatocyte has been replaced with fat and the fat dissolves out in the paraffin embedding process.

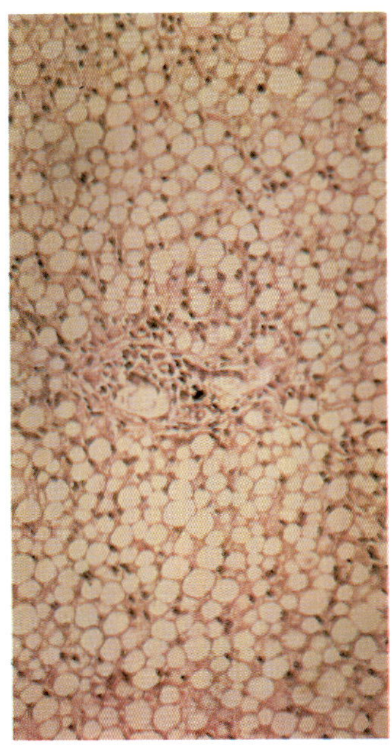

A low power magnification shows a portal triad in the center of the field and fatty metamorphosis of the hepatocytes.

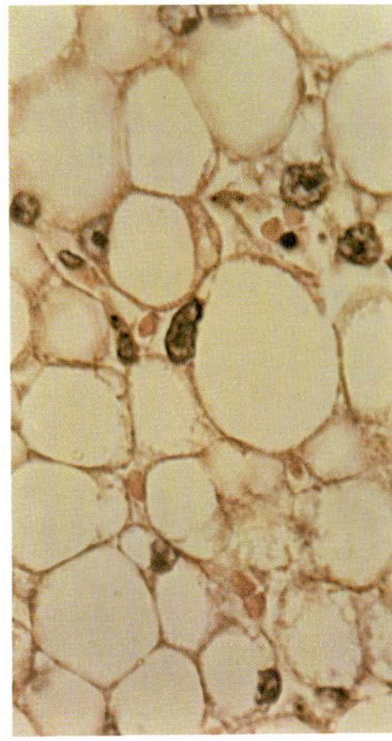

The process is seen best at higher power; the fat pushes the nuclei to the perimeter of the cells to form "signet ring" configurations.

FATTY METAMORPHOSIS OF LIVER

CLINICAL ACCOUNT 464

The patient was a Ugandan female 25 years old who was well until six months before coming to the hospital. At that time she noticed swelling of the ankles. Over the following months this spread to the legs, back, and abdomen. She gradually became weak and developed both dizziness and headaches. Her abdomen continued to swell and in the preceding month had affected her arms and face. Weakness became so pronounced that she was unable to stand.

Physical examination revealed anasarca, emaciation, and marked pallor of the skin and mucous membranes. The temperature was 37 degrees C., pulse 88, respirations 24, and blood pressure 120/60 mm. Hg. Physical findings included a systolic murmur over the tricuspid area, enlargement of the liver to three fingerbreadths below the right costal margin, and shifting dullness over the abdomen. The urine showed a trace of protein. The hemoglobin was 2.0 Gms. per 100 ml. The cells were hypochromic and microcytic with marked anisocytosis. A chest x-ray was not remarkable. The stool revealed hookworm eggs. On the second hospital day she had a bloody stool, collapsed, and died.

Autopsy examination revealed many whipworms throughout the small intestine, an intact intestinal mucosa, ascites and marked pallor of the liver suggestive of pronounced fatty metamorphosis. The heart weighed 200 Gms., lungs 330 and 420 Gms., liver 2230 Gms., spleen 160 Gms., and kidneys 90 and 100 Gms.

THE ENTITY

The most common pathologic change in the liver is the accumulation of fat in the hepatocytes. Lipids reach the liver as chylomicrons which are absorbed from the gut, and as fatty acids which are carried from the fat depots of the body. In the liver, with the help of the lipotrophic factors choline and methionine, lipoproteins are synthesized within and discharged from the hepatocytes. Thus lipid substances continually enter into and emerge from the liver cells. The mechanisms of lipid accumulation are increased deposition or impaired removal of these materials. Frequent among them are infections, congestive heart failure, and especially alcoholism which mobilizes lipid, increases its transport to the liver, and impairs the utilization of it (1). In other countries starvation, which deprives the patient of choline and methionine, is a frequent cause. The ileal bypass procedure for the treatment of morbid obesity may operate in the same way. The lipid accumulates first in the pericentral cells, gradually spreads to all parts of the lobules, and uniformly involves all of the lobules. As a consequence the liver becomes extremely large and may weigh over 5,000 gms. The cut surface is greasy and pale yellow. Burst cells release lipid and cause fat embolism. Sudden unexpected death is not uncommon (2).

1. Leevy, C.M. Fatty Liver: A Study of 270 Patients with Biopsy Proven Fatty Liver and a Review of the Literature. Medicine 41:249-278, 1962.
2. Graham, R.L. Sudden Death Associated with Fatty Livers. Bull. J. Hopkins Hosp. 74:16, 1944.

AMYLOIDOSIS OF LIVER

CLINICAL ACCOUNT 6002

The patient was a white male 63 years old who developed hepatomegaly four years before the last hospital admission. Biopsy disclosed amyloidosis. Since then his condition had steadily worsened; weight decreased and weakness developed. Diarrhea began three years before admission and seemed to follow the ingestion of meat, green vegetables, and citrus fruits. Renal disease developed eighteen months before admission and was manifested by nocturia and by intermittent swelling of the lower extremities.

The temperature was 98.2 degrees F., pulse 96, respirations 18, and blood pressure 110/70 mm. Hg. The patient was weak and emaciated. The heart and lungs were normal. The liver margin was hard, nontender, and seven fingerbreadths below the right costal margin. There was a 3 plus pitting edema of the ankles.

The urine revealed 4 plus proteinuria, a few coarsely and finely granular casts, and a small number of leukocytes. The hemoglobin was 16.7 Gm., hematocrit 51, and leukocytes 10,800 with a slight neutrophilia. The blood urea nitrogen and serum creatinine were 115 and 6.9 mg. per 100 ml., respectively. The total protein was 5 Gm. with 2 Gm. albumin and 3 Gm. globulin. The alkaline phosphatase was 200 units (normal 30-85).

On the day after admission bright red blood was passed per rectum, the blood pressure fell to 50/50 mm. Hg., and the patient died.

Autopsy examination revealed amyloidosis of the heart, liver, pancreas, kidneys, spleen, lymph nodes, bone marrow, adrenals, parathyroids, and tongue. There were also edema of the right and left lungs (900 and 875 Gm.), acute fibrinous enterocolitis that was attributed to uremia, and plasmacytosis of the vertebral bone marrow. The liver weighed 4100 Gm.

THE ENTITY

Amyloidosis occurs in a primary form involving mainly the muscles of the heart, gut, and tongue, in a secondary form involving the liver, spleen, kidneys and adrenals, in a primary distribution association with plasma cell myeloma, and in a localized tumor-like form especially in the upper respiratory tract. Hepatic involvement is equally frequent in the primary and secondary forms. The amyloid is first engulfed by the Kupffer cells, then spills out into the spaces of Disse and, with accumulation, gradually causes a pressure atrophy of the hepatocytes. The liver cells slowly undergo necrosis and eventually disappear so that in advanced cases solid masses of amyloid replace large areas of liver. As the amyloid accumulates, the liver becomes large, pale, waxy, and firm. This is a unique gross pathologic change.

Of 47 patients with liver involvement, two-thirds displayed signs of hepatic disease (1). The two most common were hepatomegaly and ascites. Other stigmata of cirrhosis were absent (cutaneous angiomas, abdominal collateral vessels, palmar erythema, gynecomastia, and testicular atrophy). Splenomegaly and jaundice were uncommon. Functional tests are often unreliable even though structural change is pronounced. The Congo red disappearance test is useful, being positive in thirteen of nineteen cases. The most reliable diagnostic procedure is needle biopsy of the liver. Death is much more often due to renal or cardiac involvement than to hepatic failure.

1. Levine, R.A. Amyloid disease of the liver. Am. J. Med. 33:349, 1962.

AMYLOIDOSIS OF LIVER

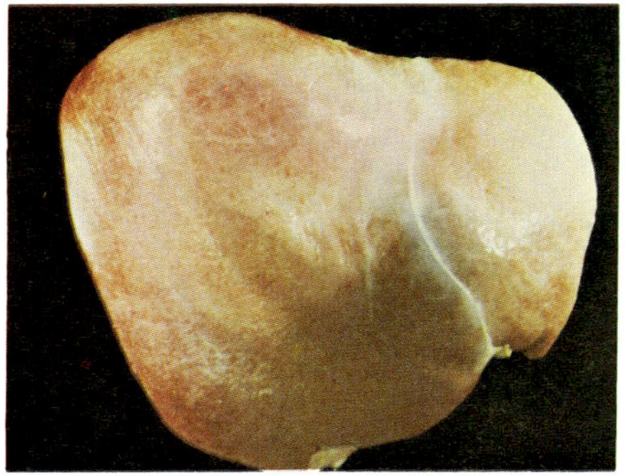

The liver is globoid, the surface is pale, and the consistency is uniformly increased.

At closer view, these observations are more apparent. Pallor and waxiness and uniform change are especially evident.

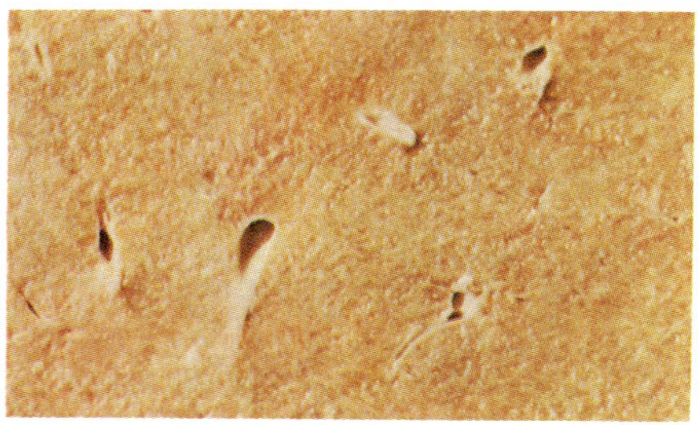

The cut surface is firm and uniformly pink and has a waxy or lardaceous aspect. Small vessels and bile ducts are not evident. The resilience of normal hepatic tissue is lost.

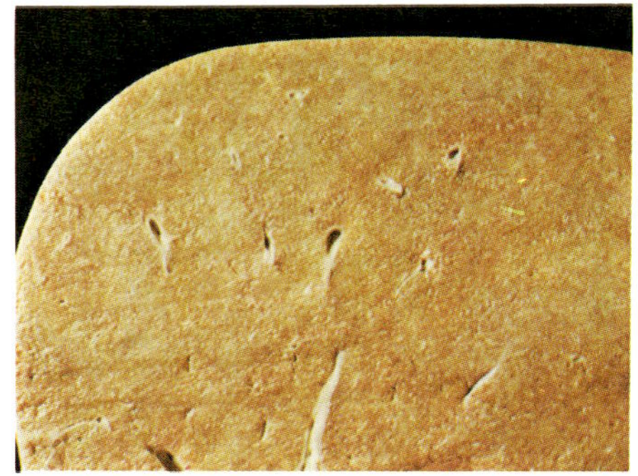

The microsection reveals a pale pink structureless material that fills the hepatic sinusoids and exerts pressure on the lining epithelial cells. As a result, the cells atrophy and disappear, leaving a scattering of hepatocytes in a broad mass of hyaline.

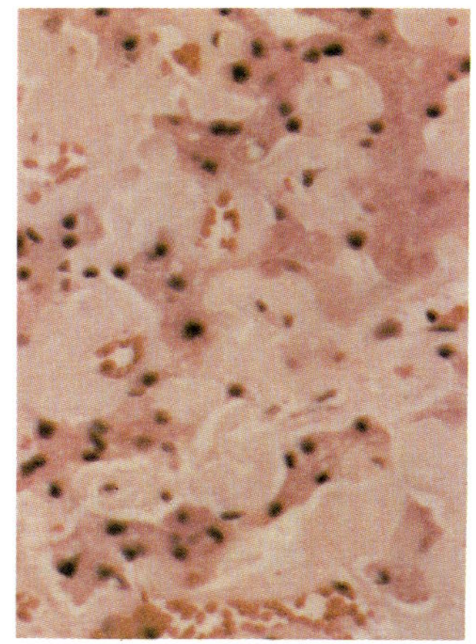

ACUTE NECROTIZING HEPATITIS

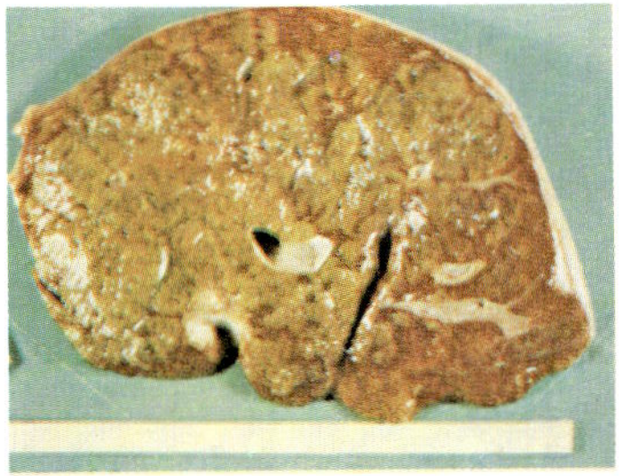

The cut surface of the liver reveals a pale greenish brown portion and a bright red portion. The former is viable if injured hepatic parenchyma. The latter is collapsed tissue in which only stroma and vessels are left.

The junction of the two is shown; masses of hepatocytes are distinct from wide bands of stroma in which bile ductules are evident.

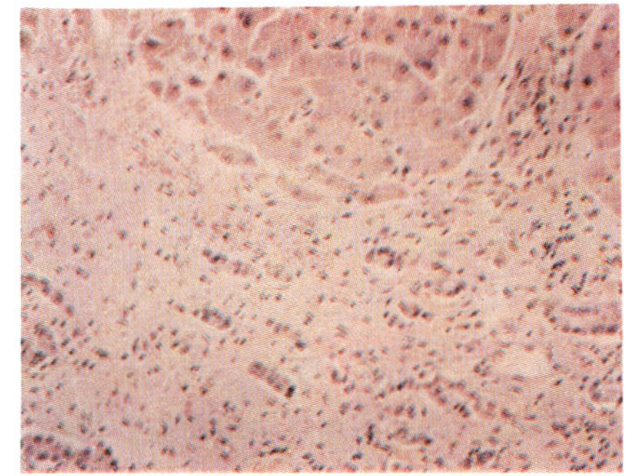

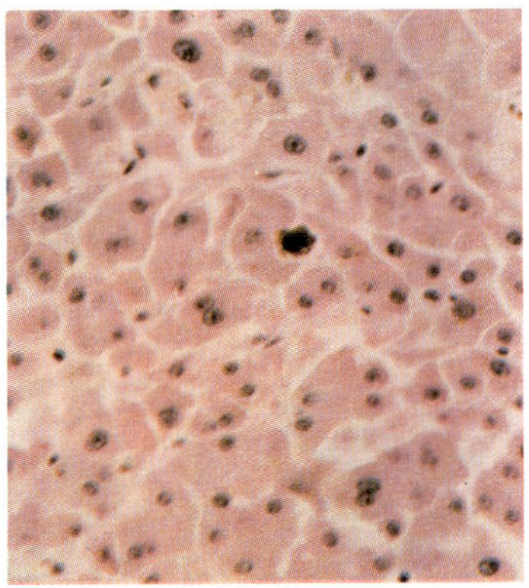

The viable parenchyma reveals pronounced variations in cell size, increased numbers of mitotic figures, and the presence of bile lakes.

In the collapsed portion, all of the hepatocytes have departed and only stroma with foci of recent hemorrhage and a scattering of bile canaliculi remain.

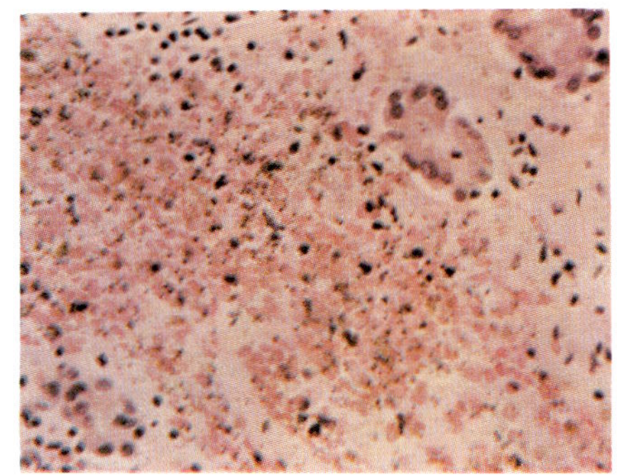

ACUTE NECROTIZING HEPATITIS

CLINICAL ACCOUNT 6602

The patient was a black male 38 years old who was well until three months before entering the hospital. At that time he noticed a slight yellow discoloration of his eyes and a brownish red discoloration of his urine. These persisted and were intermittently accompanied by dark red blood in the stool. One week before admission fatigue became pronounced, bright red blood was seen in the stool, and a physician was consulted. Resulting laboratory data indicated liver disease, and the patient was admitted to the hospital. There had been no parenteral medications, blood transfusions, or previous episodes of jaundice. However, a brother-in-law had been ill earlier in the year with jaundice and a diagnosis of hepatitis with a positive Australia antigen test had been made. The patient had been taking isoniazid for the four months preceding hospitalization because of a positive tuberculin skin test.

The temperature was 98.6° F., respirations 12, pulse 80, and blood pressure 150/80 mm. Hg. The sclerae were slightly icteric. The head, neck, and chest were not remarkable. The abdomen was soft, flat, and nontender. Bowel sounds were normal, and no organs or masses were palpated.

The urine was normal except for bile and the presence of urobilinogen in a dilution of 1:20. The blood was normal. Significant laboratory data included a prothrombin time of 18 sec. (control 13 sec.), a total bilirubin of 13 mg. (6 mg. direct) a total protein of 6.3 Gm. (2.6 Gm. albumin), a blood cholesterol of 275 mg., an alkaline phosphatase of 210 units, a glutamic transaminase of 620 units, a blood ammonia of 170 mcgm., and a serum lactic dehydrogenase of over 1500 units. Three LE cell preparations were negative, as was a test for Australia antigen.

The serum bilirubin gradually rose to 25 mg., and the patient became lethargic and then confused. The blood urea nitrogen gradually rose to 90 mg. On the twenty-sixth hospital day chest x-rays disclosed bronchopneumonia. Sputum cultures at this time revealed Gram positive diplococci. A pleural effusion developed on the right, the patient gradually lapsed into coma, and death occurred on the thirtieth hospital day.

THE ENTITY

Massive hepatic necrosis occurs in both sexes at all ages and is characterized by the sudden onset of fever, chills, weakness, anorexia, and jaundice. The liver is tender to palpation, and the serum levels of glutamic oxalic and glutamic pyruvic transaminase are markedly elevated. The serum bilirubin is also raised, and both conjugated and nonconjugated forms are present. In fulminant cases coma develops and death occurs in four to ten days after the onset.

In such cases the liver is soft, shrunken, and flabby, with a green finely wrinkled surface. The cut surface is coarsely mottled with yellow from necrosis, green from bile, and red from foci of hemorrhage. Later, the necrotic debris is carried away, the liver shrinks, and broad dark red zones of collapsed stroma alternate with soft pale green bulging masses of residual parenchyma. The margins of the viable tissue are infiltrated with segmented granulocytes. If the patient survives, fibrous tissue replaces the collapsed stroma so that the broad irregular scars of postnecrotic cirrhosis form. Early death is due to hepatic failure with or without cholemic nephrosis; late death is due to portal hypertension and occasionally the development of hepatocellular carcinoma.

Causes include a virus (infectious or serum hepatitis), mushroom poisoning (*Amanita phalloides*), toxins (carbon tetrachloride, phosphorus), drugs (chloroform, cinchophen, arsenicals, gold compounds, and possibly isoniazid), and perhaps dietary deletions (vitamin E and trace amounts of selenium). Often the cause is not apparent.

EARLY LAENNEC CIRRHOSIS

CLINICAL ACCOUNT 5954

The patient was a Negro male 47 years old who was admitted to the hospital because of nausea and vomiting. For the past fifteen years he had been an alcoholic. For the past eleven years he had had recurring pancreatitis. For the past four years he had been diabetic. Over the past two years he had passed bulky pale greasy stools. Dull epigastric pain began one week before admission, and for the two days preceding admission he had had nausea, vomiting, and a slight fever.

The temperature was 101 degrees F., respirations 34, pulse 100, and blood pressure 130/90 mm. Hg. The principal findings of the physical examination were shifting dullness in the abdomen and a liver margin 6 cm. below the right costal margin.

The patient was tachypneic, the air hunger increased, and death occurred sixteen hours after admission to the hospital. The clinical diagnosis was malabsorption syndrome.

THE ENTITY

Neither steatosis nor focal fibrosis of the liver constitutes cirrhosis. Moreover, focal fibrosis of the portal triads is insufficient for the diagnosis. When the portal connective tissue distorts the lobules, however, then the diagnosis is valid. The connective tissue reaches out from the triads to connect with adjacent triads and, less frequently, with the central veins of the lobules. The process is uniform and monolobular in distribution. When the connective tissue is young and has not yet contracted, the capsule of the liver may be smooth and the texture of the cut surface may be only slightly increased in firmness so that the gross diagnosis may be missed. Later the fibrous bands contract, the serosa becomes finely nodular, and the cut surface is so firm that the thumb cannot be pushed into the liver substance. At this stage the gross diagnosis is obvious, also the perilobular scarring reveals a widespread infiltration with lymphocytes and a conspicuous proliferation of minute bile ductules. Later, some lobules will atrophy and disappear while others will regenerate and enlarge so that the cut surface comes to be grossly distorted by small and large nodules of regenerative hepatocytes.

As this process continues, the flow of portal blood through the liver becomes obstructed. As a consequence, the portal flow reroutes into the coronary veins and thence enters the submucosal esophageal veins in which varices form. The high pressure in the splenic vein is associated with splenic enlargement due partly to chronic passive hyperemia. The peritoneal vessels draining into the portal vein are also affected, and transudation into the peritoneum occurs. Thus ascites, splenomegaly, and esophageal varices are main accompaniments of the later stages of cirrhosis.

Ascites formation is complex and involves low protein production by the injured liver with reduced intravascular osmotic pressure, relative increase in hydrostatic pressure, decreased renal perfusion, and increased levels of circulating antidiuretic hormone. Nevertheless, "weeping" of lymph from the surface of the liver has been observed directly. In an attempt to determine whether this transudation also occurs from the peritoneum of the

EARLY LAENNEC CIRRHOSIS

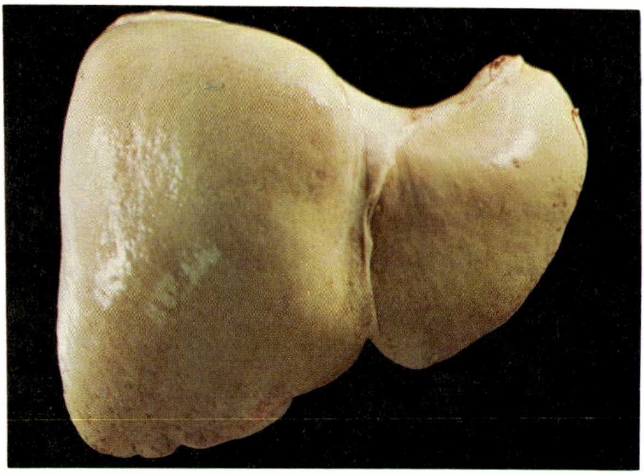

The superior surface of the liver reveals a normal contour, a pale yellow color, and an extremely fine nodularity of the serosal surface.

The gross appearance of the cut surface is not remarkable except for pallor and light yellow discoloration.

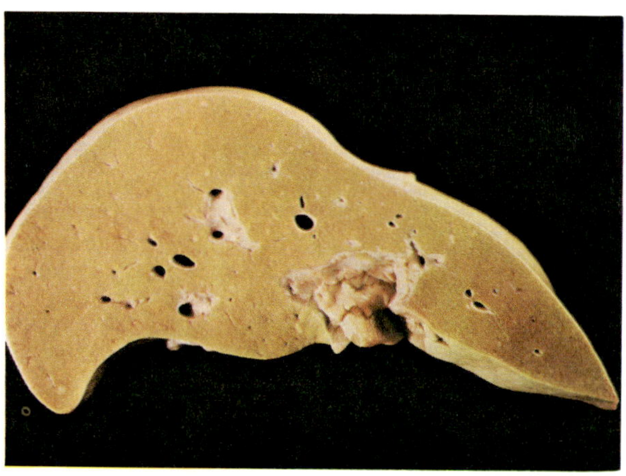

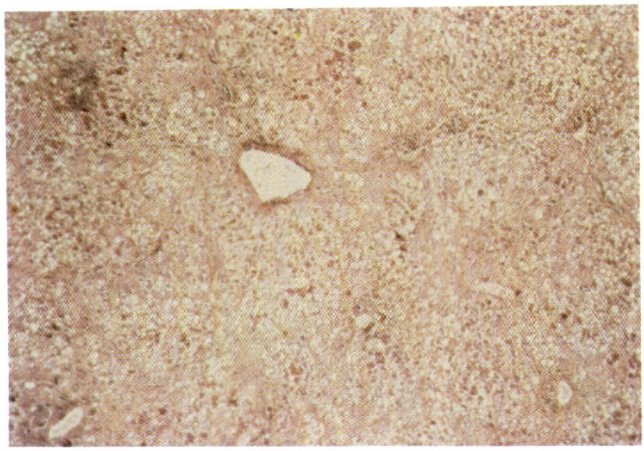

At low power magnification, extensive steatosis of the hepatic cells is evident. Also visible are proliferating bile ductules and irregular bands of fibrous connective tissue.

At higher power in the region of a portal triad, increased connective tissue, parenchymal steatosis, and a light infiltration with lymphocytes may be seen.

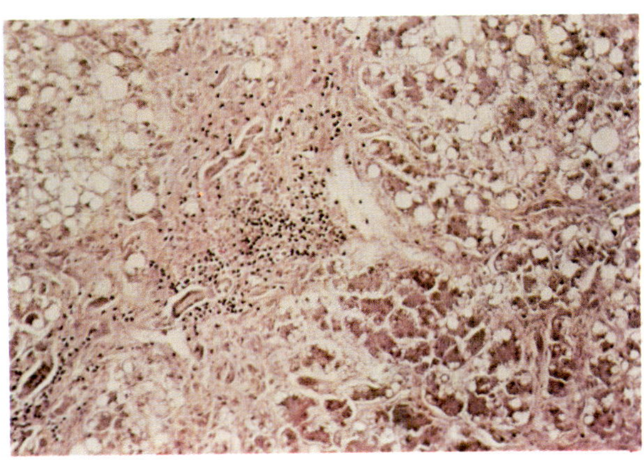

splanchnic bed, radioactive-tagged albumin was injected into the mesoappendiceal veins of rats made cirrhotic by a prolonged choline-deficient diet rich in lipids (1). Collection of fluid by absorption from the peritoneum and the surface of the liver revealed Glisson's capsule to be the more pronounced site of fluid production. Thus lymphatic obstruction in the cirrhotic liver appears to play a prominent role in ascites formation.

1. Gibson, J.D., and Smith, J.C. The origin of ascites in experimental cirrhosis in the rat. Am. J. Path. 41: 535-547, 1962.

LATE LAENNEC CIRRHOSIS

CLINICAL ACCOUNT 5867

The patient was a white male 50 years old who developed ankle edema, ascites, and muscle wasting nine years before the last hospital admission. Biopsy of the liver at that time revealed cirrhosis. Varices of the esophagus were detected by radiographic studies four years after the onset of this illness. One year before admission a cerebrovascular accident caused a right hemiparesis. Four months before the onset of symptoms, the patient was exposed to a hydrocarbon insecticide (malathion); there had been no jaundice or alcoholism prior to that time.

The patient was emaciated. The temperature was 98.6 degrees F., pulse 100, respirations 20, and blood pressure 120/80 mm. Hg. The heart and lungs were normal. Veins were prominently dilated over the lower chest, the abdomen was markedly dilated, and a fluid wave was elicited. The right arm and leg were spastic.

The urine revealed a trace of albumin, an occasional hyaline cast, and a few bacteria. The hemoglobin was 13.8 Gm., the hematocrit was 43 per cent, and the leukocytes numbered 12,000 with a moderate neutrophilia. The total serum bilirubin was 2.4 mg. with 1.2 mg. conjugated. The condition of the patient gradually worsened. He was found unresponsive and died on the eleventh hospital day.

Autopsy examination revealed Laennec cirrhosis of the liver with varices of the esophagus that had ruptured and caused a massive gastro-intestinal hemorrhage. There were also cholelithiasis, hyperemia of the spleen, atrophy of the testes, gynecomastia, and wasting of skeletal muscle. An old infarct was found in the internal capsule of the brain. Additional diagnoses were incidental. The liver weighed 750 Gms.

THE ENTITY

Cirrhosis is a chronic and irreversibly progressive disease of the liver that is characterized by pronounced scarring and slight chronic inflammation of the hepatic tissue. There are three main kinds, i.e., fatty-nutritional, postnecrotic, and biliary. Less common are three other kinds, i.e., pigmentary (hemosiderin), parasitic (schistosomiasis), and syphilitic. While the word cirrhosis embraces all of these, it was originally selected to characterize the color of fatty-nutritional or Laennec cirrhosis; it means "fawn or russet, bordering on the greenish". The hepatic fibrosis due to prolonged heart failure with marked chronic passive hyperemia is not a true cirrhosis.

Nutritional, which is also known as portal or Laennec cirrhosis, usually begins with widespread steatosis of the hepatic cells. This is followed by a fine perilobular fibrosis that uniformly affects all of the lobules. The connective tissue extends outward from the portal triads to join with adjacent triads and also, but less frequently, extends to the central veins. As the lobules become encircled, some undergo degeneration and disappear while others undergo regeneration and enlarge. Eventually an irregular distribution of small and large hepatic nodules, often measuring 4 to 6 cm. in diameter, come to replace the normal cut surface. The interlobular scars become dense but tend to remain even in width, and this feature is helpful in distinguishing advanced Laennec from postnecrotic cirrhosis. The connective tissue bands are lightly infiltrated with lymphocytes and display a proliferation of small bile ductules. As the process advances, the liver becomes small, firm, and coarsely nodular.

LATE LAENNEC CIRRHOSIS

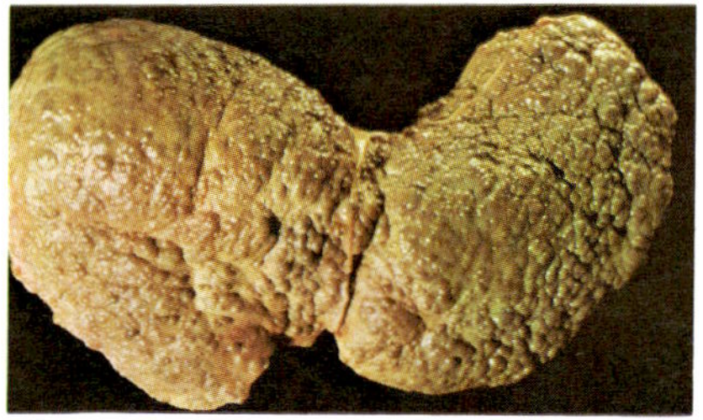

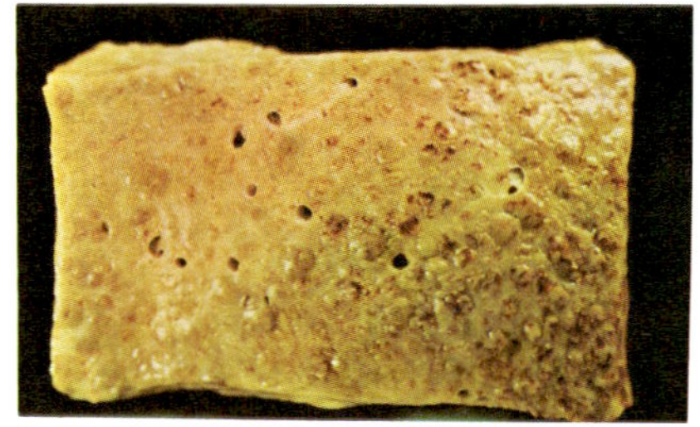

Left: The organ is small and the external surface is glistening and coarsely nodular. The nodularity is approximately uniform. **Right:** A close-up photograph of the cut surface reveals nodules of regeneration composed of hepatocytes that are surrounded by dense bands of pale gray fibrous connective tissue.

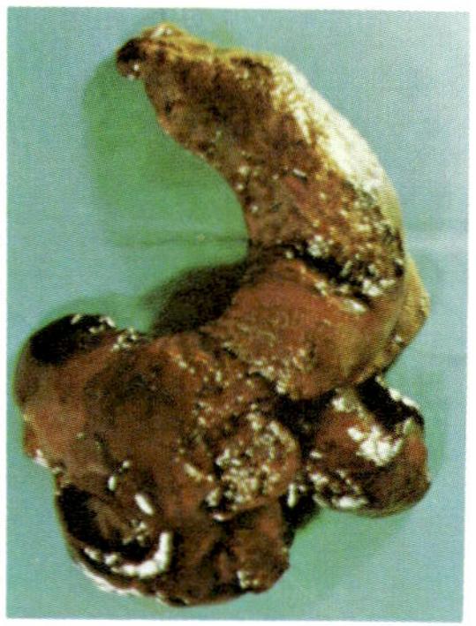

The stomach contains a massive blood clot; it forms a cast of the gastric lumen. It is the consequence of rupture of an esophageal varix which forms in the attempt to convey portal blood around the liver by diverting it to the coronary vein, esophageal veins, azygos veins, and superior vena cava.

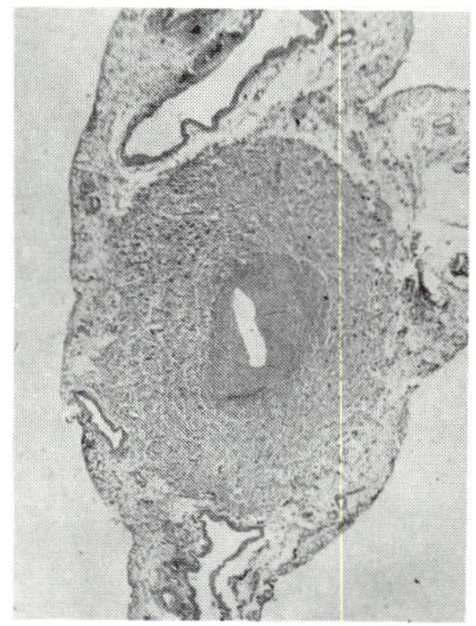

The round ligament of the liver reveals a patent lumen. It too attempts to divert portal blood around the liver by conveyance to the superficial epigastric veins of the abdominal wall and thence to the superior or inferior vena cava. Normally the round ligament is only a potential channel; its patency is another vascular adaptation to the obstructed flow of blood through the liver.

PRIMARY BILIARY CIRRHOSIS

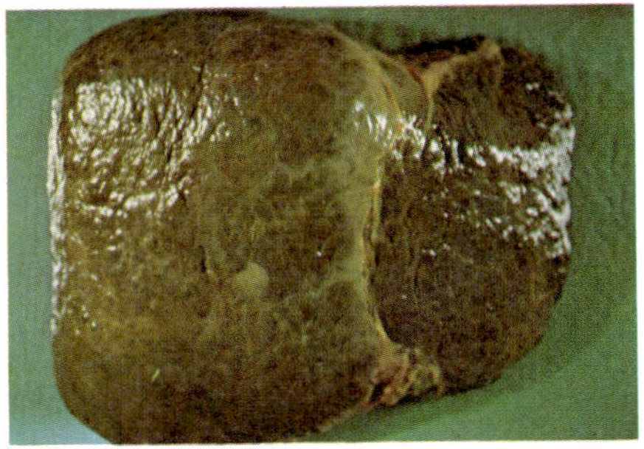

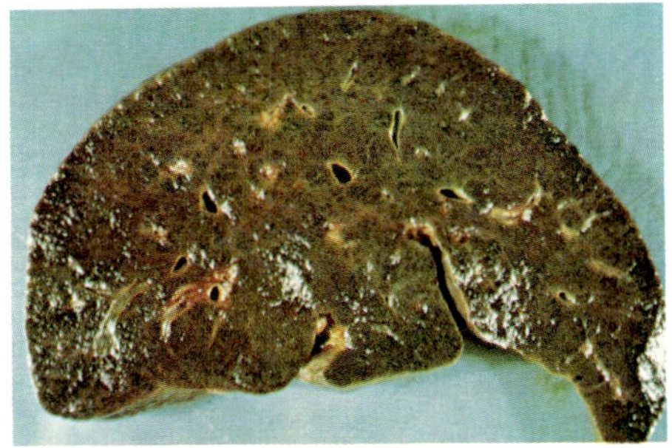

Left: The superior surface of the liver reveals a fine nodularity and a dark green coloration. **Right:** The cut surface also displays a dark green color that is characteristic of biliary cirrhosis.

Left: A close-up shows again the green parenchyma, and an increase of gray fibrous tissue that is tinged with red. **Right:** The histologic section shows connective tissue at the center and periphery of a hepatic lobule. The characteristic pronounced increase of bile ductules is not shown.

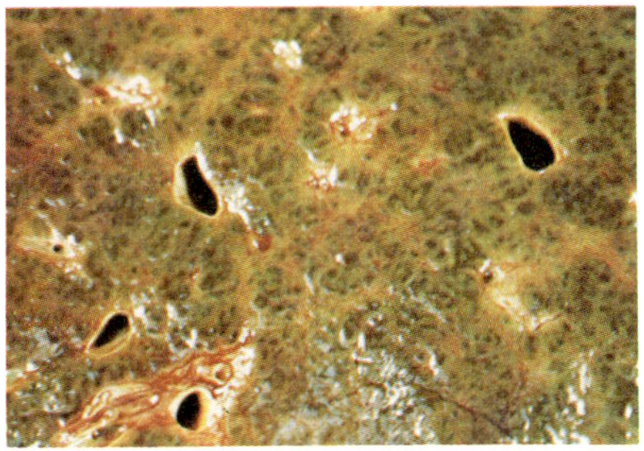

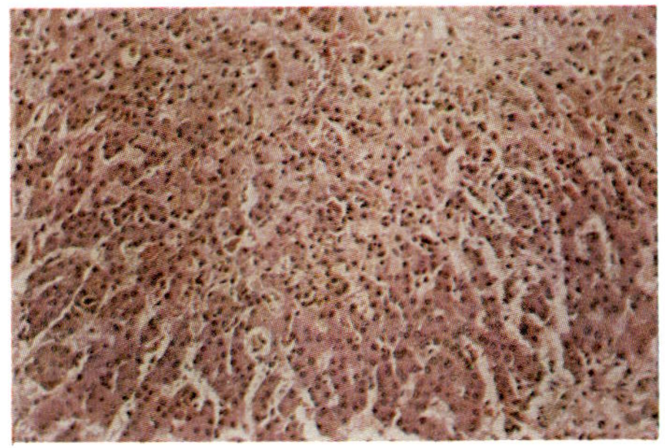

PRIMARY BILIARY CIRRHOSIS

CLINICAL ACCOUNT 7181

The patient was a black female 84 years old who was well until three years before hospital admission. At that time itching of the skin developed. This was soon followed by jaundice, dark urine, and pale stools. There had been no pain, fever, previous jaundice, blood transfusion, exposure to hepatotoxins, or recent anesthesia. A sister was thought to have primary biliary cirrhosis, and her serum revealed a positive mitochondrial antibody test. The patient underwent a cholecystectomy; no calculi were found and no improvement resulted. A liver biopsy was consistent with primary biliary cirrhosis. The patient began to lose weight. At various times over the ensuing months there were anemia, ecchymoses, ascites, periorbital edema, and swelling of the ankles. The jaundice waxed and waned, the itching persisted, and the pale yellow stools became "fluffy" and malodorous and floated.

The patient was obese and icterus was pronounced. The vital signs were normal. The abdomen was soft and protuberant, and slight shifting dullness was elicited. The spleen and liver were enlarged and the ankles were swollen.

The urine was normal except for bile. The hemoglobin was 10.5 Gms., the hematocrit was 32 per cent, and the leukocytes were normal in number and kind. The blood cholesterol ranged from 280 to 380 mgs., and the serum triglycerides were 284 mgs. (normal 10-160). The alkaline phosphatase was 316 mU., and the serum lactic dehydrogenase and glutamic transaminase were moderately elevated. A test for mitochondrial antibody was negative.

Swelling of the abdomen increased. The patient became progressively obtunded and died after twenty-six days in the hospital. The principal autopsy findings were primary biliary cirrhosis, bile nephrosis, and 1000 ml. of ascites.

THE ENTITY

Bile duct obstruction causes biliary cirrhosis which occurs in two forms. The primary form is uncommon, the obstruction is in the finest biliary radicals, and the condition is often associated with hyperlipidemia. The secondary form is common and is due to obstruction of the extrahepatic bile ducts by calculi, stenosing scars, or obstructive tumors. In infancy it may be due to congenital atresia of the biliary tract.

Primary biliary cirrhosis (Hanot's) occurs especially in dark-complected middle-aged women who first complain of prolonged pruritus. Thereafter, icterus gradually develops, the urine darkens, and the stools become light in color. The skin reveals lipid deposits in the eyelids (xanthelasma) and over the knees and elbows (xanthomas). The serum bilirubin is raised, the alkaline phosphatase is elevated, and the blood lipids are extremely high (circa 1000 mg./100 ml.). The serum albumin tends to be low, and the serum globulin is moderately raised. Antibody to a mitochondrial antigen is characteristic and aids in the distinction from secondary biliary cirrhosis. Steatorrhea and osteoporosis may develop as fats fail to be emulsified and fat-soluble vitamins (D) are not absorbed. Ascending cholangitis and pulmonary infection may be terminal events.

The liver is normal in size, dark green in color, and diffusely scarred in a monolobular pattern. Plasma cells, lipid-laden macrophages, and bile duct proliferation are conspicuous in the periportal scars. Granulomas resembling those of sarcoidosis may be present. Florid atherosclerosis affects the aorta and large arteries. While the cause is unknown, the obstruction appears to be in the smallest biliary ductules, and the condition may be autoimmune in nature.

POSTNECROTIC CIRRHOSIS

CLINICAL ACCOUNT 6262

The patient was a white male 63 years old who smoked heavily and drank alcohol excessively over a long period of time. He was known to have cirrhosis and on one occasion experienced bleeding from the upper gastro-intestinal tract. At that time, however, x-rays of the esophagus and stomach were normal. He had also experienced one bout of pneumonia. The present admission was for treatment of a fracture of the left hip suffered when the patient fell.

The vital signs were normal. Physical examination revealed "liver palms" and spider angiomas. The liver margin was palpated six fingerbreadths below the right costal margin. Except for the left hip, the remainder of the examination was essentially unremarkable.

The blood and urine were normal. The hip was pinned and recovery was uneventful. Over the following eight months anorexia, weight loss, and confusion developed. Radiographic examination revealed a mass in the mediastinum and widespread metastatic disease of bone. His condition gradually worsened, and death occurred approximately eight months after his hip fracture.

Autopsy examination disclosed a carcinoma of the right adrenal cortex with widespread metastases. Additional diagnoses included acute ulcers of the duodenum, postnecrotic cirrhosis of the liver, metastatic carcinoma of the jejunum, atrophy of the testes, passive hyperemia of the spleen, and bronchopneumonia of the upper lobe of the left lung.

THE ENTITY

Postnecrotic cirrhosis is characterized by broad flat scars, presumably due to a preceding massive necrosis, that irregularly distort the liver contour. The necrosis is presumed to be due to a fulminant viral hepatitis or to a toxin such as cinchophen, arsphenamine, or trinitrotoluene. The pronounced, coarse, irregular distortion of the hepatic contour differs altogether from the fine uniform nodularity of Laennec or biliary cirrhosis. The hepatic tissue between the broad flat scars undergoes compensatory regeneration to form small or large nodules. On section the broad scars are firm and pale gray while the intervening tissue is normal in color or mottled with green from biliary obstruction or focally red from recent hemorrhage. In the scars there are lymphocytes and plasma cells in moderate numbers; bile duct proliferation is moderate as well.

The condition occurs in adults of both sexes. It may develop after an episode of hepatitis as evidenced by fever, jaundice, vomiting, and epigastric pain; more often, it develops without a preceding illness, and occasionally it is an incidental autopsy finding. The clinical manifestations are those of nonspecific cirrhosis; the liver is usually small and the coarse scars are occasionally palpable through the abdominal wall. Portal obstruction and ascites are less frequent than with finely nodular cirrhosis. Liver cell carcinoma, however, is more frequent. The course tends to be progressive once major clinical findings appear, and death is usually due to liver failure or intercurrent infection.

POSTNECROTIC CIRRHOSIS

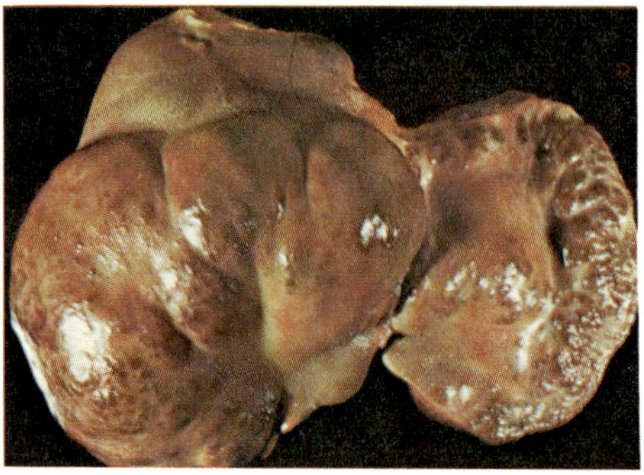

The superior surface of the liver reveals large flat irregular scars that grossly disfigure the normal contour of the organ.

The cut surface displays massive pale gray fibrous scars that extend irregularly throughout the hepatic parenchyma.

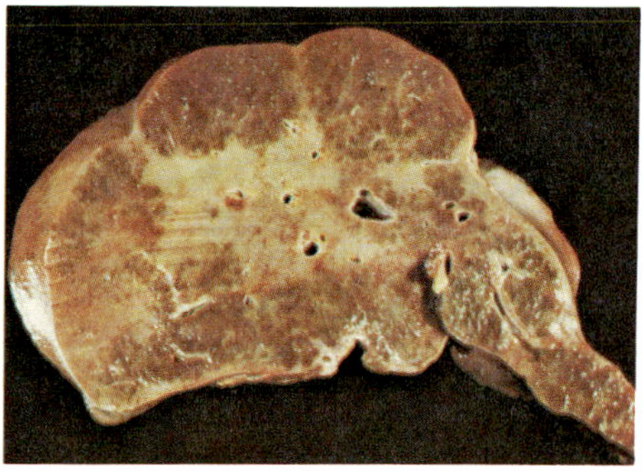

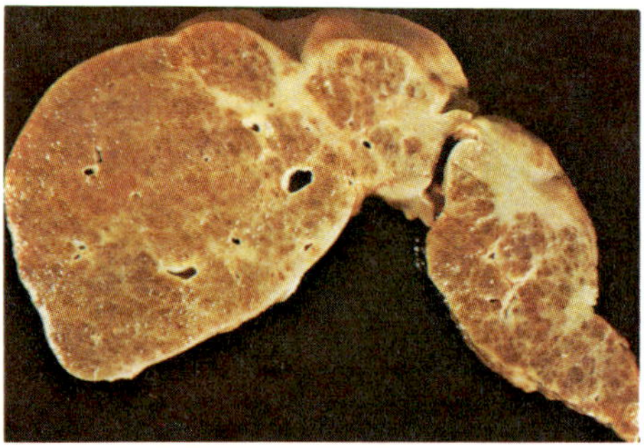

A second cut surface reveals the size, extent, and irregularity of the massive pale gray scars.

A histologic section discloses the dense fibrous connective tissue composing the gray scars in which bile duct proliferation and a small number of lymphocytes are evident.

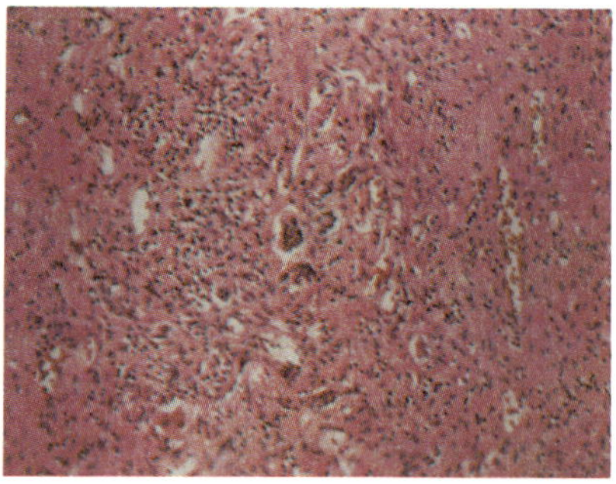

HEPATOCELLULAR CARCINOMA

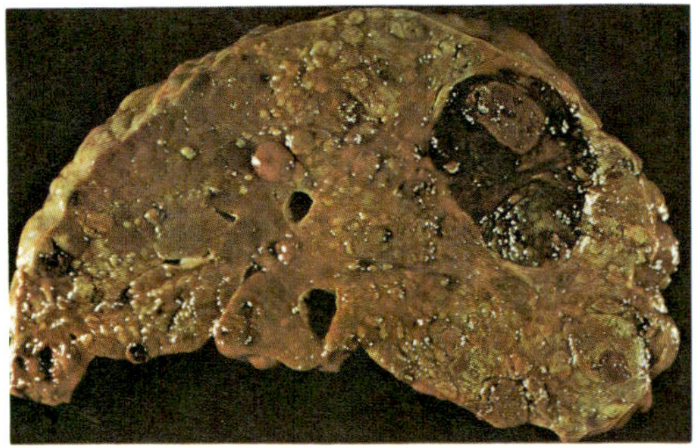

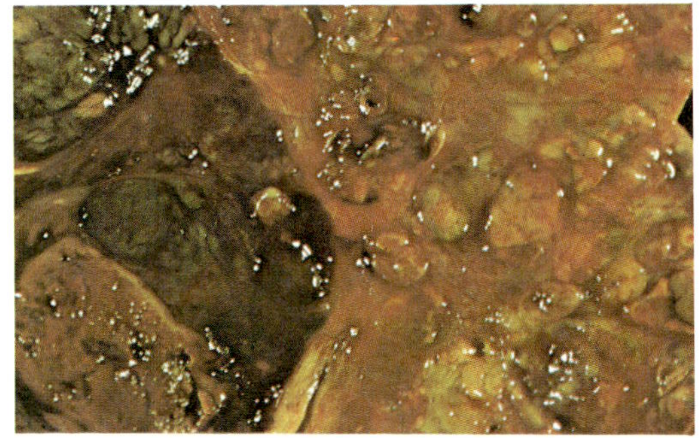

Left: The cut surface of the liver reveals the coarse nodules of advanced cirrhosis and a discrete oval focus in which bile stasis is especially pronounced. **Right:** A closer view discloses the large regenerative liver nodules, the focal intense bile staining, and the coarse bands of dense fibrous tissue.

Left: A still closer view reveals the same features again; nowhere is it possible to be certain of malignant tumor. **Right:** The microsection presents necrotic hepatic parenchyma on the left, viable liver tissue on the right, and solid masses of epithelial tumor cells in the upper middle. The tumor is an undifferentiated carcinoma arising from hepatocytes.

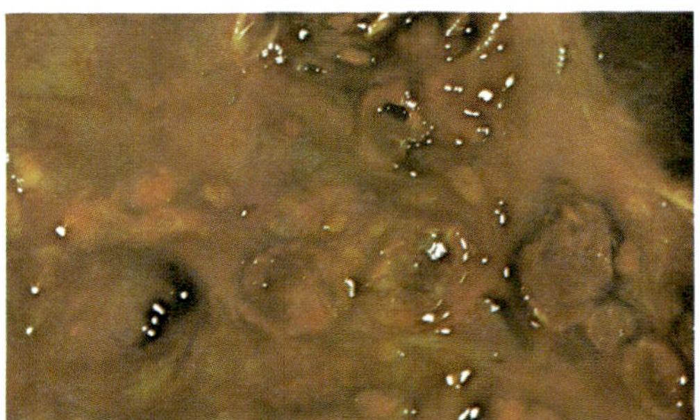

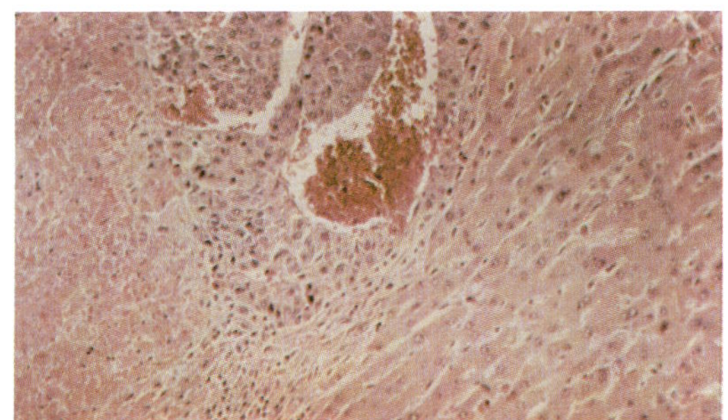

HEPATOCELLULAR CARCINOMA

CLINICAL ACCOUNT 448

The patient was a black male 35 years old who was well until four months before hospital admission. At that time he developed pain in the right hypochondrium and swelling of the abdomen. Anorexia and productive cough developed two months later. One month before admission yellow discoloration of the sclerae was first noted. Physical examination revealed jaundice, emaciation, ascites, and a nodular liver. Cytotoxic drugs were given, the patient's condition worsened, and death occurred suddenly on the tenth hospital day.

Autopsy examination revealed macronodular cirrhosis, hepatocellular carcinoma, tumor thrombus of the portal vein, ascites (2,000 ml.) and pulmonary metastases.

THE ENTITY

Carcinoma of the liver is the commonest malignant tumor in several parts of sub-Saharan Africa (1). Most are hepatocellular carcinomas, and 50 to 70 per cent arise in livers that are cirrhotic. They grow rapidly and cause large palpable masses. The cancer may consist of a single massive nodule, and it may also be multinodular and widespread, especially if cirrhosis is present. Extension of the tumor into the portal vein and to the lymph nodes of the porta hepatis is common. Death is usually due to cachexia.

The tumor occurs twice as often in males as females; most patients are between 25 and 45 years of age, and the principal complaints are pain in the right hypochondrium associated with anorexia and loss of weight. Ascites occurs in one half of the cases. Fever, progressive jaundice, and hepatic coma are uncommon. The tumor is rapidly progressive, and death usually occurs within a few weeks of the time of diagnosis. About 60 per cent of tumors produce an alpha globulin that is normally secreted only in fetal life by the liver and yolk sac. The test for this protein (alpha-fetoglobulin) is almost specific and is positive in 60 to 70 per cent of cases.

Of the cirrhotic livers harboring carcinomas, most are intermediate (posthepatitic) or macronodular in type. Etiologic possibilities of the cirrhosis, and perhaps of the carcinomas, include malnutrition, parasitic infestation, viral disease, alcoholism, and toxic substances. Malnutrition, although common in infants, is reversible; when it occurs in adults, it leads to atrophy rather than to fatty metamorphosis as a precirrhotic condition. Schistosomiasis causes "pipe stem" fibrosis but not regenerative nodules or diffuse destruction of the hepatic tissue. Although viral hepatitis may progress to cirrhosis, this is not likely common. Nevertheless, 40 per cent of Ugandans with liver cell carcinoma have a positive hepatitis-associated antigen (H.A.A.) test (2). Clinical information does not indicate that alcoholism is a major cause of cirrhosis in Africans (1). Plant toxins may damage the liver (senecid and crotaria), plant toxins abound in Africa, and aflatoxin produced by *Aspergillus flavus* causes liver cell carcinoma in experimental animals. Moreover, aflatoxin is present in Ugandan foodstuffs. Thus, while the cause of cirrhosis and liver cell carcinoma in Africa remains unknown, the possibilities favor viral inflammation and mycotoxins.

1. Shaper, A.G., Kibukamusoke, J.W., and Hutt, M.S.R., Editors. Medicine in a Tropical Environment, British Medical Association, London, 1972.
2. Vogel, C.L., Mody, N., Anthony, P.P., and Baker, L.F. Hepatitis associated antigen in Ugandan patients with hepatocellular carcinoma. Lancet 2:621-624, 1970.

PYOGENIC ABSCESS OF LIVER

CLINICAL ACCOUNT 6898

The patient was a white male 24 years old who was well until one year before hospital admission. At that time a routine physical examination revealed hepatomegaly. This persisted and his present admission was for investigation of this finding. Past history revealed that the patient had developed ulcerative colitis at age 17 and had been treated since then with adrenocortical steroids. He had also had Raynaud's disease for several months preceding hospitalization.

The temperature was 37.0 degrees C., pulse 120, respirations 18, and blood pressure 160/110 mm. Hg. The thyroid was diffusely enlarged. Physical examination was not remarkable except for hepatomegaly, a small amount of ascites, and blue discoloration of the finger tips.

The urine was normal. The blood revealed a hemoglobin of 14.9 Gm., and a leukocyte count of 10,100 with a differential count that included 18 per cent eosinophils, and 12 per cent atypical lymphocytes. A liver scan showed focal decreased concentration in the right lobe. A T-3 test was consistent with hyperthyroidism. Biopsy of the liver revealed cirrhosis. Sigmoidoscopy disclosed relatively inactive ulcerative colitis. A total colectomy was performed. In the second postoperative week spiking fever developed and blood culture revealed bacteroides organisms. Septic shock developed. Laparotomy revealed pus in the peritoneum, for which drainage was instituted. The patient died five days after the laparotomy.

Autopsy examination revealed abscesses of the liver, acute fibrinopurulent peritonitis, micronodular cirrhosis, widespread organizing arterial thrombi, bilateral hemorrhagic bronchopneumonia, and candidiasis of the heart, lungs, kidneys, stomach and small intestine. Cultures of the hepatic abscesses disclosed bacteroides. The thyroid weighed 28 Gms. and revealed hyperplasia on microscopic examination.

THE ENTITY

Hepatic abscesses are often due to biliary obstruction with ascending cholangitis. As the inflammation ascends, exudate escapes from the small biliary channels into the hepatic parenchyma. Abscesses formed in this way are almost always multiple, small, and widely spread (1). The obstructing conditions include cholecystitis, stone in the bile ducts, post-inflammatory fibrosis, and carcinoma of the head of the pancreas. Multiple abscesses may also be due to bacteremia from pyelonephritis, bacterial endocarditis, or suppurative disease of the lungs.

Single abscesses of the liver are almost always associated with abdominal infection and acute pylephlebitis. The infections include appendicitis, diverticulitis, ulcerative colitis, and such surgical manipulations as plication of a gastric or duodenal ulcer. Single abscesses are usually in the right lobe, the size is variable, and the margins are shaggy, friable, and greenish or yellowish gray. When close to the surface, perforation may cause subhepatic or subphrenic extension. While many abscesses are sterile, the organisms usually recovered are *E. coli,* staphylococci, streptococci, or some combination of these.

Clinical features include a septic febrile course with shaking chills, drenching sweats, and a dull aching pain over the liver, which is often enlarged and occasionally tender. There may also be nausea, vomiting, lethargy, and subclinical jaundice. Leukocytosis with neutrophilia is constant. A liver scan is the most useful diagnostic procedure. The diagnosis is often missed and the mortality is high. Multiple abscesses are treated with antibiotics and relief of the biliary obstruction. Single abscesses must be surgically drained or they terminate fatally (1).

1. Pyrtek, L.J., and Bartus, S.A. Hepatic pyemia. New Eng. J. Med. 272:551-554, 1965.

PYOGENIC ABSCESS OF LIVER

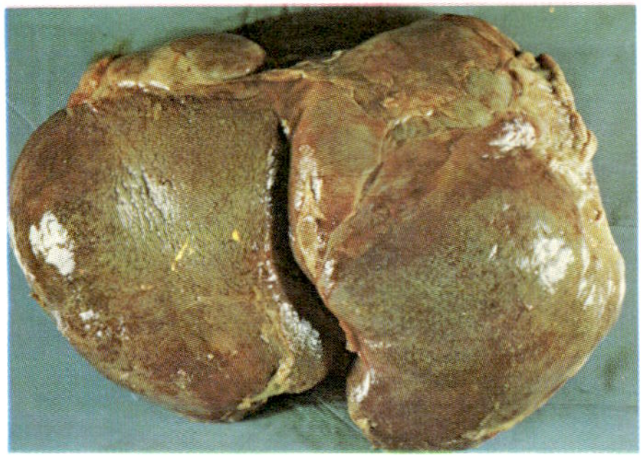

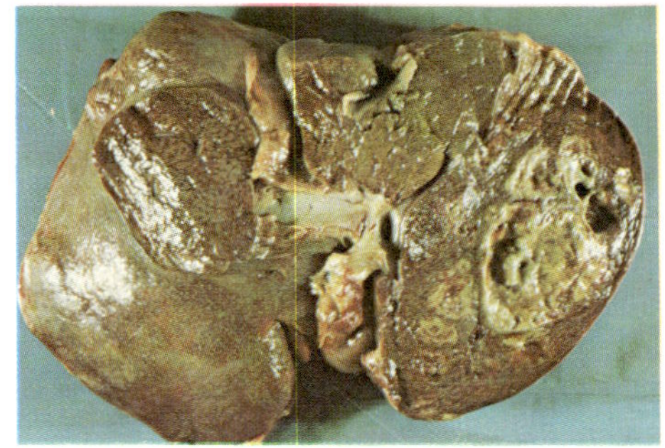

Left: Portions of the hepatic surface are finely wrinkled and elsewhere focally discolored dark brownish red. **Right:** Section of the undersurface reveals a large multiloculated abscess in the right lobe.

Left: A close-up view discloses the shaggy friable greenish gray lining margin that is altogether different from the reddish brown surface of the amebic abscess. **Right:** A low power microsection reveals the abscess cavity on the right, viable liver on the left, and necrotic hepatic tissue with massive exudate in the center.

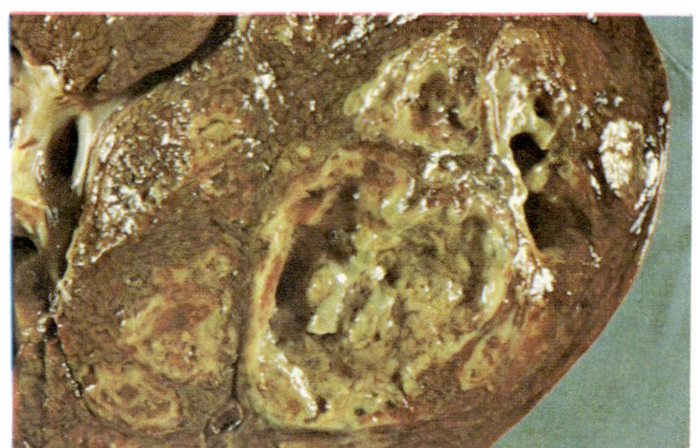

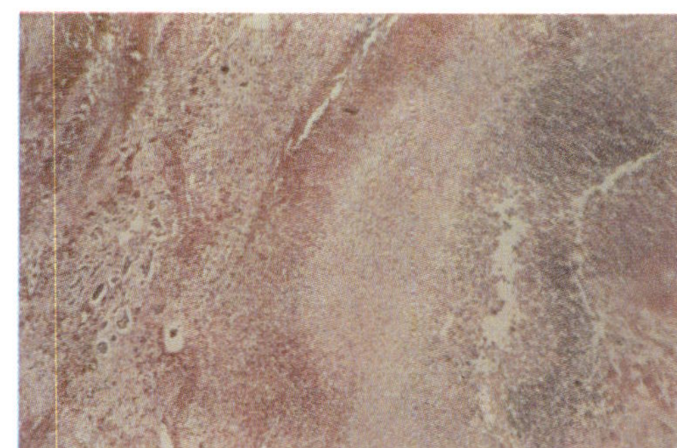

AMEBIC ABSCESS OF LIVER

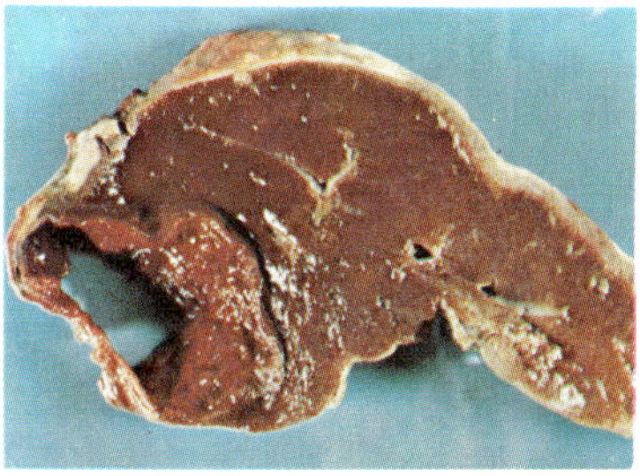

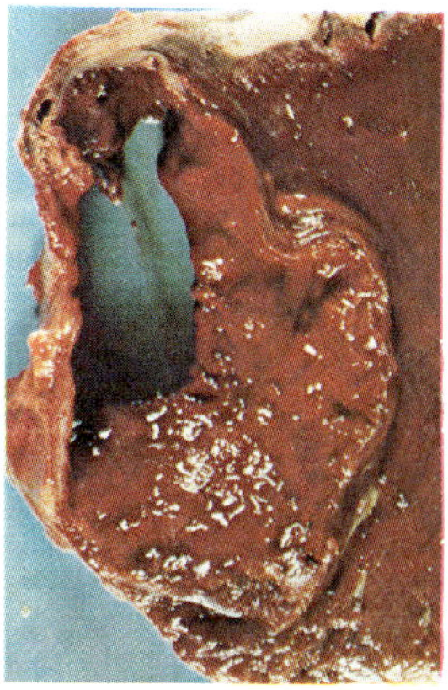

Left: The hepatic cut surface reveals a large cavity of the right lobe. The pale gray margin on the upper surface of the liver is due to partial fixation of the tissue in formalin. **Right:** A close-up of the cavity discloses the paste-like composition and brownish red coloration of the shaggy material lining the cavity. This material has been likened to anchovy paste, and it is characteristic of amebic "abscesses."

Left: Section discloses the amorphous debris lining the cavity and the dense underlying connective tissue margin. It is useful to observe that leukocytes are not present in this lesion. **Right:** At higher power a trophozoite may be made out in the lining debris. Hemosiderin, free and within macrophages, gives the brown tinge to the gross color of the lesion.

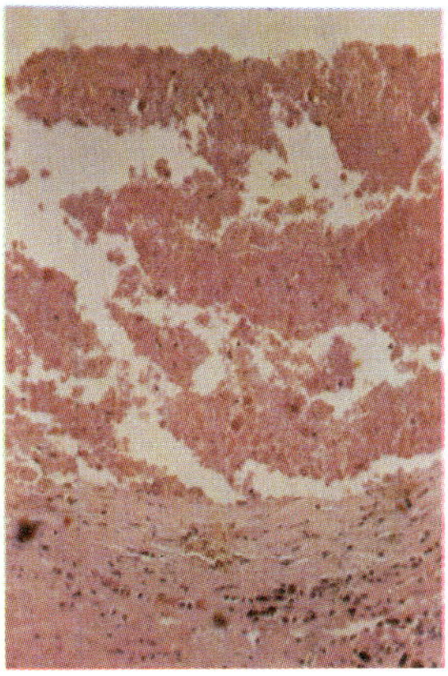

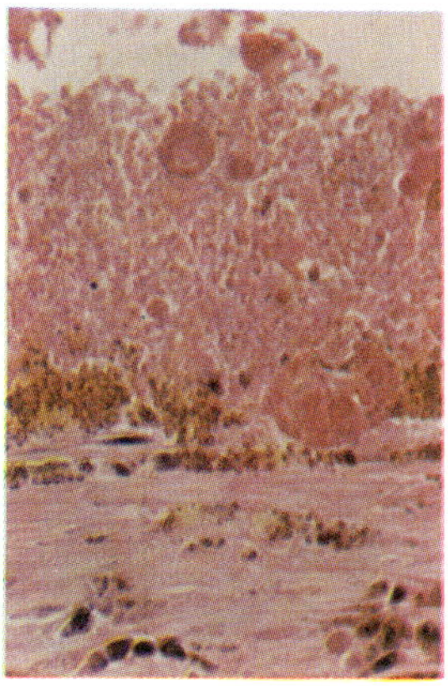

AMEBIC ABSCESS OF LIVER

CLINICAL ACCOUNT 7314

The patient was a black female 69 years old who was admitted to the hospital because of constipation and distension of the abdomen. Eleven months previously a carcinoma of the ovary had been treated by total abdominal hysterectomy and bilateral salpingo-oophorectomy. Six months before admission x-radiation of the pelvis was given for recurrence of the tumor. Thereafter a clear vaginal discharge was noted, and about one month before coming to the hospital the discharge turned brown in color and had a fecal odor. Constipation began two weeks before hospitalization, and abdominal distension had been noted for the four days prior to admission.

The temperature was 37.1 degrees C., pulse 130, respirations 18, and blood pressure 112/70 mm. Hg. Physical examination revealed distension of the abdomen, induration of the pelvic tissues, and a rectovaginal fistula.

The urine disclosed bacteria and leukocytes. The hemoglobin was 8.8 Gms., hematocrit 27.5 per cent, and the leukocytes numbered 7,000 per cmm. with a normal differential count. An x-ray of the abdomen revealed distended loops of ileum with air-fluid levels. Therapy with a Cantor tube failed to relieve the obstruction. A perirectal abscess formed. The patient refused a colostomy. She died after forty-two days in the hospital.

Autopsy examination revealed metastatic carcinoma of the peritoneum, fibrous adhesions of the peritoneum with stenosis and obstruction of the ileum and colon, a right subphrenic abscess, and a rectovaginal fistula. There was also an amebic abscess of the liver.

THE ENTITY

Endameba histolytica resides in the intestines of asymptomatic carriers who are occasionally food handlers. The organisms pass from the gut as cysts which are hardy, and infestation takes place by ingestion of the cysts through careless habits of hygiene. The capsules of the cysts resist the acid of the stomach, excystation takes place in the ileum, and four trophozoites emerge. The organisms pass into the colon, secrete a proteolytic enzyme, and burrow into the mucosa to form small shallow ragged ulcers that are associated with dysentery which tends to be chronic.

The burrowing also carries the trophozoites into the venules of the portal system in which they are moved to the liver, where abscesses are prone to develop. The abscesses are usually single, most often in the right lobe, and frequently measure 15 to 20 cm. in diameter. The lining surfaces are composed of shaggy necrotic debris that is chocolate brown in color and resembles anchovy paste. The cavity is usually sterile, leukocytes are not present in the wall, and the lesion is not technically an abscess. The "abscess" may become quiescent but has a tendency to perforate the right hemidiaphragm to form a hepatobronchial fistula.

The lesion occurs more often in men than women and develops almost exclusively in adults (1). The clinical features are pain and tenderness in the right upper quadrant of the abdomen associated with respiratory disturbance at the base of right lung. Fever, anemia, and leukocytosis are common. Stool examination for trophozoites is usually negative. Fluoroscopy reveals a fixed elevated right hemidiaphragm, and hepato-scanning discloses the size and position of the cavity. Aspiration yields a chocolate brown paste in which neither bacteria nor trophozoites are often found. Anti-amebic therapy frequently provides prompt and dramatic relief so that surgical intervention is seldom required.

1. Turrill, F.L., and Burnham, J.R. Hepatic amebiasis. Am. J. Surg. 111:424-430, 1966.

METASTATIC CARCINOMA OF LIVER

CLINICAL ACCOUNT 5940

The patient was a Negro male 45 years old who entered the hospital because of increasing shortness of breath. For the past six years he had had dyspnea on exertion, nocturnal paroxysms of dyspnea, and slight pain in the chest. The pain was especially prominent over the right hemithorax. The patient was a chronic alcoholic and had been hypertensive for the past twenty-three years.

The blood pressure was 140/110 mm. Hg. The conjunctivae were flushed and the buccal membranes were cyanotic. The right optic disc was blurred. The subcutaneous tissues of the face and neck were full and thick. The neck veins were distended and firm. A venous pattern over the chest was not described. The abdomen was distended, and the remainder of the examination was not remarkable. An x-ray of the chest disclosed an enlarged right hilar shadow. Biopsy of a bronchus and a right supraclavicular lymph node revealed undifferentiated carcinoma at both sites. The patient died after two weeks in the hospital.

Autopsy examination revealed an undifferentiated carcinoma of the right main bronchus that extended into the superior vena cava and caused stenosis of that vessel with production of the superior caval syndrome. The cancer metastasized widely. There were also hypertrophy of the heart, bronchopneumonia of both lungs, and bronchiectasis of the right lung. The liver weighed 2810 Gm.

THE ENTITY

The liver is the most frequent site of metastatic growths (1). These originate especially in organs drained by the portal vein, i.e., the colon, pancreas, stomach, and esophagus. Extraportal sites include the lung, breast, prostate, and uterus. The mechanisms are embolization of the portal vein or hepatic artery, and retrograde lymphatic flow from tumor in lymph nodes at the porta hepatis. The metastases may be single or multiple, small or large, localized or diffuse, and soft or hard. No gross pattern suggests a specific site, and "streamlining" of portal flow so that cancers from the left side of the abdomen spread to the left lobe of the liver, and vice versa, is discounted (2). Melanoblastomas produce black metastases; chorioepitheliomas produce metastases that are soft, succulent, dark red, and hemorrhagic. The metastases tend to grow outward in all directions so that most are spherical in shape. Necrosis allows the centers to collapse; for this reason surface lesions tend to become umbilicated. Massive diffuse intrasinusoidal involvement occurs especially with melanoblastomas, and occasionally with carcinomas of the breast, lung, or stomach (3). Tumor cells invade the hepatic venous outflow tract and embolize the lungs; this spread also occurs by lymphatic flow and embolization of the thoracic duct.

Extremely widespread involvement may occur without functional loss that is detectable. Tumor obstruction of the portal vein, however, especially when associated with low serum proteins, may cause ascites, and tumor obstruction of the bile ducts may cause jaundice. The serum alkaline phosphatase tends to be elevated when bile flow is obstructed.

1. Willis, R.A. The Spread of Tumors in the Human Body. Butterworth & Co., London, 1952.
2. Cole, J.W., Krohmer, J., Bonte, F.J., and Schatten, W. An experimental study of intrahepatic distribution of portal blood. Surg., Obstet., & Gynec. 102:43, 1956.
3. Smith, J.C. Diffuse intrasinusoidal metastatic cancer of the liver. Ann. Int. Med. 54:104, 1961.

METASTATIC CARCINOMA OF LIVER

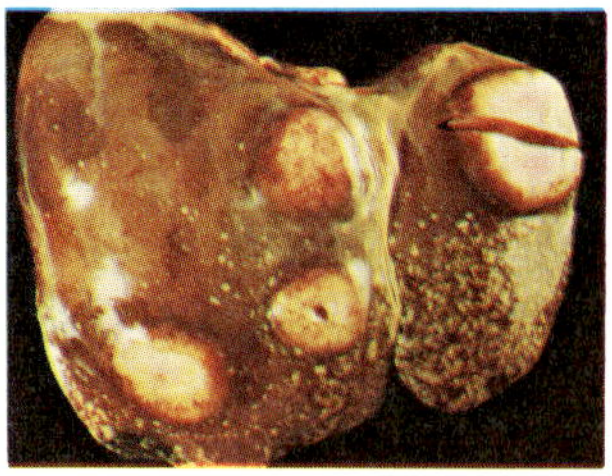

The serosal surface reveals small and large nodules of metastatic disease. In large nodules, necrosis causes the central portions to shrink. When large nodules are present on the serosa, the central shrinkage, or umbilication, may be seen grossly or occasionally felt clinically. Umbilication thus indicates secondary rather than primary tumor.

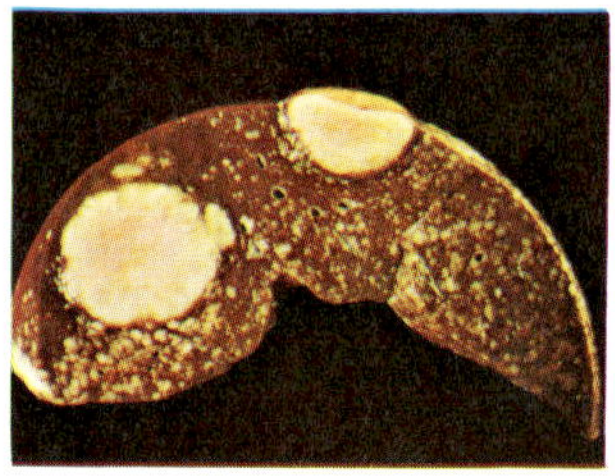

The metastatic nodules are evident on the cut surface. The serosal aspect of the larger nodule reveals umbilication. Metastatic disease in liver is often silent; blockage of bile ducts, however, causes an elevation of serum alkaline phosphatase and this may be followed by jaundice.

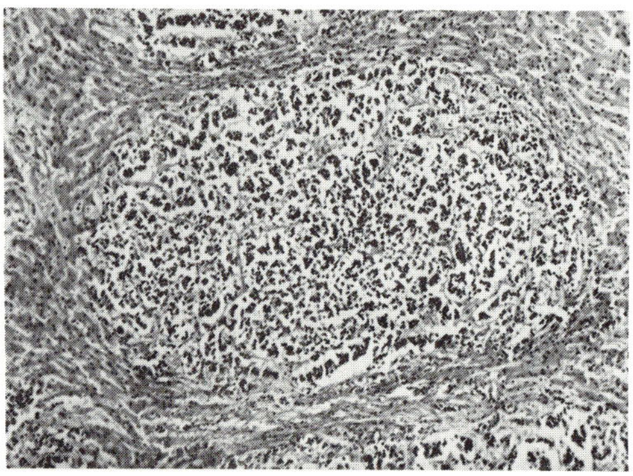

The unmagnified section shows the distribution of metastatic tumor. For such a lesion to develop, it is necessary for tumor cell emboli to come to rest in a sinusoid, attach to an endothelial cell surface, find a favorable growth environment, and invade the tissue.

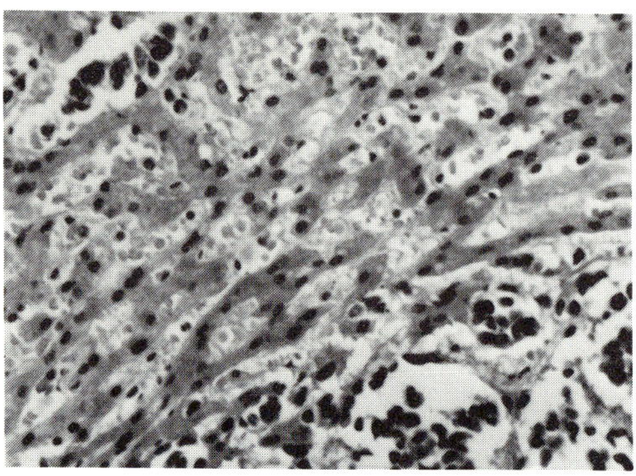

The magnified section reveals metastatic tumor growing in hepatic tissue. It is likely that the tumor destroys the hepatic cells in this process.

AORTICO-DUODENAL FISTULA

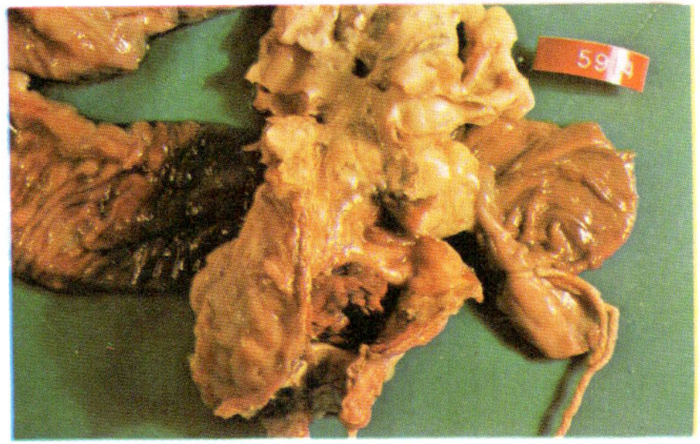

Viewed from the duodenal surface, the opening of the fistula is visible.

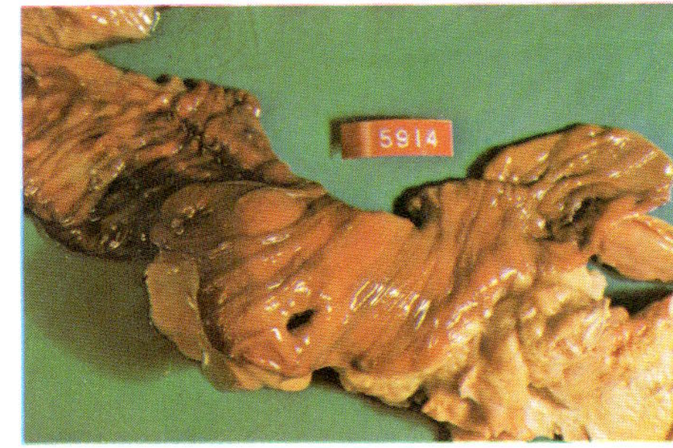

Above: The aorta is opened from the posterior aspect so that the duodenum lies anterior to it. Atherosclerosis is evident in the aortic wall. The orifice of the aneurysm, partially occluded by mural thrombus, can be seen.

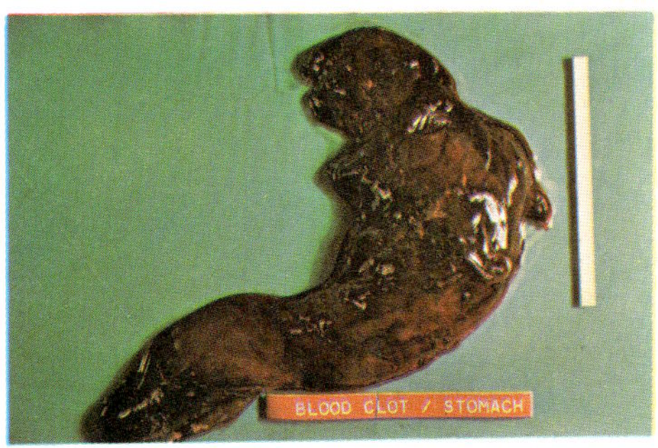

The blood clot produced by this massive hemorrhage filled the stomach and formed a cast of that chamber.

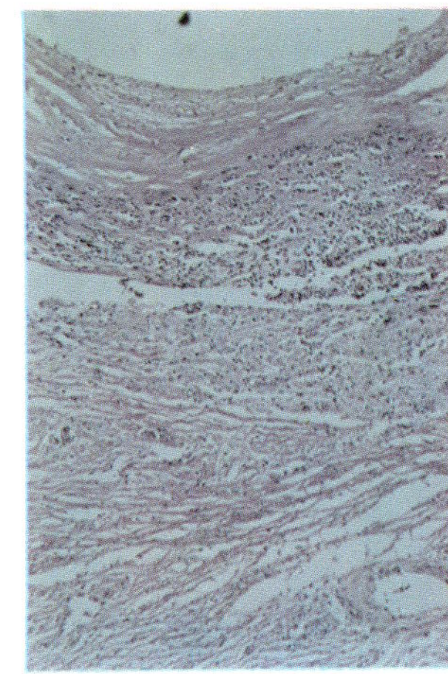

A microsection of the aortic wall at the site of rupture reveals a fragile structure with layers of fibrin and an infiltration with neutrophilic leukocytes.

AORTICO-DUODENAL FISTULA

CLINICAL ACCOUNT 5914

The patient was a white male 66 years old who vomited bright red blood and passed a black tarry stool on the day of admission to the hospital. This happened while he was defecating on the morning of that day. He noticed that his skin was cool and moist. He returned to bed and vomited about one pint of bright red blood in which clots were seen. In the afternoon a second bowel movement produced another tarry stool. He sought medical attention and was advised to enter the hospital. He had had no previous gastro-intestinal complaints.

The temperature was 98.6 degrees F., pulse 90, respirations 24, and blood pressure 130/74 mm. Hg. The heart and lungs were not remarkable. The abdomen was soft, nontender, and slightly protuberant. A pulsatile mass was present in the epigastrium. Bowel sounds were high-pitched in the right upper quadrant but normal elsewhere. Rectal examination was negative; the stool was guaiac positive.

The hemoglobin was 11.6 Gm., hematocrit 34, and leukocytes 7,000 with a normal differential count. On the day after admission he felt well and passed a black tarry stool. On the next day an x-ray study of the stomach was undertaken; the patient suddenly vomited 500 ml. of bright red blood, and the study was discontinued. A transfusion was given. On the third day he felt well although hematologic examination revealed a hemoglobin of 9.9 Gm. and a hematocrit of 29 per cent. On the fourth day the patient died quietly.

Autopsy examination revealed a saccular aneurysm of the abdominal aorta, a perforation of the aneurysm into the duodenum, and a massive recent intestinal hemorrhage that extended into the stomach and formed a cast of it. The aorto-enteric fistula contained a large recent thrombus. Additional diagnoses included hypertrophy of the heart (550 Gm.), arteriolar nephrosclerosis, and a cortical adenoma of the left adrenal.

THE ENTITY

Aneurysms of the aorta are most common in the abdominal portion. They are usually saccular and are almost always located below the renal arteries. They are attributed to arteriosclerosis. When less than 5 cm. in diameter, they are usually asymptomatic. Over 7.5 cm., pain is often produced, a pulsatile mass is usually felt, and rupture is likely. The clinical diagnosis is aided by lateral x-ray films of the abdomen which show curved lines of calcium that denote the aneurysmal wall. No medical treatment is effective. Resection is nearly always possible; the operative mortality ranges from three to ten per cent (1).

Rupture occurs especially at four sites; the retroperitoneum, the peritoneal cavity, the inferior vena cava, and the gut, in this order. In the gut, the most common site is the duodenum. Of 91 aorta-enteric fistulas, the sites of rupture were esophagus 11, stomach 8, duodenum 63, jejunum 5, ileum 3, and colon 1 (2). The conspicuous clinical manifestation is sudden, and often massive, hematemesis.

1. Darling, R.C. Peripheral artery surgery. New Eng. J. Med. 280:141, 1969.
2. Foster, J.H., and Vetto, R.M. Aortic intra-aneurysmal abscess caused by sigmoid-aortic fistula. Am. J. Surg. 104:850, 1962.

MECKEL'S DIVERTICULUM OF ILEUM

CLINICAL ACCOUNT 7348

The patient was a white male 61 years old who was well until eight months before entering the hospital. At that time he noted weakness of his right hand. Over subsequent weeks this spread to his entire right side and was accompanied by a regression of mentation. Six months before admission biopsy revealed a glioblastoma multiforme of his right cerebral hemisphere. Focal radiation therapy was given and the patient improved. Two months before admission, weakness recurred and was accompanied by dizziness and headache.

The vital signs were normal. Physical examination was not remarkable except for neurologic function, i.e., the right side was weak, the Romberg test was positive, and the deep tendon reflexes on the right were increased. In addition, the patient forgot words, could not write, could not subtract, and could not hold a train of thought. Cranial nerve and sensory function were physiologic.

The blood and urine were normal. A left carotid arteriogram and a brain scan revealed left parietal changes consistent with recurrent tumor. The patient's condition progressively deteriorated, and he died after two months in the hospital.

THE ENTITY

Meckel's diverticulum is the commonest anomaly of the intestinal tract, being found in about 2 per cent of autopsies. It is a blind pouch 2 to 12 cm. in length located on the anti-mesenteric side of the small intestine about 1 meter proximal to the ileocecal junction. The mouth is wide, the lumen is large, and the wall contains all of the normal structures of the small intestine. The mucosa is usually ileal, but pancreatic tissue and gastric mucosa may be present, especially at the tip. That the diverticulum is a remnant of the duct between the gut and yolk sac was first pointed out in 1808 by Meckel, a German professor of anatomy (1).

Although the tip of the diverticulum is usually free and unattached, a fibrous cord may connect it to the umbilicus. Occasionally the diverticulum may extend to the umbilicus and even open onto it so that an ileo-umbilical fistula is formed. Less frequently the umbilical end is open and the intestinal end is closed with a fibrous cord attaching the latter to the ileum. Thus a vitelline sinus is formed that secretes a scanty mucous discharge onto the abdominal wall. Least frequent is a vitelline cyst that is connected to the umbilicus on the one side and to the ileum on the other by separate fibrous cords. Of course only a fibrous cord from umbilicus to ileum may constitute the duct remnant.

The symptomatic conditions of the diverticulum are common in infancy and childhood, and especially in males. Acid secretion of the ectopic gastric mucosa may form peptic ulcers that occasionally perforate the wall. Symptoms may also arise from intestinal obstruction (volvulus or intussusception), non-specific diverticulitis (concretions or foreign bodies), herniation of the diverticulum (umbilical or inguinal), and benign or malignant tumors including carcinoma.

1. Soderlund, S. Meckel's diverticulum. Acta chir. scand., Supplement 248, 1959.

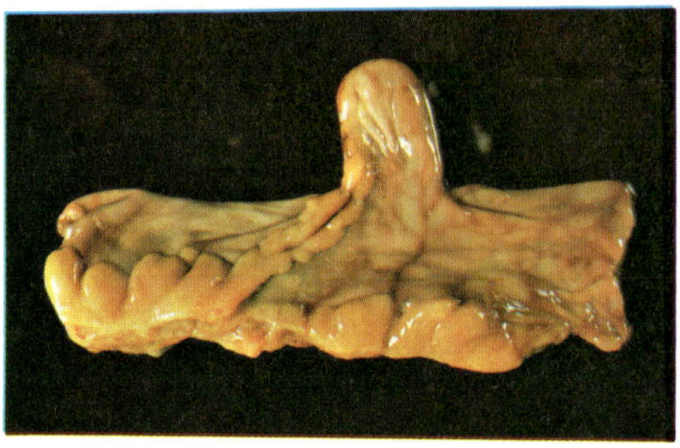

The Meckel's diverticulum extends downward from the normal ileum. The mesenteric border of the ileum is at the upper margin of the picture; the diverticulum regularly emerges from the antimesenteric side.

The opened gut shows the wide mouth of the diverticulum, the large circumference of it, and the mucosa which is similar to that of the ileum. Neither pancreatic tissue nor gastric mucosa is evident at the tip.

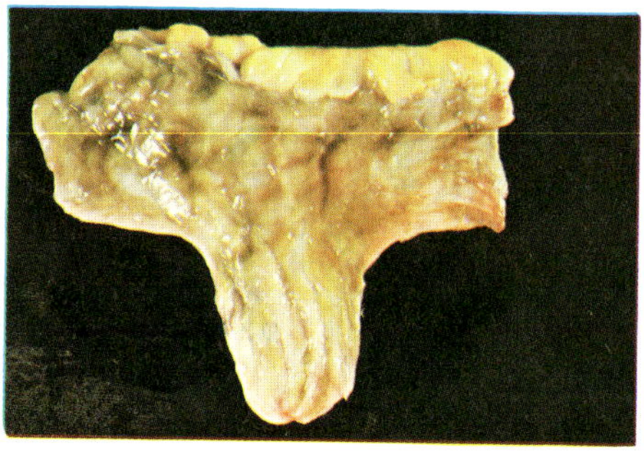

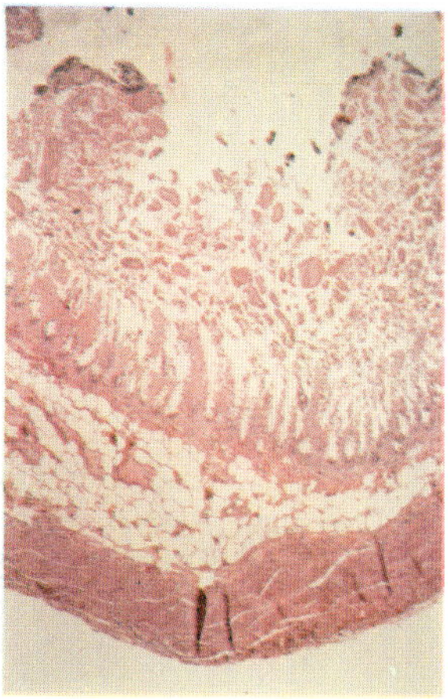

The wall of the diverticulum includes all of the structures of the normal ileum.

Autolysis has affected the mucosa; neither gastric mucosa nor pancreatic tissue is present here.

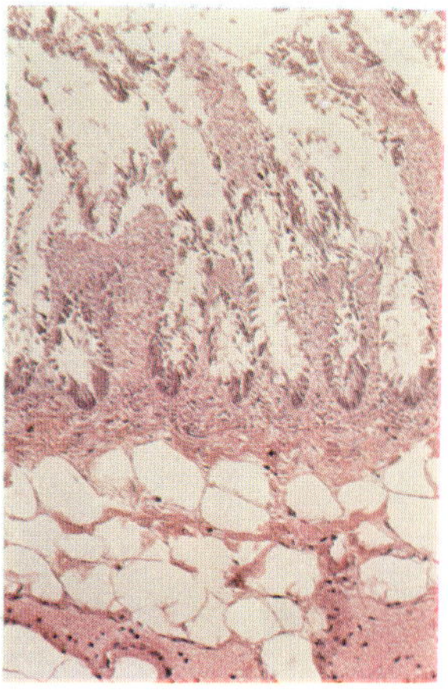

KWASHIORKOR

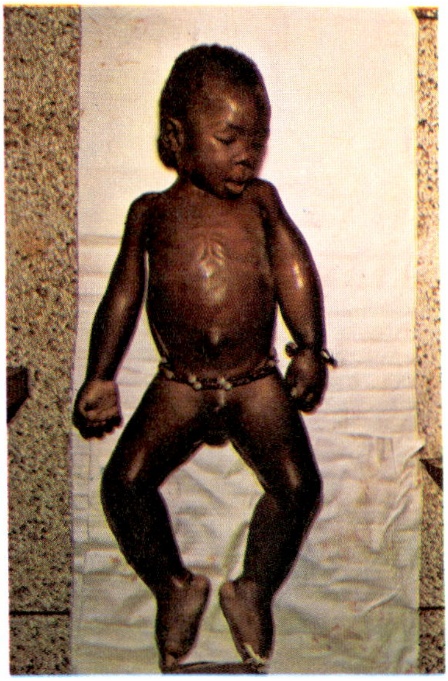

The only external signs of protein starvation are the dorsal edema of the hands and feet.

The opened small intestine is so thin as to be translucent. The mucosal side faces the viewer.

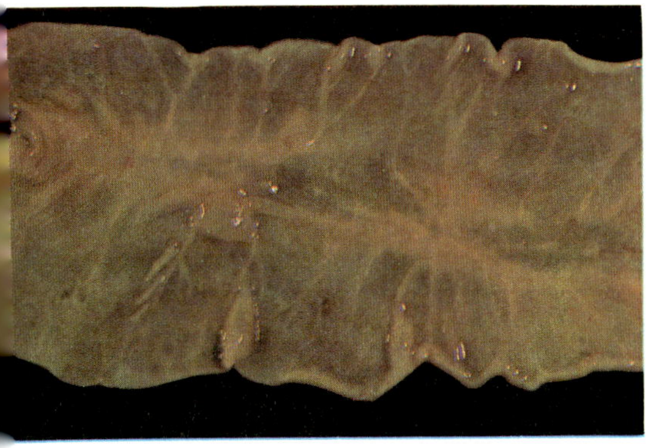

At higher power the atrophic changes are more evident, especially in the mucosa where only an occasional nest of epithelial cells remains.

A histologic section of ileum reveals the thin wall, the mucosal atrophy, and the absence of villi.

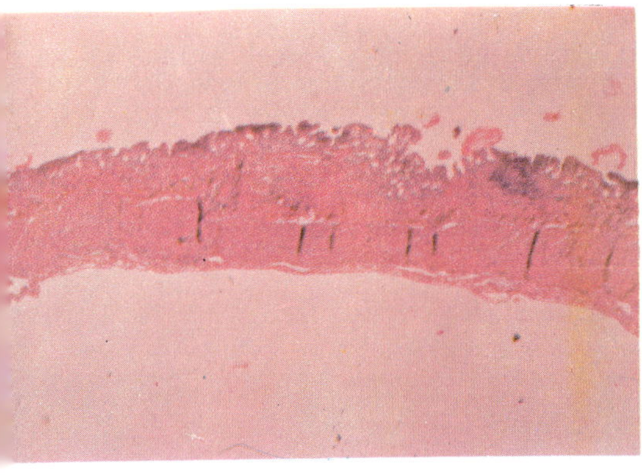

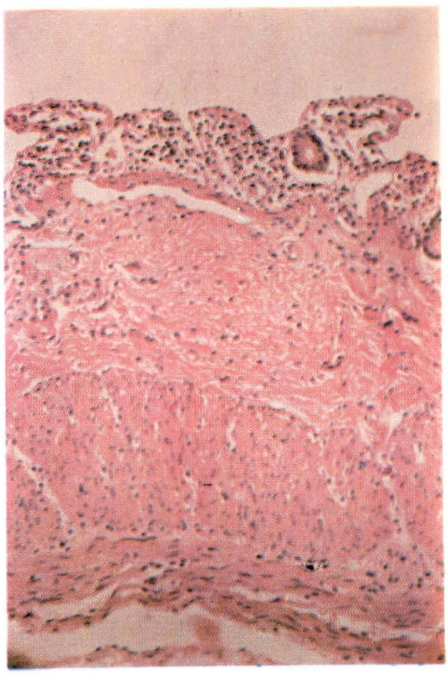

KWASHIORKOR

CLINICAL ACCOUNT 471

The patient was an 18-month-old Ugandan male child who was referred from another hospital with a diagnosis of severe kwashiorkor and bronchopneumonia. The patient was afebrile. The skin and mucous membranes were pallid. Edema was conspicuous in the subcutaneous tissues of the hands and feet. The respirations were grunting in character. The hemoglobin was 5.6 Gms. per 100 ml. A transfusion of whole blood (250 ml.) was given. The child died on the day after admission.

Autopsy examination revealed cachexia, bronchopneumonia, pigmentation of the liver and spleen characteristic of malaria, and atrophy of the other organs consistent with kwashiorkor. With expected data in parentheses, the following were found: body length 69 cm (78), body weight 8.4 Kgm (12.2), heart 38 (52), lungs 130 each (72, 65), liver 270 (345), spleen 36 (30), kidneys 32 each (42, 40), and brain 870 (1042). The pancreas weighed 9 Gms.

THE ENTITY

Kwashiorkor means "deposed one". It is a protein-calorie malnutrition that begins when the infant is weaned, usually because of a subsequent pregnancy. Thus the infant is "deposed" from the mother with breast milk of high nutritional value to the available foods such as cassava root and matoke (plantain banana) of low nutritional content. Gradual protein starvation then begins and the clinical effects tend to appear at two to three years of age. The condition carries a considerable mortality and is endemic in the developing countries. In Egypt and Guatemala, for example, the death rates for 1- to 4-year-olds are 25 times greater than in developed countries (1).

Constant clinical features include failure of growth, wasting of muscles, subcutaneous edema, and psychologic changes manifested by apathy, misery, and dejection. There are also often lightening of the hair, pallor of the skin, moon facies, and diarrhea. Occasionally there are hepatomegaly, "flaky-paint" rash of the skin, infections, and vitamin deficiencies. The body temperature may be abnormal due to inability of the basal metabolic rate to respond to changes in the environmental temperature.

The urine reveals a reduced excretion of hydroxyproline due to a low turnover of collagen associated with the failure of growth. The blood discloses a moderate anemia; the hemoglobin, however, may be under 6 Gms. per 100 ml. if malaria or hookworm disease co-exist. The plasma proteins are low, and the blood sugar is often in the 20 to 40 mg. range. The bone marrow tends to be hypoplastic, and the stools frequently reveal steatorrhea.

Organ changes consist of hepatomegaly due to fatty metamorphosis, atrophy of the pancreas, and flattening of the intestinal mucosa. Treatment consists of giving enough protein and calories to restart growth. Most steadily improve although the mortality is 10 to 15 per cent. All of the organ changes revert to normal. Factors associated with therapeutic failure include age under 18 months, plasma proteins under 3 Gms., and rectal temperature under 96 degrees F. or 35.5 degrees C. Heart failure due to fluid overload in early treatment may develop. When therapy succeeds, full recovery is usual although interference with learning ability and behavioral development may persist.

1. Shaper, A.G. Kibukamusoke, J.W., and Hutt, M.S.R. Medicine in a Tropical Environment. British Medical Association, London, 1972.

METASTATIC CARCINOMA OF ILEUM

CLINICAL ACCOUNT 6262

The patient was a white male 63 years old who was admitted to the hospital because of weakness, lethargy, and confusion. He had been well until six months previously, when he suffered a pathologic fracture of the left femur. A chest x-ray disclosed a mass in the mediastinum that extended into the right upper lung field. Bronchoscopy, scalene node biopsy, and cytologic examination of aspirated pleural fluid failed to reveal tumor cells. The mediastinal mass enlarged and a superior vena caval syndrome developed. After radiation therapy the syndrome subsided. Later, additional x-rays revealed metastases in ribs and in dorsal and lumbar portions of spine. The patient had been told fifteen years previously that he had cirrhosis. Since then there had been several episodes of abdominal swelling.

The patient was cachectic. The vital signs were normal. Physical examination revealed slight enlargement of the liver, a fluid wave in the abdomen, and dilatation of the veins over the abdomen. The spleen was not palpable.

Urinalysis was not recorded. The hemoglobin was 12.6 Gm., the hematocrit was 39 per cent, and the leukocytes numbered 8,000 with a normal differential count. A serologic test for syphilis was negative. A chest x-ray revealed massive enlargement of the mediastinum. An electrocardiogram disclosed low voltage in the main leads. Serum electrolytes, glutamic transaminase, and urea nitrogen were normal. The serum lactic dehydrogenase was 1650 units per 100 ml. The stool was 4 plus guaiac positive. The patient's condition worsened, and he died after nine days in the hospital.

Autopsy examination revealed a carcinoma of the right adrenal with metastatic disease of the lungs, left adrenal, spine, abdominal wall, ileum, and lymph nodes (bronchopulmonary, mediastinal, and para-aortic). Bronchopneumonia was pronounced in the upper lobe of the left lung. The liver weighed 1475 Gm., and revealed postnecrotic cirrhosis. No metastases were found in the hepatic tissue.

THE ENTITY

Primary cancers of the small intestine are so rare that it is advisable to exclude secondary malignant disease before accepting the diagnosis. Metastatic carcinoma of the ileum is suggested by the symptoms of intestinal obstruction and the radiographic findings of ileal involvement in a patient who has previously had a malignant tumor. The most common intra-abdominal primary sites are the stomach, colon, and ovary (1). The most common extra-abdominal sites are the uterine cervix with squamous carcinoma, and the skin with melanoblastoma. Primary sites above the diaphragm are rare although cancer of the lung is known to metastasize to ileum (2). The tumor cells lodge in the submucosa, break through the surface, and produce a sessile ulcer that encircles the lumen or angulates the bowel. The lesions are often single. Intussusception may occur.

1. Constante, A., Dockerty, M.B., and Mayo, C.W. Metastatic tumors of the small intestines. Surg., Gynec. & Obstet. 105:159, 1957.
2. Burns, W.A., and Matthews, M.J. Metastatic mucosal tumors of the small intestine. Med. Ann. Dist. Columbia 39:8, 1970.

METASTATIC CARCINOMA OF ILEUM

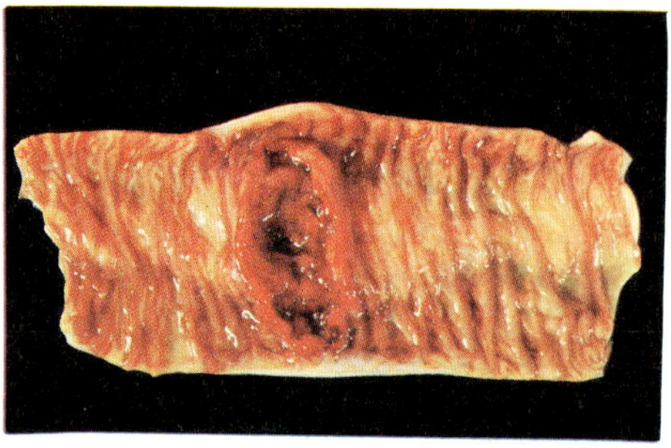

The photograph reveals the mucosal surface of ileum with a central ulcer about which the margins are raised and firm.

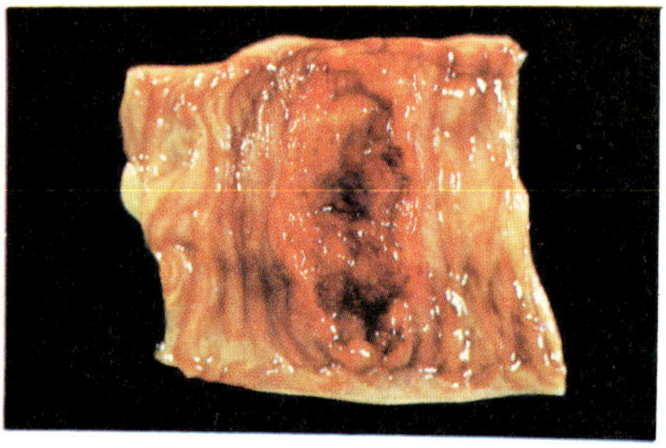

The magnified section reveals tumor lining the ulcer above, muscularis in the middle, and tumor extending to peritoneum below.

The cross section discloses deeply basophilic tumor cell masses lining the ulcer surface and extending through the wall to reach the overlying peritoneum. This suggests that perforation would have occurred had the patient lived.

A close-up view of a second ulcer reveals a similar appearance. The transverse orientation to the long axis of the ileum indicates that the lesion is not arising in a Peyer's patch which is orientated with its long axis parallel to that of the bowel.

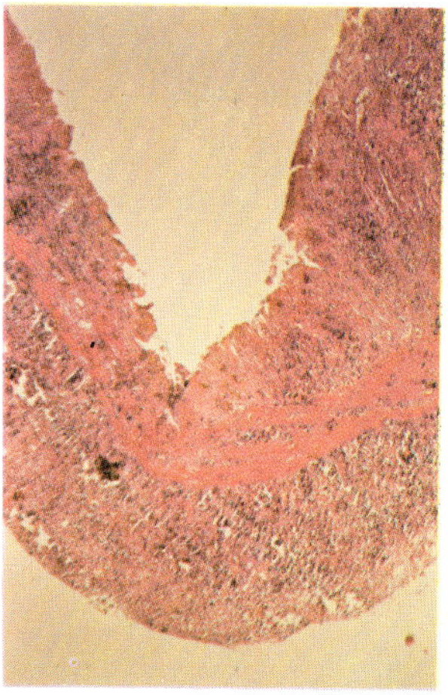

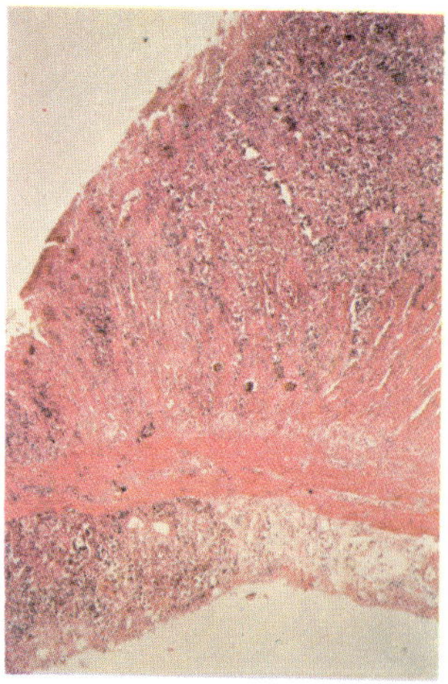

ASCARIS LUMBRICOIDES

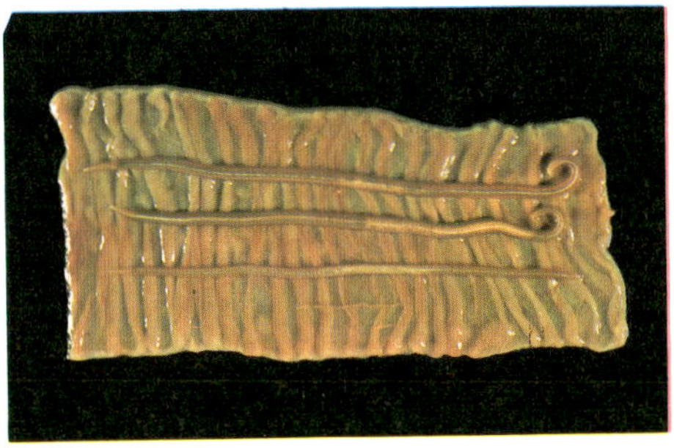

Three adult ascaris worms are stretched out on the mucosa of the ileum.

A closer view reveals the size of the worms as compared with the transverse folds of the ileal mucosa.

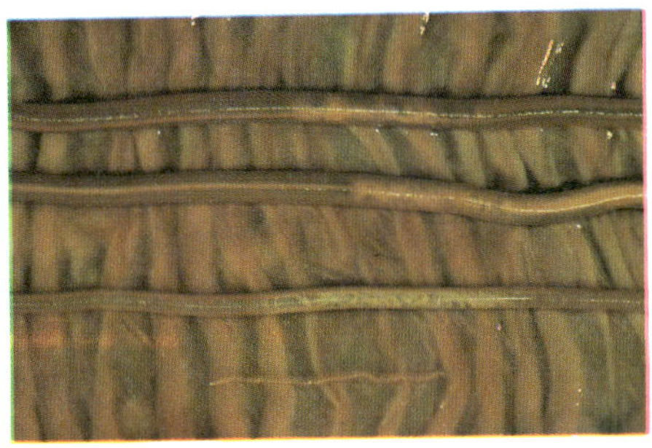

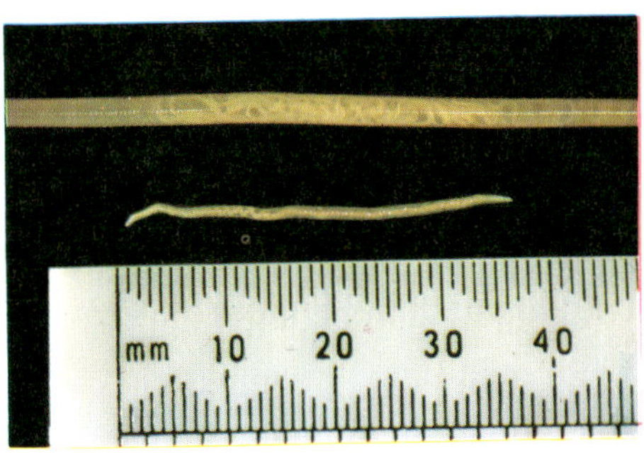

An immature worm and a mature worm are aligned with a millimeter ruler.

All of the worms from the patient lie in a single tangle and cluster. It can be seen that such a mass could easily obstruct the intestine.

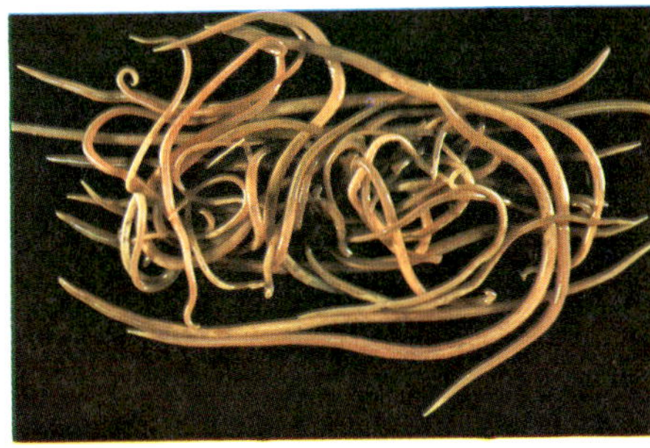

ASCARIS LUMBRICOIDES

CLINICAL ACCOUNT 454

The patient was a Ugandan female 24 years old who was well until three months before admission to the hospital. At that time she developed exertional dyspnea.

The temperature was 37.4 degrees C., pulse 116, respirations 22, and blood pressure 100/70 mm. Hg. The lung fields disclosed crepitant rales. There was a gallop rhythm and a slight systolic murmur. The fingers were clubbed, and the lower legs revealed pitting edema. Before treatment could be started, the patient suddenly died.

Autopsy examination revealed endomyocardial fibrosis with a mural thrombus of the left ventricle. The heart weighed 380 Gms.

THE ENTITY

Ascaris is a large human roundworm. Over the world it infects more than 600 million people, and in some countries over 90 per cent of the population is infected (1). Infection is most pronounced in those regions where vegetables are fertilized with human excreta, farm produce is eaten fresh, and hygienic practices are substandard. These conditions prevail especially in Asia, Africa, and Central and South America. It is estimated that 3 million Americans harbor *Ascaris lumbricoides*. Infection is especially pronounced in infants and children who are too young to be careful about what is put into the mouth.

The adult worm inhabits the jejunum, where it does not suck blood from the mucosal surface but nourishes itself from the succus entericus. The worm measures about 15 to 30 cm. in length, and the time of intestinal residence is about six months to a year. The male fertilizes the female, and the female produces about 200,000 eggs per day. The eggs are oval, mammillated, golden brown, and measure 75 microns in greatest dimension. The eggs are not infective when passed per rectum; they become so about six weeks later after embryonating in warm shady soil. If these conditions are not found, the egg remains dormant for long periods in its tough and mammillated shell.

With ingestion, the larva emerges from its shell in the jejunum. It then penetrates the mucosa, gains the venous circulation, and passes to the liver in the portal vein and thence to the right heart and lungs. In the pulmonary tissue the larva escape the capillaries, ascend the bronchi, and surmount the epiglottis to move down the esophagus, through the stomach, and back to the jejunum. The transit time is nine to twelve weeks. In the jejunum the larvae mature to adulthood.

As the larvae make the pulmonary passage, there may be fever, dyspnea, cough, blood-tinged sputum, slight eosinophilia, and radiographic changes so pronounced as to suggest bronchopneumonia. These clinical effects are known as Loeffler's phenomenon. The symptoms last one to ten days. After the worm reaches adulthood, it has two outstanding features: the first is to explore all openings and the second is a tendency to wrap itself around other worms to produce tight bundles. The latter causes intestinal obstruction, usually of the ileocecal region. The former causes the worm to enter the appendix, the uterine tubes, the ampulla of Vater, and the pancreatic or common bile ducts. A variety of acute syndromes follow these peregrinations.

1. Marcial-Rojas, R.A., Editor. Pathology of Protozoal and Helminthic Diseases, The Williams and Wilkins Co., Baltimore, 1971.

REGIONAL ENTERITIS

CLINICAL ACCOUNT 07271

The patient was a Negro female 49 years old who had experienced pain in the abdomen associated with intermittent vomiting and diarrhea for the past three years. Two weeks before admission her stools became firmer than usual and bowel movements became less frequent. For the past three days, all food and liquid were vomited and bowel movements ceased altogether. On the day before admission the abdominal pain became pronounced, and distension of the abdomen was noted. Physical examination revealed the abdomen to be tympanitic, slightly tender, and moderately distended. The hemoglobin was 14.3 Gm., the hematocrit was 41, and the leukocytes numbered 13,400. A tube was passed, the abdomen was decompressed, and contrast studies indicated an obstruction of the mid-ileum. On the seventh hospital day the abdomen was surgically explored.

Exploration of the abdomen revealed thickening of the distal four feet of the terminal ileum. Within this length there were two "skip" areas or uninvolved segments. The affected portions were thick and stenosed. The attached mesentery was short and thick, and the enclosed lymph nodes were large and soft. The diseased ileum, normal cecum, and portion of ascending colon were excised, and an end-to-end ileocolic anastamosis was performed. The pathologic diagnosis was regional enteritis.

THE ENTITY

Regional enteritis was described by Crohn and associates in 1932 (1). It is a chronic intermittent granulomatous inflammation, usually of the terminal ileum, of unknown cause, that tends to begin during young adulthood. Clinically there are nausea, vomiting, anorexia, loss of weight, pain in the abdomen, cramps, and especially constipation and diarrhea. Contrast radiographs show a characteristic "string sign" at the sites of involvement. "Skip areas" are also characteristic between the affected segments. The condition subsides and recurs and lasts for many years.

The inflammation is sharply segmental, the mucosa is ulcerated, and the submucosa is massively fibrosed. About half of the cases reveal tuberclelike structures in the exudate. The inflammation penetrates the wall and extends to the mesentery, regional lymph nodes, serosa, and adjacent structures such as the colon, abdominal wall, and adjacent loops of ileum with which fistulae tend to form. The process causes stenosis and obstruction, frequently hemorrhage, and occasionally perforation with diffuse peritonitis or localized abscess. Sharply segmental involvement, deeply penetrating tendency, and granulomatous nature thus characterize the condition.

1. Crohn, B.B., Ginzburg, L., and Oppenheimer, G.D. Regional ileitis; pathologic and clinical entity. JAMA 99:1323-1329, 1932.

REGIONAL ENTERITIS

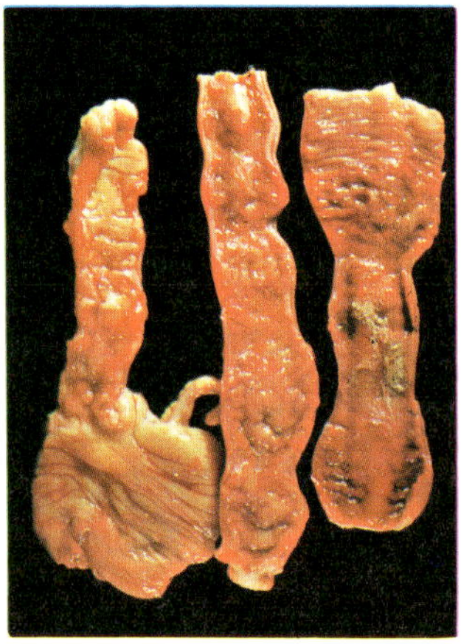

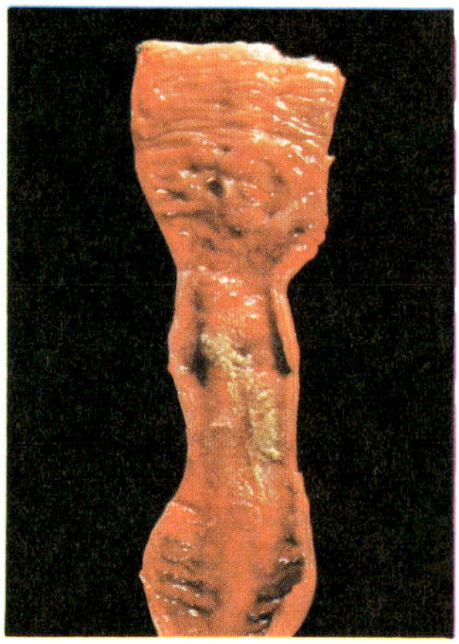

Left: The photograph shows three segments of distal ileum with cecum and appendix attached to one. "Skip" areas are present on each end of the segment on the right. All segments reveal focal stenosis, ulceration of the mucosa, and thickening of the wall. A sharp margin between normal and abnormal tissue is especially evident in the segment on the right. **Right:** A closer view reveals two characteristics of regional enteritis, i.e., the lesion is sharply demarcated from uninvolved bowel, and the inflammation is deeply penetrating so that the wall is regularly thickened and the serosa is roughened by fibrous adhesions which tend to attach to some adjacent structure.

Left: A close-up shows an ulcer covered with fibrin. The wall is markedly thickened with dense fibrous connective tissue. The mucosa on each side of the ulcer is inflamed, edematous, and nodular. **Right:** Section reveals the ulcerated mucosa, the fibrosed submucosa, and the inflammation which extends through the muscle layers to the mesentery. Necrosis of intestinal wall and penetration of the inflammatory process often lead to perforation with peritonitis or the formation of fistulas to adjacent structures. In more than half of the cases, the inflammation is granulomatous with multinucleated giant cells in the inflamed sites.

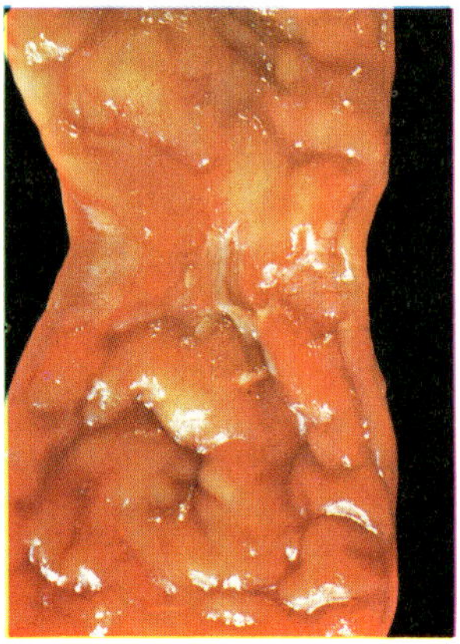

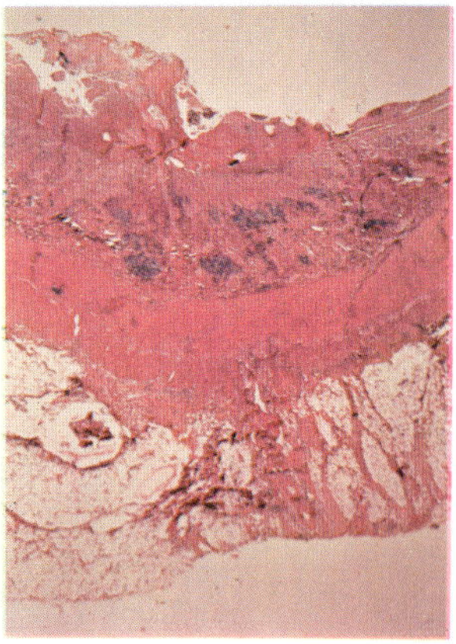

ACUTE APPENDICITIS

The appendix lies with the cut end on the left and mesoappendix above. The serosa is hyperemic, dull, and roughened by elastic, friable, pale yellow strands of fibrin.

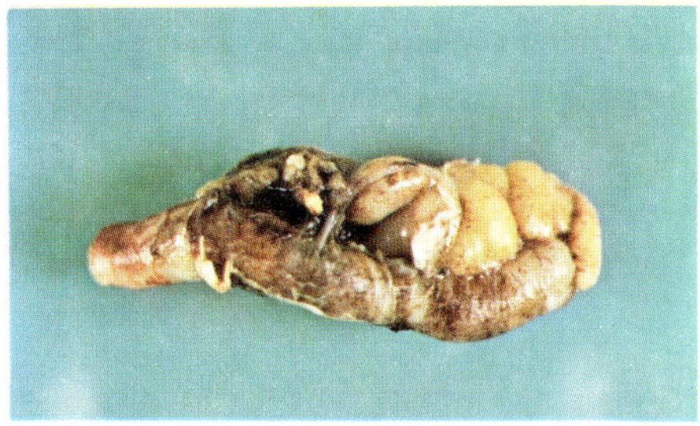

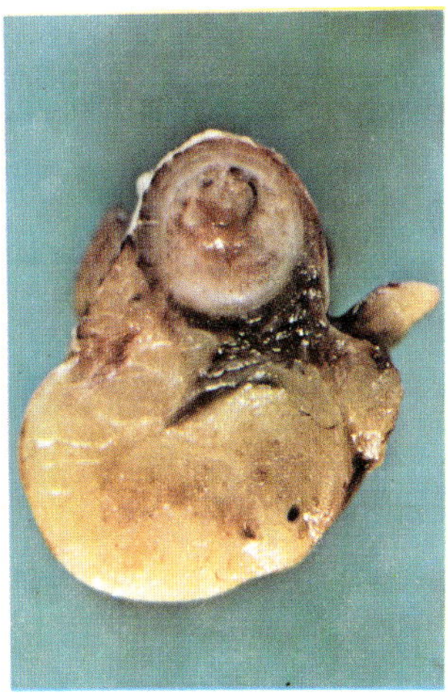

Section reveals fibrin on the serosa above, and the adipose tissue of the mesoappendix below. The lymphoid tissue of the submucosa is markedly hyperplastic so that the lumen is reduced to a narrow marginal crescentic slit.

The unmagnified microsection reveals serosal roughening with fibrin, basophilia of the external muscle layers due to rich leukocytic infiltration, and submucosal lymphoid hyperplasia that is so pronounced as to obscure the lumen.

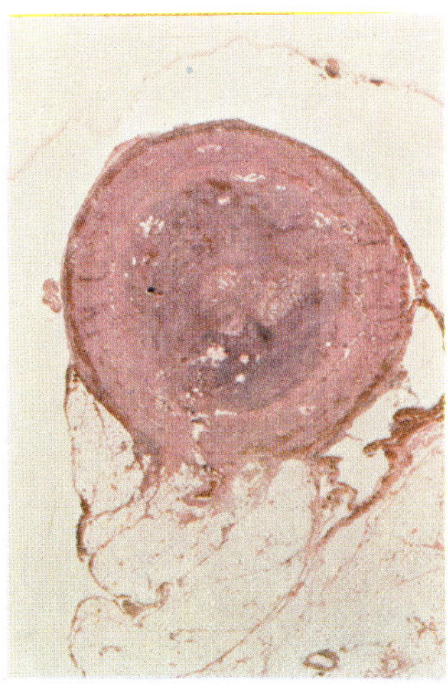

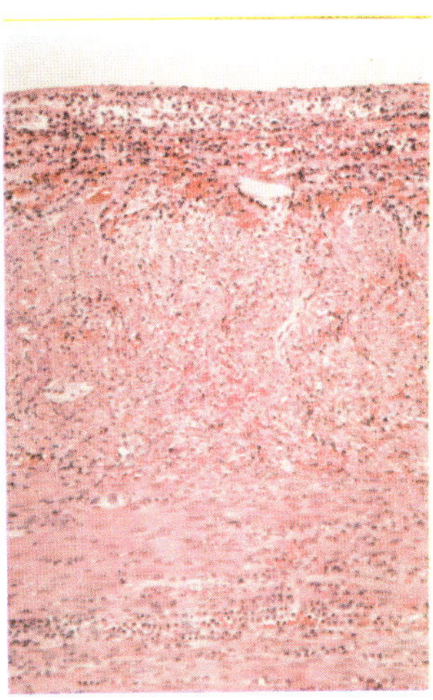

At higher power, segmented neutrophilic granulocytes can be seen extending through the external muscle layers to the serosa.

ACUTE APPENDICITIS

CLINICAL ACCOUNT U6746

The patient was a white male 27 years old who was well until the night before admission to the hospital. He experienced generalized abdominal discomfort and was unable to sleep. In the morning he had no appetite. Later in the day the abdominal discomfort changed to pain in the right lower quadrant. He was admitted to the hospital at 5:30 P.M.

The temperature was 37.2°C, pulse 86, respirations 20, and blood pressure 110/70 mm. Hg. The head, neck, and chest were not remarkable. The abdomen disclosed tenderness that was most pronounced just below McBurney's point. The pain was increased by extension of the right leg (psoas sign). In addition, gentle steady pressure over the abdomen, when suddenly released, also caused sharp exacerbation of the pain (rebound tenderness). Rectal examination elicited slight tenderness that was referred to the right lower abdomen.

The urine was normal. The hemoglobin was 16.1 Gms., and the leukocytes numbered 11,400 per cmm. with 83 segmented neutrophils, 1 band cell, and 16 lymphocytes per 100 cells counted. X-rays of abdomen and chest revealed clear lung fields and neither focal calcification nor intestinal obstruction.

Appendectomy, 7:45 P.M. The patient recovered uneventfully.

THE ENTITY

Acute appendicitis is the most common cause of "acute surgical abdomen" (1). It occurs at all ages but most commonly affects children and young adults. Over half of the cases are due to obstruction which increases the pressure within the lumen so that the veins are compressed, ischemia develops, the mucosa ulcerates, and bacterial invasion of the wall follows. The principal cause of the obstruction is hyperplasia of the submucosal lymphoid follicles which is most pronounced in children and young adults. Viral diseases causing lymphoid hyperplasia, such as measles, are associated with acute appendicitis. Other causes of obstruction are inspissated feces (fecalith), pin worms (*Enterobius vermicularis*), and fruit pits. In about 40 per cent of cases no obstruction is found and the cause is obscure.

Morphologic features, as first recognized by Fitz in 1888, are ulceration of the mucosa and suppurative inflammation of the muscle layers that extends to the serosa, which is covered by fibrin and exudate. As necrosis develops, the wall ruptures. If this takes place gradually, the omentum seals off the site and a periappendiceal abcess forms. If the perforation takes place rapidly, diffuse peritonitis develops and shock and paralytic ileus often follow. Additional complications include wound infection at the incision site, pelvic or subphrenic abscess formation, and acute pylephlebitis with septicemia, portal thrombosis, or hepatic abscesses.

McBurney described the clinical features in 1889. They include fever, loss of appetite, and abdominal pain followed by vomiting. In the beginning the pain is intermittent, colicky, and epigastric or peri-umbilical. Later it localizes in the right lower quadrant and becomes constant. Rupture causes sudden relief as the pressure drops. The abdomen reveals tenderness at McBurney's point, 2 inches inside the anterior iliac spine on a line from that spine to the umbilicus. The blood discloses a leukocytosis with a neutrophilia. An x-ray of the abdomen rules out a calcified ureteral calculus, an x-ray of the chest rules out a right lower lobe pneumonia, and a urinalysis excludes renal infection by the absence of pyuria. Surgical excision of the appendix is curative.

1. Davis, L. Christopher's Textbook of Surgery, Ninth Edition, W.B. Saunders Co., Philadelphia, 1968.

TRICHOCEPHALUS TRICHURIS (WHIPWORM)

CLINICAL ACCOUNT 460 OR 464.72

The patient was a Ugandan female 25 years old who had been well until six months before coming to the hospital. At that time she noticed swelling of the ankles. Over the following months this spread to the legs, back and abdomen. Her abdomen continued to swell and in the month before hospitalization affected her arms and face. Weakness became so pronounced that she was unable to stand.

Physical examination revealed anasarca, emaciation, and marked pallor of the skin and mucous membranes. Physical findings included a systolic murmur over the tricuspid area, enlargement of the liver, and shifting dullness over the abdomen. The hemoglobin was 2.0 Gms. per 100 ml. The cells were hypochromic and microcytic. A chest x-ray was not remarkable. The stool revealed whipworm eggs. On the second hospital day she had a bloody stool, collapsed, and died.

Autopsy examination revealed whipworms throughout the ileum, ascites, and marked pallor of the liver suggestive of fatty metamorphosis. The heart weighed 200 Gms., liver 2230 Gms., and kidneys 90 and 100 Gms.

THE ENTITY

The whipworm gets its name from a long whiplike extremity. Originally thought to be the tail, the extremity gave rise to the generic name *Trichuris*, which means "hairlike tail." Later it was discovered that the whip portion consists of a long esophagus attached to the head. Hence the generic name *Trichocephalus,* meaning "hairlike head," came into use.

Trichocephalus trichuris inhabits the cecum, appendix, and colon. The female is slightly larger than the male and measures 3.5 to 5.0 cm. in length. The worms burrow into the mucosa and lie parallel to the surface often with the tail projecting into the lumen. The morphologic effects include necrosis of epithelial cells at the sites of the head attachments, and chronic inflammation that lies above the muscularis mucosa. The affected parts are usually normal grossly. The female releases many eggs which are barrel-shaped and yellowish brown with an opening at each end that is closed with a transparent plug of mucus. The eggs pass through the rectum, fall to the ground, and embryonate in warm moist shady soil in about 21 days. Infection begins with ingestion of the embryonated eggs through unsanitary practices. These hatch in the small intestine, the larvae pass to the cecum, and maturation to adulthood takes place at that site.

In the rural tropics, 75 per cent of the population may be infected. The infections may be slight and asymptomatic or massive and symptomatic. How the worms harm the host is not clear, although inflammation and necrosis at the site of head attachment, and nerve irritation with increased peristalsis have been suggested. Whichever, the patient experiences nervousness, insomnia, headache, and anorexia. The blood reveals an eosinophilia. When the infection is massive, tenesmus, mucoid diarrhea with blood-streaked stools, and occasionally rectal prolapse may be experienced. In addition, there are often weakness, anemia, and weight loss. The diagnosis is established by stool examination and identification of the characteristic eggs.

TRICHOCEPHALUS TRICHURIS (WHIPWORM)

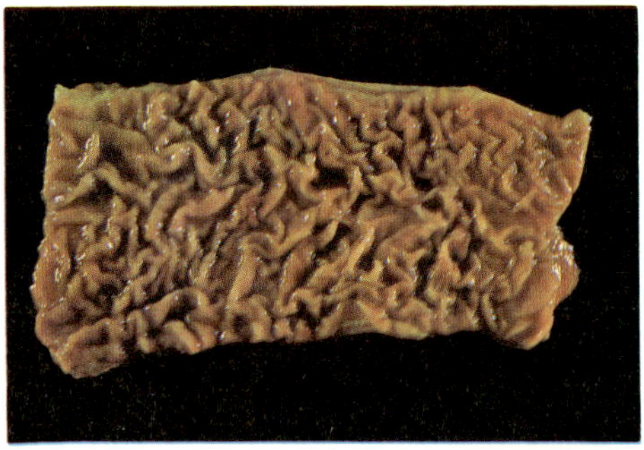

The organism is small and slender, so it is not conspicuous against the mucosal folds of the small intestine.

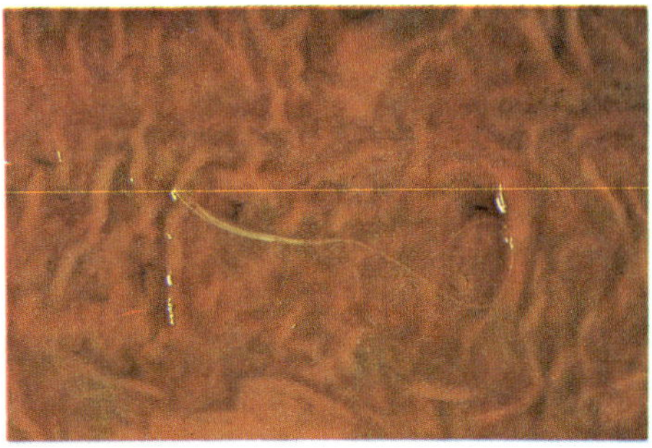

A closer view reveals the hair-like extremity which consists of the esophagus that connects the head with the rest of the body.

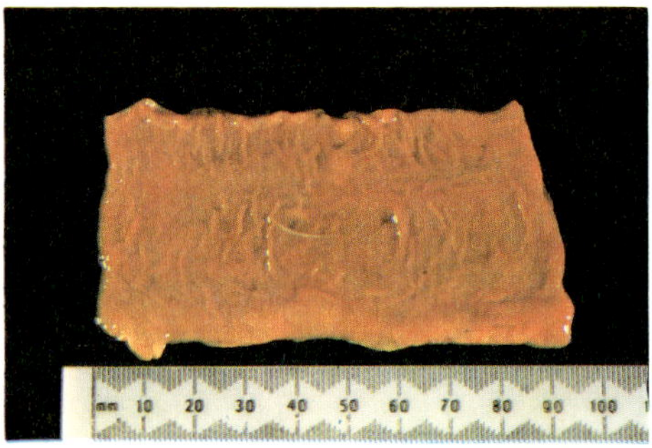

Again lying on the ileal mucosa, size can be estimated from the millimeter rule.

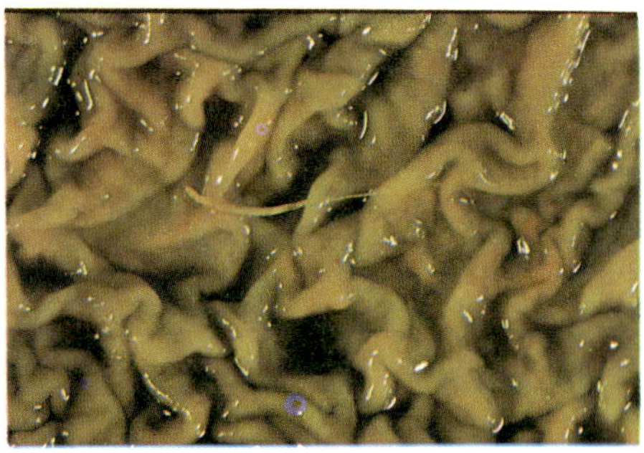

A close-up of the same worm reveals the body and the long hair-like esophagus; the head is too small to see without magnification.

ANCYLOSTOMA DUODENALE (HOOKWORM)

The hookworm is very small and is not conspicuous on the mucosa of the small intestine.

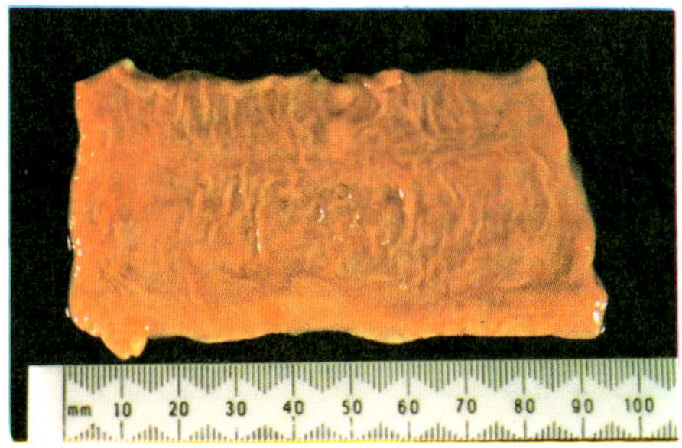

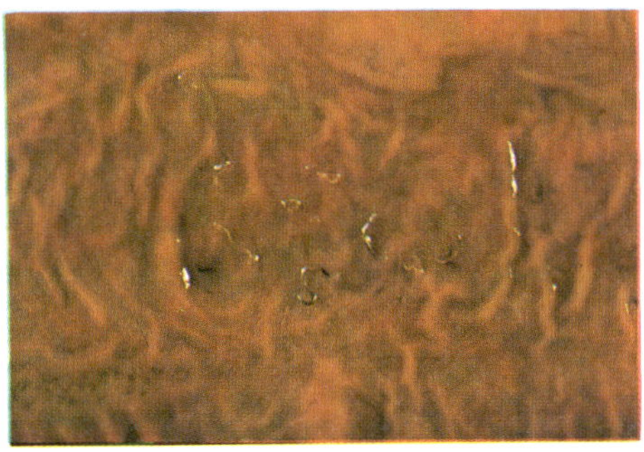

A closer view reveals the short curled worms.

After partial fixation the adult worms are more clearly seen.

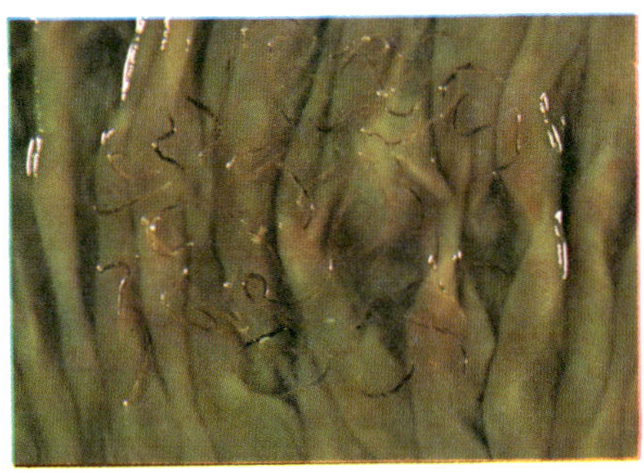

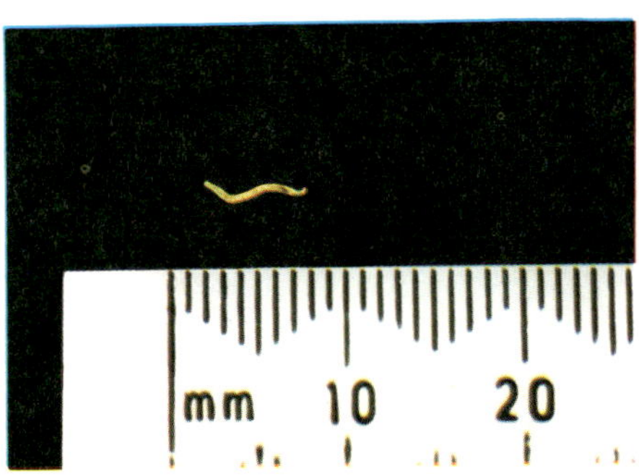

Against a millimeter rule, the size of the worm can be seen.

ANCYLOSTOMA DUODENALE (HOOKWORM)

CLINICAL ACCOUNT 444

The patient was a black male 48 years old who was epileptic and fell from his bed one week before admission to the hospital. He sustained an injury to his forehead and then became somnolent and was thought to have a subdural hematoma. The patient died in a comatose state. Autopsy examination revealed a subdural hematoma, pulmonary edema, and fatty degeneration of the myocardium suggestive of prolonged anemia. The jejunal mucosa appeared intact, and on the surface there were a large number of hookworms.

THE ENTITY

The European hookworm, *Ancylostoma duodenale,* parasitizes man only, inhabits the jejunum, and attaches itself to the gut with two large curved teeth. From this "bite" the worm sucks blood, which causes a pronounced hypochromic microcytic anemia. Combined with malnutrition, common in the tropics, a state of advanced inanition gradually develops.

The male hookworm measures 1.0 cm. in length, the female 1.3 cm. Both are cylindrical and pale pink or yellowish gray. The female produces 15,000 to 20,000 eggs per day. Each egg measures 60 x 40 microns, possesses a transparent shell, and contains an embryo composed of four to seven blastomeres. Within 24 hours of stool passage the blastomeres develop into motile rhabditiform larvae. These then undergo two additional molts over the next five days to become filariform larvae that thrive in warm moist soil and are infective for man. The filariform larva does not take food but subsists on the nutrients in the epithelial cells of its own midgut. It remains viable in soil for about nine weeks. During this time it is infective for man by an ability to penetrate the skin of the barefoot walker, which causes a transient "ground itch." The organism invades capillaries and passes to the pulmonary vessels, where it migrates through the alveolar walls, proceeds up the bronchi and over the epiglottis to reach the intestine by way of the esophagus and stomach. The passage from skin to jejunum may take as little as 24 hours. In the intestine the filariform larvae undergo three more molts to become adult worms with sexual organs and a pathogenic effect. The time from skin invasion to the fecal passage of eggs is about eight weeks. Adult worms persist in the gut for only a few months, but reinfection is common and chronic ancylostomiasis is usual. Infected patients frequently become asymptomatic carriers of the worm. The pathologic changes range from none to minute jejunal ulcerations with chronic inflammation and submucosal fibrosis. Anemia develops, and in heavy infections the worms may cause the loss of 100 ml. of blood per day. The clinical consequences include malaise, weakness, diarrhea, loss of weight, and persistent pain or discomfort in the hypogastrium. Antihelminthic treatment relieves all symptoms (1).

1. De Leon, E., and Maldonado, J.F. Uncinariasis, in Pathology of Protozoal and Helminthic Diseases, P. 734, Williams & Wilkins Co., 1971.

TENIA SAGINATA (TAPEWORM)

CLINICAL ACCOUNT 440

The patient was a black male adult, age unknown, who was brought to the hospital because of vomiting blood on the previous night. At the time of admission the patient collapsed and died.

Autopsy examination revealed pleural effusions of 500 ml. on each side, acute fibrinous pleuritis, and bronchopneumonia of the right and left lungs, which weighed 1220 and 830 Gms., respectively. The ascending aorta disclosed a saccular aneurysm. The heart weighed 440 Gms. The aorta revealed intimal wrinkling suggestive of syphilitic aortitis. An incidental finding was a tape worm, *Tenia saginata*, of the small intestine.

THE ENTITY

Tenia saginata is the most widespread of the long worms (1). It inhabits man, who is the only host, and only one worm is ordinarily found per person. The head of the worm (scolex) attaches to the duodenum and produces repeating segments (proglottids) that extend down the small intestine. An adult worm consists of 700 to 900 proglottids and measures 5 to 10 meters in length. The scolex is equipped with four suckers that provide for attachment to the mucosa and ingestion of intestinal nutrients. The head is minute, the proglottids of the neck are extremely small, and those of the mid-portion are large and approximately square. At the distal end, the proglottids are large and oval or elongated. The tapeworm nourishes itself by passing nutrients from the suckers of the head to the proglottids of the tail through a series of canals that extend the length of the worm.

Each proglottid contains a uterus and testis. It is self-fertilizing, and as maturity is reached, the gravid uterus contains about 80,000 eggs. Each day eight or nine new proglottids are produced by the head, and eight or nine gravid proglottids are released by the tail. Thus the worm discharges nearly three quarters of a million eggs daily. The detached proglottids contract and expand, eventually discharging the eggs through a rent in the wall caused by this squeezing action. Although the eggs may be discharged within the intestine, most are released onto the peri-anal skin. Scotch tape pressed against the peri-anal skin is more effective than stool examination in identifying the discharged ova.

Cattle ingest the eggs from the soil, the shell is digested off and the liberated larvae penetrate the mucosa, enter the capillaries, and encyst in the skeletal muscle. In three to four months the larvae develop into cysticerci that measure 6 to 8 mm. in diameter. Ingestion of undercooked beef containing these cysticerci causes the infestation in man. The injurious effect is not pronounced although weakness, loss of weight, and excessive appetite may develop. Eosinophilia may persist. These effects may be due to the absorption of a toxin that sensitizes the host. A skin reaction to the intradermal injection of a worm extract may be elicited.

1. Swellengrebel, N.H., and Sterman, M.M. Animal Parasites in Man. D. Van Nostrand and Company, Inc., 1961.

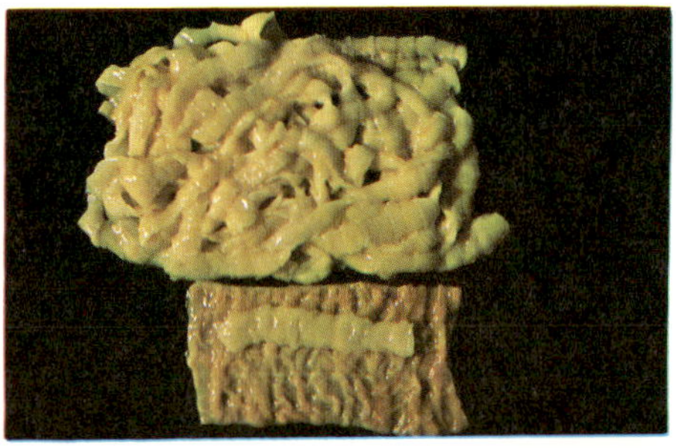

An entire single tapeworm lies as a mass of proglottids adjacent to a short strip of small intestine. A short segment of worm is stretched out on the mucosal surface of the small intestine.

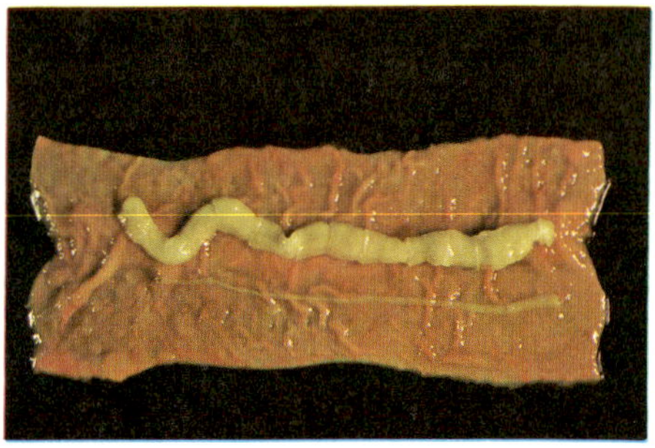

A longer strip of ileum reveals two segments of worm, i.e., the upper segment is composed of mature proglottids, the lower consists of the head at the left with the immature proglottids of the neck following to the right.

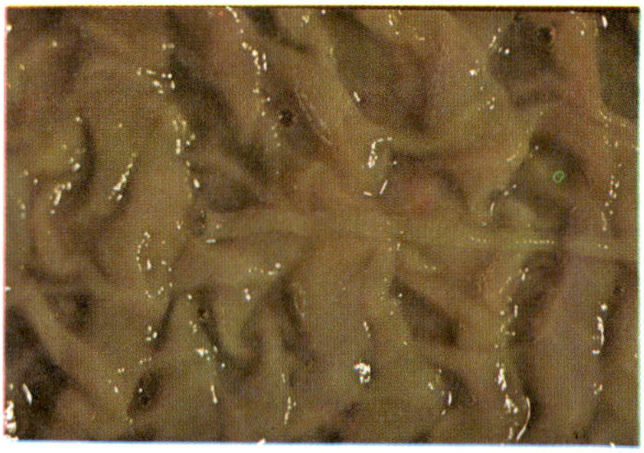

A closer view displays the head and the "new" proglottids of the neck.

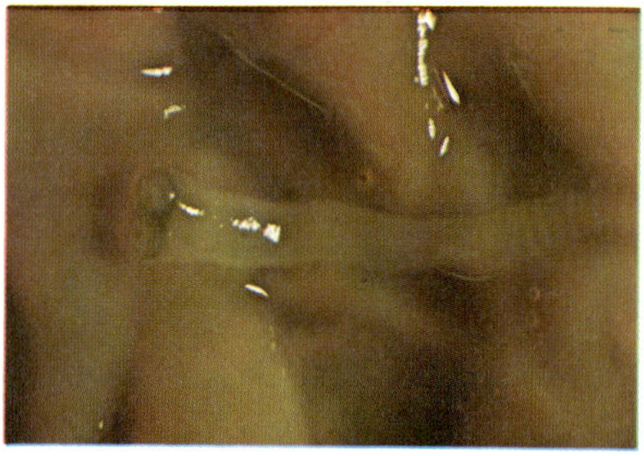

A close-up view of the head reveals two of the four suckers through which the worm takes in nutrients.

CARCINOMA OF CECUM

Right:

The opened cecum (right lower portion), the terminal ileum (vertical portion), and the ascending colon (horizontal portion) are shown. The tumor is round, slightly raised, and occupies the central portion of the cecum.

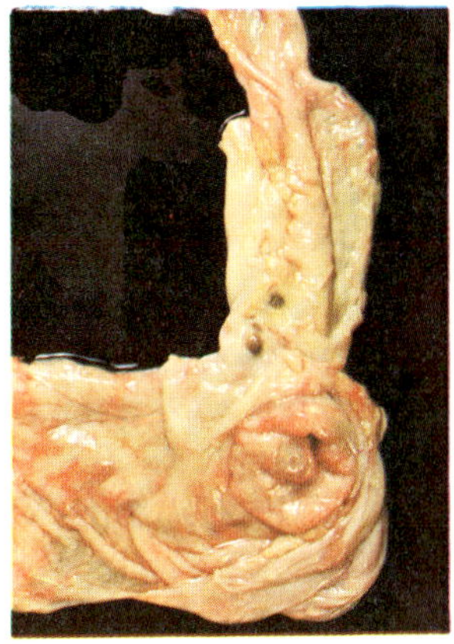

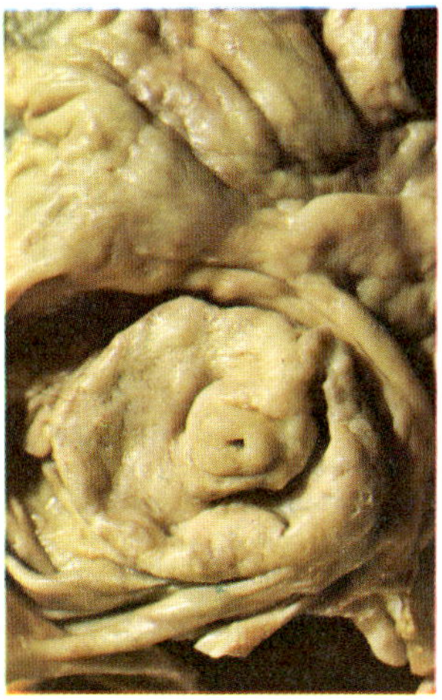

Left:

At closer range the surface of the carcinoma is better seen. The surface is raised, granular, and ulcerated. A unique feature of this case is the growth of the tumor about the base of the appendix. The dimple in the center of the cancer is the appendiceal orifice.

Right:

Section reveals the appendiceal lumen in the center of the picture on the right; the cancer infiltrates the wall of the cecum on both sides of this lumen. The serosal surface of the cecum is on the left. Carcinomas of the right colon tend to extend into the lumen ("fungate"), rather than penetrate the wall and infiltrate the adjacent tissues.

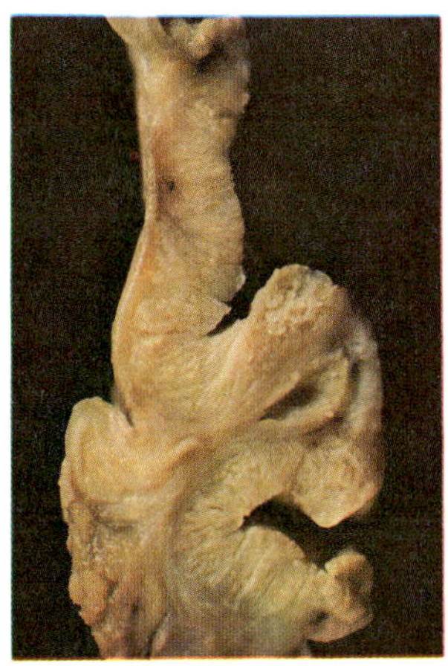

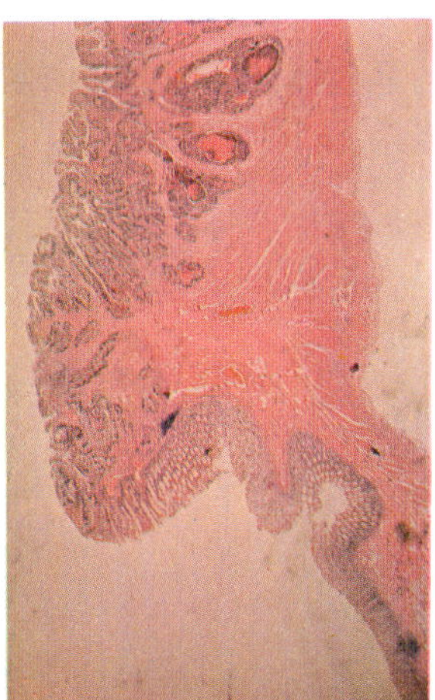

Left:

The photomicrograph shows the deeply basophilic glands of irregular size and shape penetrating the muscle layers of the colonic wall on the right. The surface is ulcerated, and oozing of blood takes place from it. Hypochromic microcytic anemia of obscure cause is a clinical characteristic of carcinoma of the cecum and adjacent ascending colon. Normal mucosa is at the top of the photograph.

CARCINOMA OF CECUM

CLINICAL ACCOUNT 6166

The patient was a Negro male 69 years old who was admitted to the hospital because of aphasia and weakness of the left arm and leg. He was well until six months previously, when discomfort in the chest was diagnosed as arteriosclerotic heart disease because of premature ventricular contractions. For the past three days he had experienced anorexia, occasional vomiting, and gradual clouding of the sensorium. On the evening of admission he was aphasic, and with muscle weakness in the extremities on the left.

The temperature was 98.6 degrees F., pulse 100, respirations 20, and blood pressure 150/50. Physical findings included 3 plus deep tendon reflexes on the left, 1 plus on the right, and a positive Babinski reflex on the left. There was no papilledema or nuchal rigidity.

The urine was yellow, cloudy, pH 6, and specific gravity 1.012 with a 2 plus reaction for glucose and negative tests for albumin and acetone. The sediment revealed 3 leukocytes and a rare epithelial cell; there were no casts or erythrocytes. The hemoglobin was 6.9 Gm., hematocrit 25, and leukocytes 11,800 with a normal differential count. The blood sugar and blood urea nitrogen were 100 mg. and 23 mg. respectively. The cerebrospinal fluid was normal. A radio-isotope scan of the brain was normal. The mental condition of the patient rapidly deteriorated and death occurred on the third hospital day.

Autopsy examination revealed bronchopneumonia of the right and left lungs. Other diagnosis were incidental including a small carcinoma of the cecum. The brain weighed 1125 Gm. and was not unusual externally except for slight edema of the meninges. After fixation, sections disclosed a recent infarct of the right half of the pons.

THE ENTITY

The distribution of cancer of the colon is indicated by the tabulation of Jackman and Beahrs (1). They found 34 cancers of the cecum, 30 of the ascending colon, 19 of the hepatic flexure, 44 of the descending colon, 140 of the sigmoid, and 377 of the rectum. Thirty additional cancers were anorectal.

Carcinomas of the cecum and right colon are characterized by anorexia, weakness, and pain in the abdomen. The pain is often slight and may be no more than postprandial discomfort and a sense of fullness. Anorexia induces a loss of weight. The surface of the cancer ulcerates and slowly bleeds so that the patient complains of weakness and pallor marks his skin. The bleeding induces a hypochromic anemia that may be pronounced. The blood mixes thoroughly with feces in its passage through the colon so that blood at defecation is not visible to the patient but the stool is regularly positive to guaiac. In over half of patients a mass is palpable in the right side of the abdomen.

Cancers of the right colon grow slowly, and they grow into the lumen. The lumen is capacious, the wall is distensible, and the fecal stream is semiliquid. For these reasons obstruction is late and a change of bowel habit is rare.

1. Jackman, R.J., and Beahrs, O.H. Tumors of the Large Bowel. W.B. Saunders Company, Philadelphia, 1968.

CHRONIC ULCERATIVE COLITIS

CLINICAL ACCOUNT P9613

The patient was a Negro female 24 years old who was well until two years before hospital admission. At that time cramping pain in the abdomen and diarrhea began. The stool was liquid and contained blood and mucus. A diagnosis of chronic ulcerative colitis was made. The patient was then in her eighth month of pregnancy; after delivery steroid enemas were given and her condition improved. Ten months later the symptoms recurred and a brief hospitalization was required. Four months after that another hospitalization was necessary. Six months later the original symptoms recurred and more treatment was given. The present admission was two months later and was necessitated by widespread cramping pain in the abdomen and diarrhea with six to eight bowel movements per day. The stool was soft and brown with streaks of red blood and gray mucus. Physical examination revealed a systolic ejection murmur heard best at the apex, tenderness to deep palpation of the abdomen, and bowel sounds that were normal. A barium study and sigmoidoscopic examination revealed chronic ulcerative colitis. On the thirty-seventh hospital day a total colectomy was performed. Except for an episode of psychosis, recovery was uneventful.

THE ENTITY

Chronic ulcerative colitis affects the sexes equally, usually the 20-40 age group, and occasionally occurs in children. The onset is often sudden with cramping abdominal pain, tenesmus, and diarrhea that characteristically includes blood, pus, and mucus. The inflammatory process begins in the rectosigmoid, progresses proximally toward the terminal ileum, and displays proximal and distal margins that are poorly defined, i.e., the transition to normal mucosa is gradual. The wall is edematous and hyperemic, and the mucosa is ulcerated and covered by exudate. Longitudinal "ulcer streaks" are characteristic. The inflammation is superficial, the external muscle layers are hypertrophic, and the wall becomes a rigid tube. Microscopically the inflammation is exudative with micro-abscesses, necrosis, and fibrin thrombi within vessels. Projection of nubs of nonulcerated mucosa forms pseudopolyps. There are no granulomas, giant cells, or tubercles.

The course is prolonged, intermittent, and associated with nutritional failure and gradual wasting. Anemia, hypoproteinemia, and electrolyte imbalance are common. Five complications include stricture which usually occurs in the rectosigmoid, hemorrhage which may be massive, perforation which is rare, pseudopolyp formation which is common, and carcinoma which tends to be multiple, mucus-secreting, and highly malignant. The last tends to arise about a decade after the onset of the disease.

The condition differs pathologically from regional enteritis by ill-defined margins of involvement, exudative inflammation that is superficial, absence of fibrosis of the wall, lack of necrosis and penetration of the ulcers, absence of granulomatous foci, and a tendency to carcinomatous transformation.

The cause is unknown. Treatment is symptomatic for the diarrhea, and prophylactic (colectomy) for the complications.

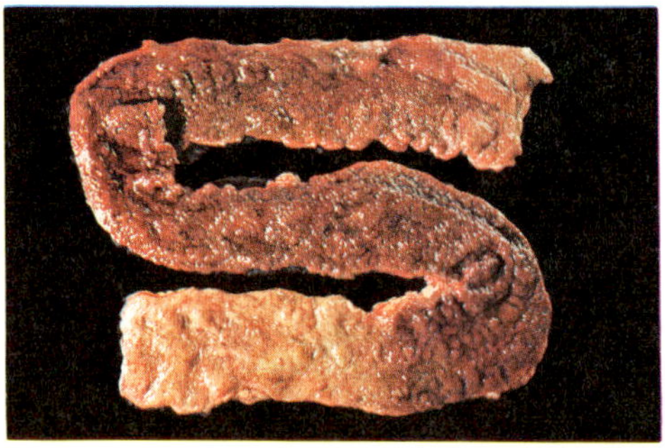

A large portion of opened color reveals the hyperemic, edematous, and ulcerated mucosa with gradual transition to normal or less affected surface at either end.

Markedly involved mucosa is on the left with much less altered mucosa on the right.

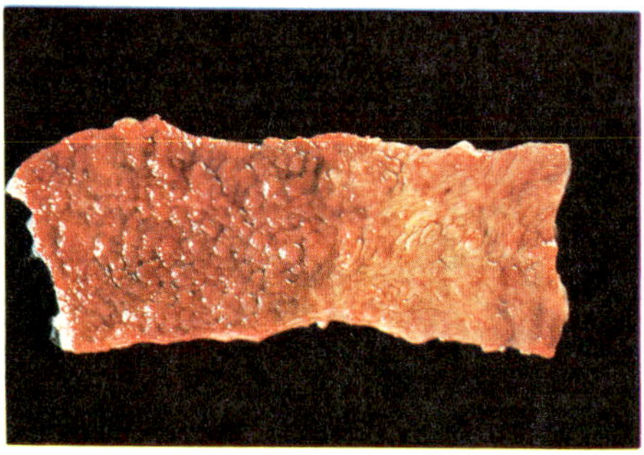

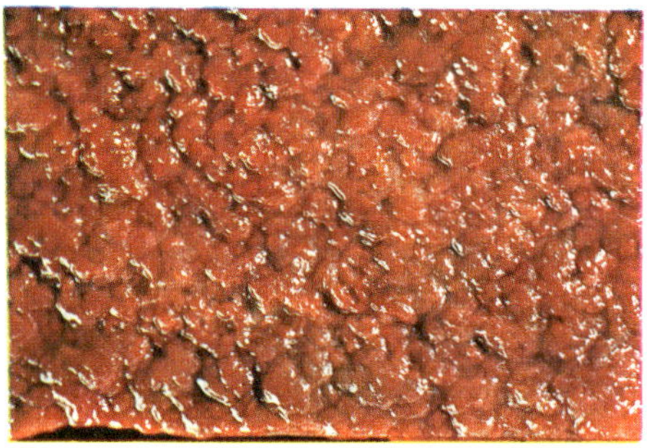

A close-up discloses the coarse nubs of inflamed mucosa between which tortuous winding ulcers are in evidence.

An unmagnified histologic section reveals thickening of the external muscle layers, irregular ulceration of the mucosa, and limitation of the exudate to the superficial layers of the wall.

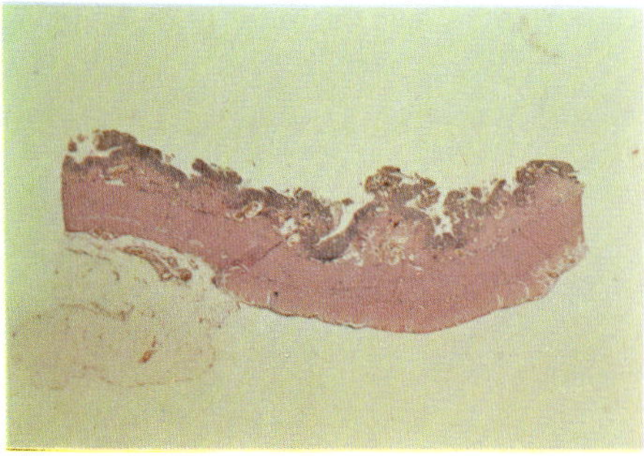

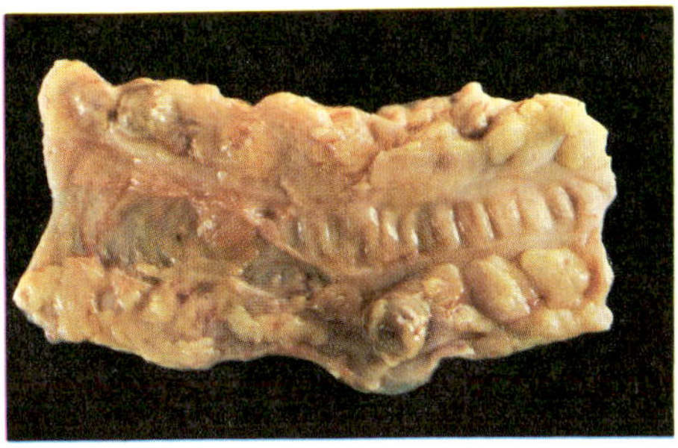

The serosal surface shows two diverticula, one in the middle of the photograph on the right, the other at the lower left portion of the picture.

The mucosal surface reveals two rows of diverticula. Fecal material extrudes from the orifices of some. None is inflamed. The "mouths" are often smaller than the lumens so that inspissated fecal material tends to be incarcerated within them.

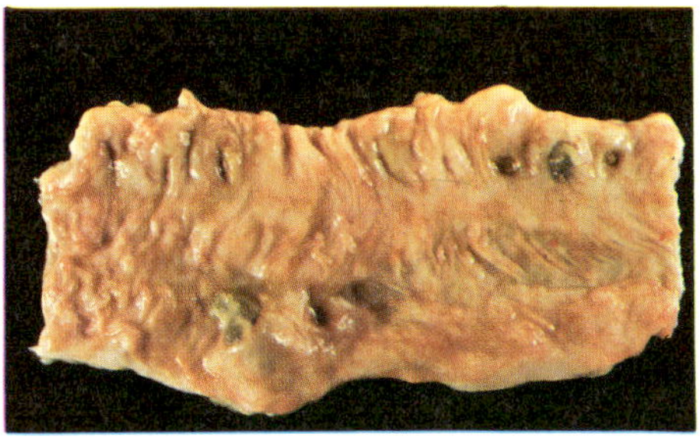

A close-up of the cut surface reveals a somewhat laminated mass of fecal material within a diverticulum. Note that the wall of the evagination is extremely thin as compared with the intact colonic wall.

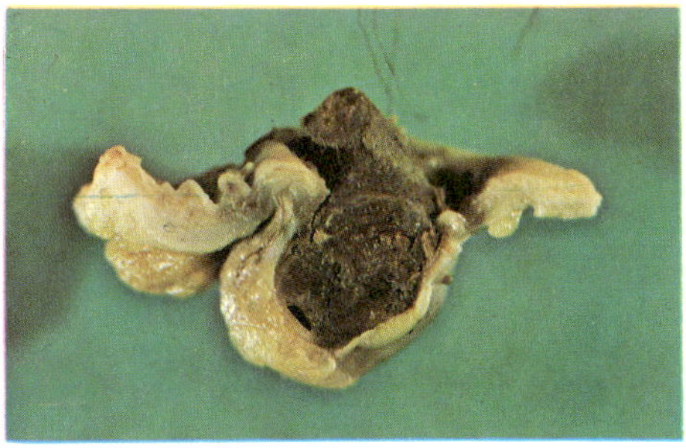

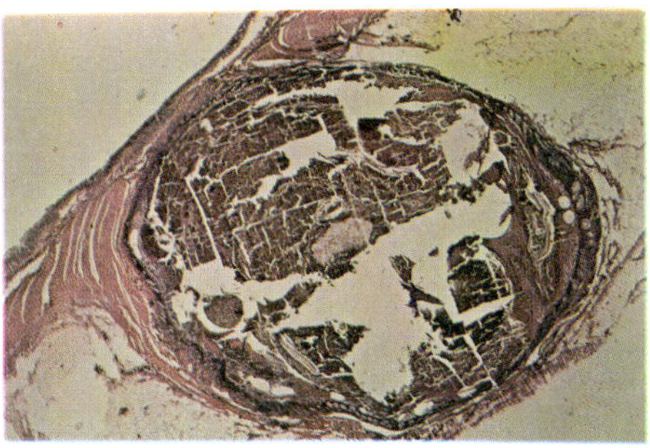

The diverticulum consists only of mucosa and a few strands of connective tissue. This is due to the pulsion nature of the structure; it is an evagination of mucosa through the external muscle layers of the colonic wall.

DIVERTICULA OF COLON

CLINICAL ACCOUNT 6117

The patient was an obese white male 64 years old who had taken nitroglycerine for angina pectoris for several years. On the day of admission, after a big dinner, the patient suffered acute anterior chest pain, vomited, and collapsed. An electrocardiogram disclosed bradycardia, heart block and recent infarction. The blood pressure was 170/100. His skin was cool and moist. He was admitted to the emergency room, where cyanosis and Cheyne-Stokes respirations were observed. The blood pressure fell to 60-70 systolic and the heart rate increased to 130 per minute. Heart sounds were faint, and rales were audible over all lung fields. He was given Dilaudid, atropine, and Aramine. He died two hours after entering the hospital.

Autopsy examination revealed a recent infarct of a papillary muscle of the left ventricle, an old infarct of the myocardium, marked arteriosclerosis of both coronary arteries, and edema of the lungs. There were also chronic pyelonephritis, calculi of the left renal pelvis, and a cyst of the left kidney. The diverticula of the colon were incidental. Some were present in the descending portion and most were present in the sigmoid.

THE ENTITY

Diverticula of the colon occur equally in the sexes, are uncommon before 35 years of age, and increase thereafter so that two thirds of the population over 80 have them. Most occur in the sigmoid colon; they are common in the descending colon, but are uncommon on the right. They occur between the tenia, close to and parallel with the attachment of the colon to the mesentery. They are multiple, globular in shape, and contain inspissated fecal material. The communications with the colonic lumen are often narrow so that fecaliths are incarcerated within them. They tend to arise at the sites of vessel penetration of the muscle layers of the wall.

Hard fecaliths abrade the mucosa, ulcers form, and inflammation follows. Abscesses occur in the fibroadipose tissue or adhesions form on the serosal surfaces. Exudative inflammation is usual; chronic granulomatous inflammation follows extrusion of foreign (fecal) material. Inflammation affects only single diverticula; the clinical manifestations are recurrent episodes of fever and pain, especially in the left lower quadrant of the abdomen.

The common complication is obstruction of the colon from pericolic inflammation and fibrosis. Hemorrhage from granulation tissue in the inflamed base of a diverticulum is uncommon. Extension of a pericolic abscess into the urinary bladder to form a vesicolonic fistula with pneumaturia and cystitis is uncommon. Perforation is rare.

CHRONIC ULCERATIVE COLITIS

CLINICAL ACCOUNT 6200

The patient was a white male 25 years old who was well until six months before admission to the hospital. At that time diarrhea began. The stools were loose, then watery, and finally bloody. During the first two months there were as many as twenty bowel movements per day. The diarrhea then gradually subsided. Ten days before admission unpleasantness in his home was followed by extreme nervousness and recurrence of the diarrhea. The patient's weight had dropped from 220 to 160 pounds. Two years previously he had seen a psychiatrist for "anxieties."

The patient lived with his parents. He was employed by his father, who was described as wealthy, demanding, and intolerant. The patient was hospitalized; the hemoglobin was 5.4 Gm., the hematocrit was 23, and the leukocytes numbered 11,400 with a neutrophilia. A barium enema revealed ulcerative colitis from sigmoid to cecum. Transfusions were given. He was discharged to see a psychiatrist.

Two months later he was re-admitted with acute fulminant ulcerative colitis. On the fifth day decompression of the colon was undertaken by cecostomy. Two days later cardiac arrest occurred, and on the following day the patient died.

Autopsy examination revealed bronchopneumonia, pulmonary thrombo-emboli, and recent infarcts of both lungs. There were also an acute esophagitis, atrophy and fibrosis of the pancreas, fatty metamorphosis of the liver, and Zahn infarcts of the hepatic tissue. An organizing thrombus was present in the right renal vein. The mucosa of the colon was ulcerated from the rectum to the cecum.

THE ENTITY

Chronic ulcerative colitis affects the sexes equally, usually the 20-40 age group, and occasionally occurs in children. The onset is often sudden with cramping abdominal pain, tenesmus, and diarrhea that characteristically includes blood, pus, and mucus. The inflammatory process begins in the rectosigmoid, progresses proximally toward the terminal ileum, and displays proximal and distal margins that are poorly defined, i.e., the transition to normal mucosa is gradual. The wall is edematous and hyperemic, and the mucosa is ulcerated and covered by exudate. Longitudinal "ulcer streaks" are characteristic. The inflammation is superficial, the external muscle layers are hypertrophic, and the wall becomes a rigid tube. Microscopically the inflammation is exudative with micro-abscesses, necrosis, and fibrin thrombi within vessels. Projection of nubs of nonulcerated mucosa forms pseudopolyps. There are no granulomas, no giant cells, and no tubercles.

The course is prolonged, intermittent, and associated with nutritional failure and gradual wasting. Anemia, hypoproteinemia, and electrolyte imbalance are common. Five complications include stricture which usually occurs in the rectosigmoid, hemorrhage which may be massive, perforation which is rare, pseudopolyp formation which is common, and carcinoma which tends to be multiple, mucus secreting, and highly malignant. The last tends to arise about a decade after the onset of the disease.

The cause of chronic ulcerative colitis is unknown; the treatment is symptomatic for the diarrhea, and prophylatic (colectomy) for the complications.

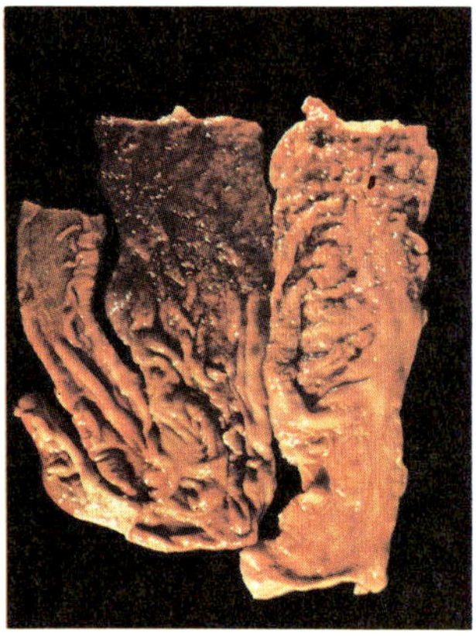

The photograph shows the gradual transition from normal to ulcerated mucosa in the ascending colon on the left, and at the rectal junction on the right. This gradual transition of the margin of the lesion is a characteristic of ulcerative colitis.

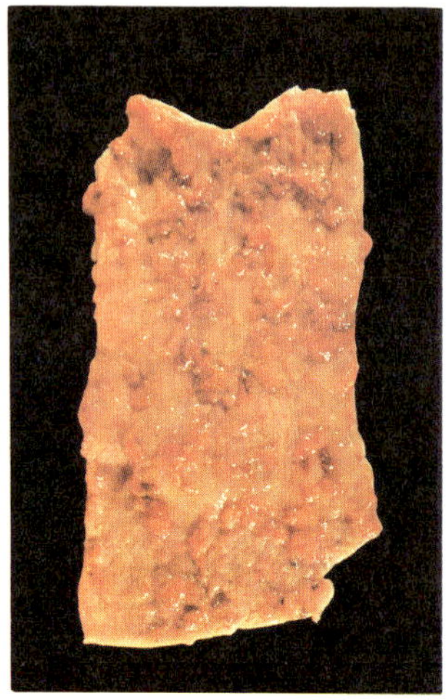

A close-up view reveals extensive ulceration with small nubs of remaining mucosa that resemble polyps and are hence called pseudopolyps.

Left: A pseudopolyp is shown at scanning power. The submucosa is largely absent, the muscle layers are only slightly thickened, and the inflammation tends not to penetrate the muscularis. **Right:** The pseudopolyp is composed of glands and stroma that are markedly inflamed. The inflammation is regularly exudative. The absence of massive fibrosis, the superficial location of the inflammation, and the exudative nature of the inflammation all differ from the main features of regional enteritis.

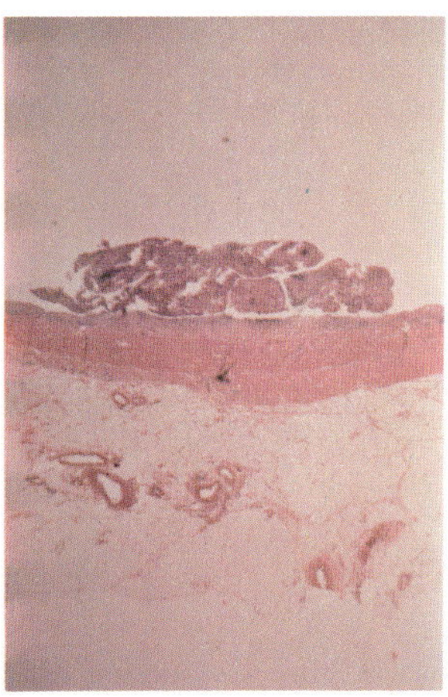

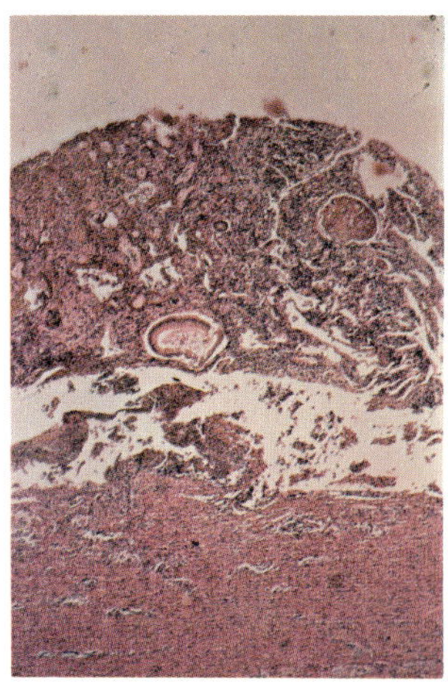

The surgical specimen revealed segments of extensive involvement and intervening "skip" areas of normal bowel. The inflamed mucosa is thick, edematous, and nodular. The junction of involved segments with normal mucosa is quite sharply defined.

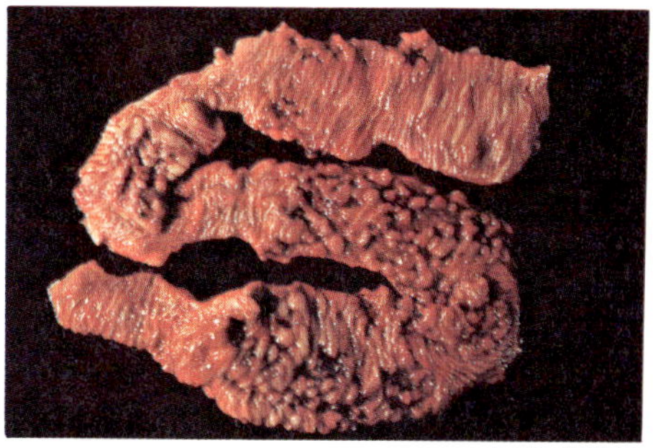

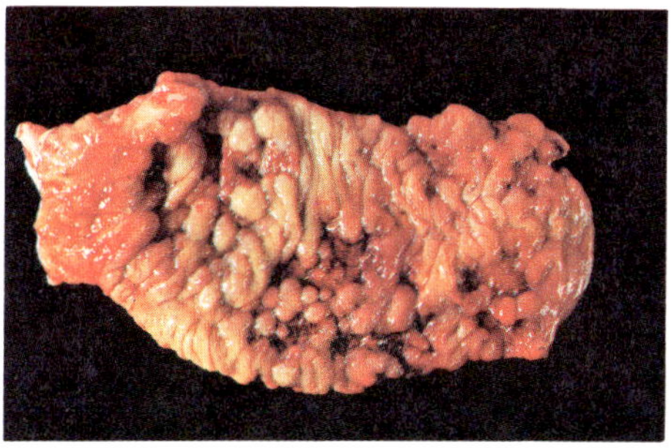

A close-up view of an involved segment reveals deep ulcers and a nodular, inflamed, and markedly edematous adjacent mucosa.

A still closer view shows the ulcer covered with blood and pus, and the intervening nodules of inflamed and edematous mucosa.

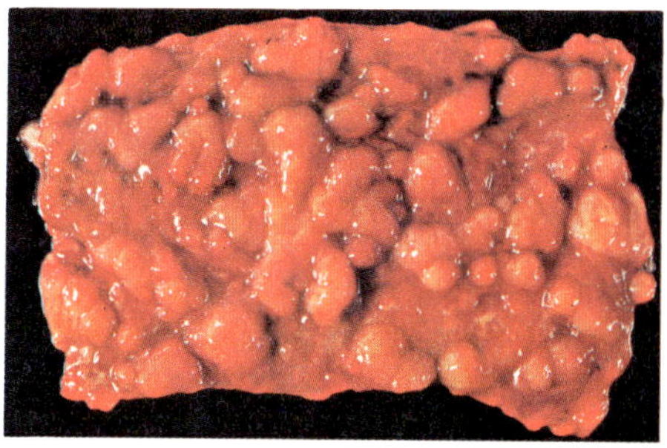

A histologic section reveals that the inflammation is granulomatous. It resembles tuberculosis, but culture, special stains, and other techniques have failed to identify acid-fast organisms or another specific causative agent. The condition is thus a granulomatous inflammation of unknown cause that affects the colon and resembles the process of regional enteritis.

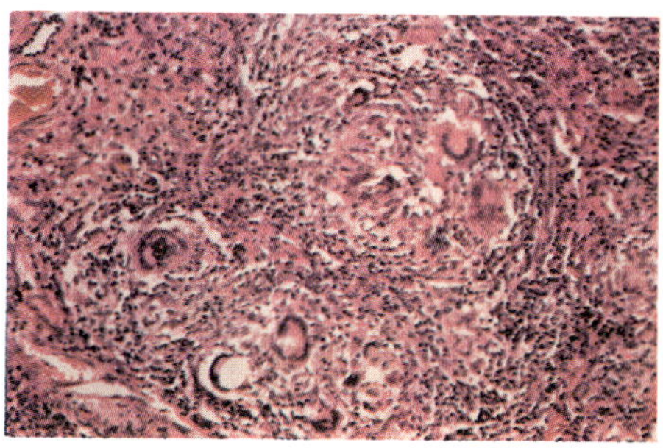

GRANULOMATOUS COLITIS

CLINICAL ACCOUNT 09351

The patient was a white female 25 years old who was well until eleven months before hospital admission. At that time diarrhea began. The stools were watery, without blood, and there were five to fifteen bowel movements per day. The diarrhea was accompanied by some anorexia and some intermittent crampy abdominal pain. Her weight had decreased from 125 to 100 pounds. During the past month there had been slight pain in the joints of the hands, feet, knees, and elbows.

The vital signs were normal. The patient was thin and anxious, and displayed a soft abdomen and a red maculo-papular rash over the dorsum of both feet. The urine was normal. The hemoglobin was 11.6 Gm., the hematocrit was 36, and the leukocytes numbered 7,800. On the third hospital day the terminal ileum, cecum, ascending colon, and appendix were removed, and an ileo-colic anastomosis was performed. The laboratory diagnosis of the specimen was "Granulomatous Inflammation." The patient was discharged after nine days in the hospital.

THE ENTITY

When the disease of Crohn and colleagues involves the colon, it is called granulomatous colitis. It affects young persons and clinically resembles ulcerative colitis. The process affects large portions of the colon; there is sharp segmental involvement with intervening "skip" areas, the mucosa displays ulcers and deep fissures, the submucosa is massively fibrosed so that the involved segments are thick and rigid, the process is transmural with extension to mesentery and lymph nodes, and abscesses and fistulae, especially of the pelvis and perineum are common. Microscopic examination usually reveals tubercles. Carcinoma is regarded as uncommon, although this is unsettled (1). These features differ from ulcerative colitis which is diffuse, superficial, exudative, unassociated with segmental fibrosis of the submucosa, less often associated with paracolic complications, and more often associated with carcinoma.

Uninvolvement of the rectum, and "skip" areas on radiographs, help distinguish the condition clinically from ulcerative colitis.

1. Perret, A.D., Truelove, S.C., and Massarella, G.R. Crohn's disease and carcinoma of the colon. Brit. Med. J. 2:466, 1968.

ADENOMA OF COLONIC MUCOSA

CLINICAL ACCOUNT 6136

The patient was a white male 56 years old who was admitted to the hospital because of severe chest pain. The pain began in the morning of the day of admission and was substernal in location with radiation to the back, neck and left arm. It was accompanied by apprehension, diaphoresis, and a feeling of weakness. The patient had had several episodes of severe angina pectoris in the year prior to the present illness and had otherwise been well.

The temperature was 97.4 degrees F., respirations 22, pulse 108, and blood pressure 100/70 mm. Hg. The neck veins were not distended. Fine rales were heard over both lung bases. The pulse was regular, the heart was not enlarged, and no murmurs were heard.

The patient was unable to void. The hemoglobin was 16.8 Gm., hematocrit 52, and leukocytes 15,400 with a moderate neutrophilia. The blood cholesterol was 275 mg., the serum glutamic transaminase was 60 u/ml., and the lactic dehydrogenase was 400 u/100 ml. A chest x-ray showed no cardiac enlargement, and slight pulmonary congestion. An electrocardiogram revealed a posterior myocardial infarct.

On the second hospital day the serum glutamic and lactic enzymes rose to 242 and 2040 units, respectively. The patient was nauseated and vomited. The pain persisted. A pacemaker was inserted. His condition regressed and death occurred after the patient had been in the hospital for five days.

Autopsy examination revealed a recent thrombus of the right coronary artery, marked arteriosclerosis of the right and left coronary arteries, and recent and old infarcts of the myocardium. Acute passive hyperemia was evident in lungs, liver, and spleen. Additional diagnoses were incidental. The colonic adenoma was an incidental finding.

THE ENTITY

The most common tumor of the colon is the adenoma. The lesion is sessile at the outset and tends to become pedunculated as peristalsis tugs at the mucosa. Most are in the distal colon, 70 per cent within reach of the sigmoidoscope. They are slightly more common in men and increase with age so that the incidence is 20 per cent over the age of 60 years. They are often multiple. Excision of one may be followed by the development of others.

The adenoma is globoid with a light red granular surface creased by fine fissures. Most measure less than 1 cm. in diameter although some are 2 to 3 cm. and a few are larger. Microscopically the cells display large nuclei that are hyperchromatic and scant cytoplasm that is nearly devoid of mucin. Mitotic figures are regularly present, and atypical epithelial pattern is not unusual. The potential for malignant transformation increases with the size of the lesion (1). Simple excision is adequate treatment when the stalk is uninvaded by tumor cells.

Adenomas coincide with carcinomas of the colon with respect to age of patient and location within the bowel. Satellite adenomas are often seen adjacent to carcinomas. All stages of transition from adenomas to carcinomas are observed, and such transformation regularly takes place in familial polyposis. For these reasons the colonic adenoma is widely regarded as a premalignant lesion.

1. Jackman, R.J., and Bears, O.H. Tumors of the Large Bowel. W.B. Saunders Co., Philadelphia, 1968.

ADENOMA OF COLONIC MUCOSA

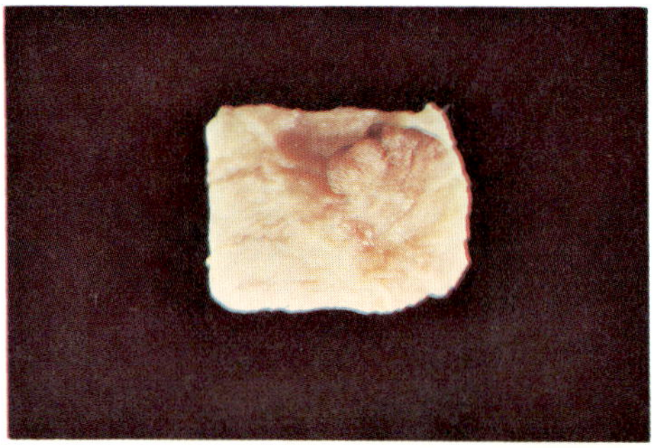

The mucosal surface of the adenoma is pale pink and finely fissured. It measures 1 cm. in diameter and is present in the sigmoid portion.

The adenoma is pedunculated, and the cut surface reveals the stalk. The surface of the stalk is covered with normal mucosa; the tip is expanded into a globular (polypoid) cluster of neoplastic epithelial cells that are benign.

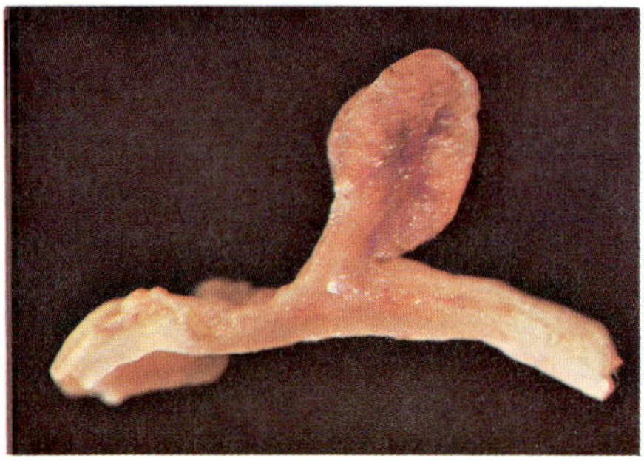

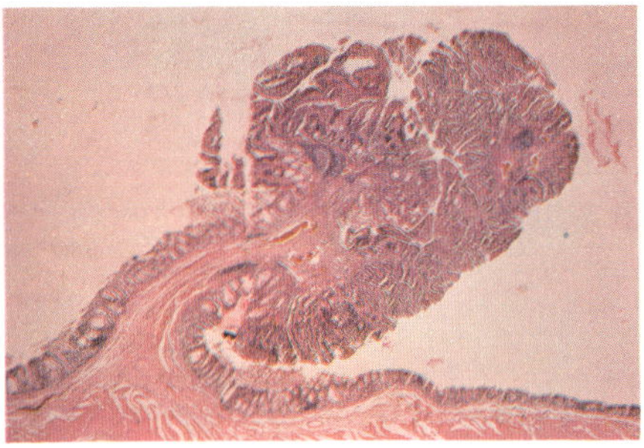

Histologic section discloses the globular mass of gland-forming mucosa at the tip of a narrow connective tissue stalk. Basophilia is conspicuous in the mucosa of the adenoma as compared with that of the normal surface covering the stalk.

A magnified microview reveals that the benign tumor cells have not invaded the connective tissue stalk in this plane of examination. Without anaplasia or such invasion, the evidence of malignant transformation is wanting. Simple excision is curative.

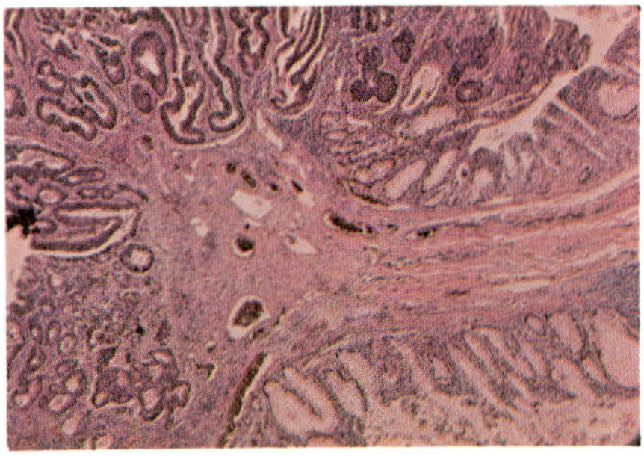

CARCINOMA OF SIGMOID

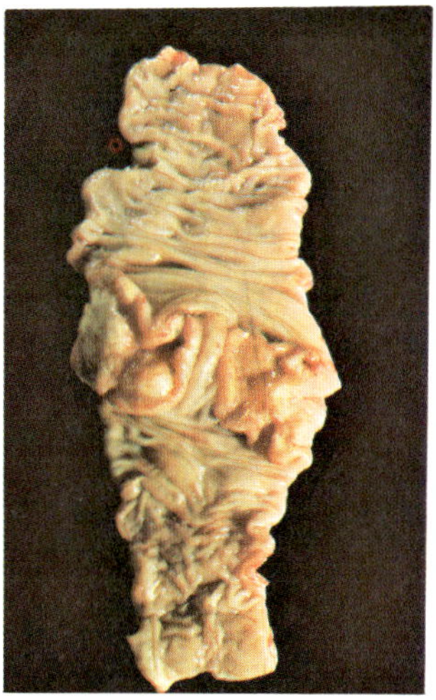

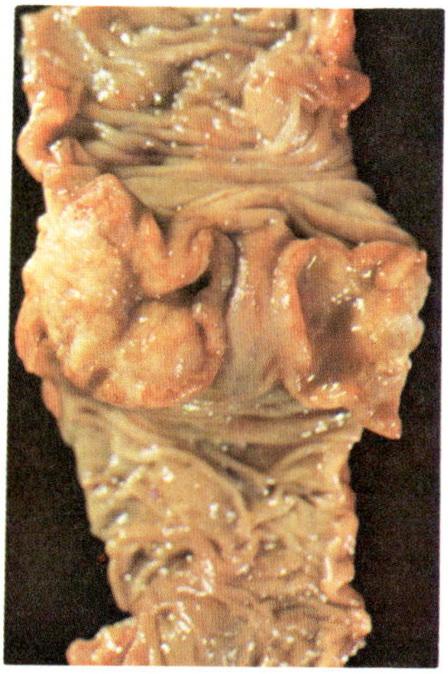

Left: The surgical specimen consisted of a left colon. The photograph reveals an ulcerating carcinoma that has encircled about ¾ of the circumference of the lumen. The tumor has caused a gradually increasing obstruction that is indicated by dilatation of the proximal segment (upper) as compared with the distal segment (lower). The obstruction was not clinically evident, perhaps because of compensatory work hypertrophy of the former part. **Right:** A close-up view reveals the character of the cancer. The margins are rolled, raised, and firm. The ulcerated base is flat, pale gray, and granular. The uninvolved mucosa is soft, moist, and normally folded. All mucosal cancers ulcerate; from such ulcers all cancers of the colon discharge usually small amounts of blood into the lumen. Occult blood is regularly present in the stool.

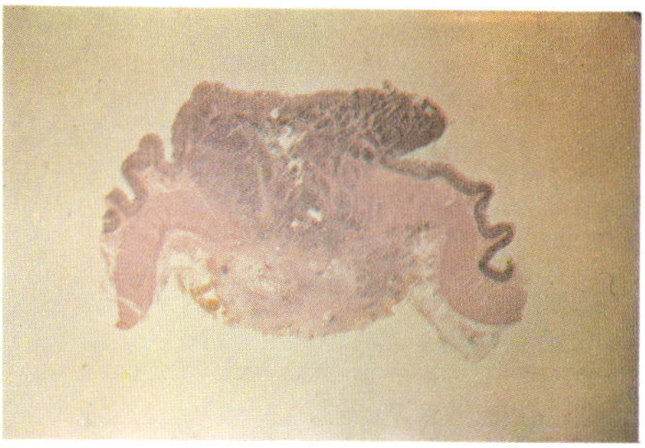

The unmagnified histologic section reveals the raised margins, the ulcerated center, and the penetration into the muscle layers of the wall and through them into the attached mesentery.

The microsection discloses irregular gland formation, loss of polarity of lining cells, bizarre nuclei, and frequent mitotic figures. These observations, in addition to the previously observed invasion of the wall, certify that the lesion is a carcinoma, and that it is a gland-forming tumor or adenocarcinoma.

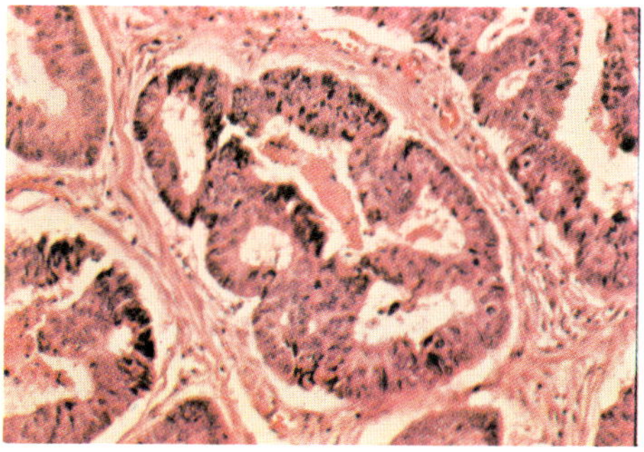

CARCINOMA OF SIGMOID

CLINICAL ACCOUNT P6497

The patient was a white female 57 years old who was last well six months before admission to the hospital. At that time she became aware of a fullness in her left flank. She delayed seeing a physician for the ensuing five and one-half months. He felt a mass in the left lower quadrant of the abdomen and ordered an x-ray study of the colon with a barium enema. The radiographs revealed a constricting lesion of the colon consistent with carcinoma. The patient was then admitted to the hospital. An 8-pound loss of weight had been noted over the past six months. There was no complaint specifically referable to the digestive tract. Physical examination revealed a nontender movable mass in the left lower quadrant of the abdomen. The blood and urine were normal except for a leukocyte count of 16,400 per cmm. Total protein, albumin-globulin ratio, serum bilirubin, phenolsulfonphthalein excretion, alkaline phosphatase, and prothrombin time were normal. On the fourth hospital day a left colectomy was performed. The specimen revealed a carcinoma of the sigmoid colon. No metastases were identified in the mesenteric lymph nodes. The post-operative course was uneventful, and the patient was discharged from the hospital after fifteen days.

THE ENTITY

Carcinoma of the colon is a common tumor of man. It is especially frequent in the sixth decade. It occurs equally in the sexes except for the distal part (rectum), where it is twice as common in men. Half of all colon cancers are within reach of the examining finger, a fourth more may be visualized by the sigmoidoscope, and the remaining fourth are equally distributed throughout the rest of the colon. On the left (descending and sigmoid), cancers infiltrate the wall, ulcerate the mucosa, and encircle the lumen. For these reasons blood is grossly evident in the stool, obstruction of the colon is common, and no mass may be palpated in the abdomen. On the right (cecum and ascending), the lumen is larger, the wall is distensible, and the stool is semiliquid. Moreover, right colon cancers tend to fungate into the lumen rather than infiltrate the wall. Right colon cancers are therefore characterized by a palpable mass in the abdomen, occult blood in the stool, and hypochromic anemia. Rate of growth is indicated by the observation that about one year is required for a three fourths encirclement of the lumen. Most are adenocarcinomas; some are undifferentiated. Colectomy may be curative. Outlook depends on tumor cell distribution at the time of treatment. Classification of Dukes: A, tumor localized to intestinal wall; B, tumor spread through wall into mesentery; and C, tumor present in wall and regional lymph nodes. For carcinomas of the rectum, the five-year rate of survival decreases according to these categories, i.e., from 81 to 64 to 27 per cent (1).

1. Dukes, C.E., and Bussey, J.J.R. The spread of rectal cancer and its effect on prognosis. Brit. J. Cancer 12:309, 1958.

NORMAL KIDNEY

CLINICAL ACCOUNT 6166

The patient was a Negro male 69 years old who was admitted to the hospital because of aphasia and weakness of the left arm and leg. Three days preceding admission he had experienced gradual clouding of the sensorium. On the evening of admission he was aphasic with muscle weakness in the extremities on the left.

The temperature was 98.6° F., pulse 100, respirations 20, and blood pressure 150/150. Physical findings included 3 plus deep tendon reflexes on the left, 1 plus on the right, and a positive Babinski reflex on the left.

The urine was yellow, cloudy, and specific gravity 1.012 with a 2 plus reaction for glucose and negative tests for albumin and acetone. The hemoglobin was 6.9 Gm., hematocrit 25, and leukocytes 11,800 with a normal differential count. The blood urea nitrogen was 23 mg. The mental condition of the patient rapidly deteriorated, and death occurred on the third hospital day.

Autopsy examination revealed bronchopneumonia of the right and left lungs. Other diagnoses were incidental. The right and left kidneys weighed 125 and 130 Gm., respectively.

THE ENTITY

Each normal adult kidney weighs about 150 Gm. and contains about 1.5 million nephrons. Each nephron consists of a glomerulus, a proximal convoluted tubule, a loop of Henle, a distal convoluted tubule, and a collecting duct. The renal tissue is perfused with over 1 liter of blood per minute, which amounts to about 20 per cent of the cardiac output. Nearly all of this passes through the glomerular capillaries, which are unique because they lie between two arterioles, i.e., an afferent bringing blood in and an efferent carrying it away. The pressure in the glomerular capillaries is 65 mm. Hg.; elsewhere it is closer to 20 mm. Hg. This high pressure "squeezes" water and solutes out of the glomerular capillaries into Bowman's space, which connects with the proximal convoluted tubules. Blood leaving the glomeruli again enters capillaries which are peritubular. Thus, glomerular blood supplies the tubules, and whatever affects the glomerular capillaries also affects the renal tubules.

The glomerulus is the interface between the circulating blood and the beginning of the excretory process. The interface consists of three layers: endothelial, basement membrane, and epithelial. The internal endothelial layer is porous and is called the "lamina fenestra." The basement membrane appears solid. The external epithelial layer is attached to the basement membrane by cytoplasmic extensions resembling foot processes; the cells are called "podocytes." Open spaces lie between these processes. This interface structure suggests that the basement membrane is the dialyzing filter of the glomerulus. So-called mesangial cells form the stalk of the glomerulus.

The glomeruli filter 125 ml. of fluid per minute into the tubules. Most of this is reabsorbed from the proximal convoluted tubules into the peritubular capillaries; some solids are also reabsorbed and some fluids are secreted by the tubules into the lumens. The net result of these three processes of filtration, reabsorption, and secretion is the formation of about 1.5 liters of urine per 24 hours.

When renal function fails, blood urea nitrogen rises. It is estimated that about 75 per cent of the nephrons must fail before this happens (1). The functional reserve of the kidney is thus large.

1. Franklin, S.S., and Merrill, J.P. The kidney in health; the nephron in disease. Am. J. Med. 28:1, 1960.

NORMAL KIDNEY

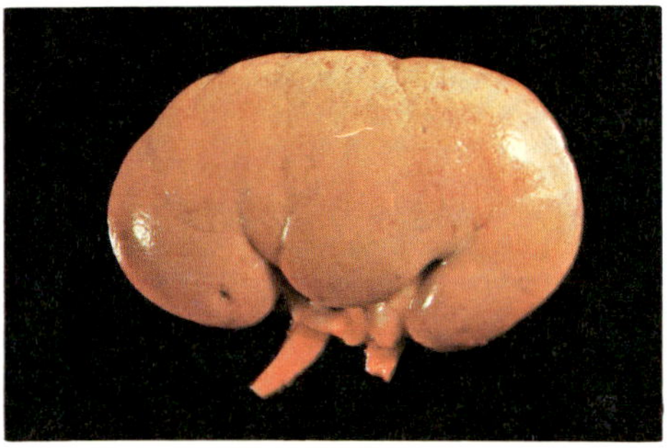

The contour and size are normal. The external surface is smooth and light red. The vessels and ureter at the hilum are normal.

The cut surface reveals a cortex of normal thickness over which the cortical striations are distinct and the corticomedullary junction is well delineated. The renal pyramids are not remarkable. The parapelvic adipose tissue is not excessive. The mucosa of the calyces and pelvis is thin, smooth, and pale gray. The pelvic chamber is not dilated, and the ureter is of normal diameter.

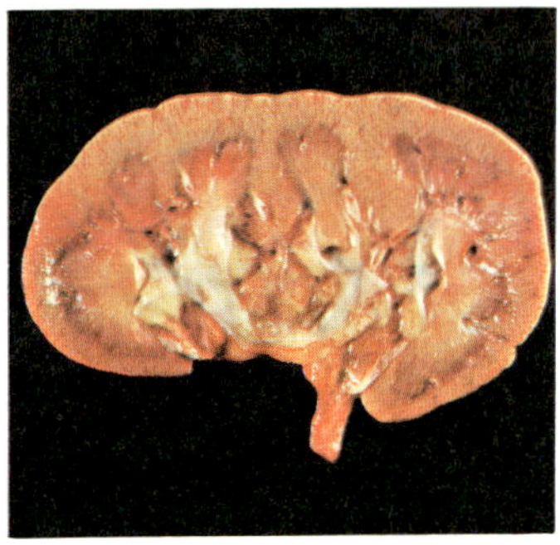

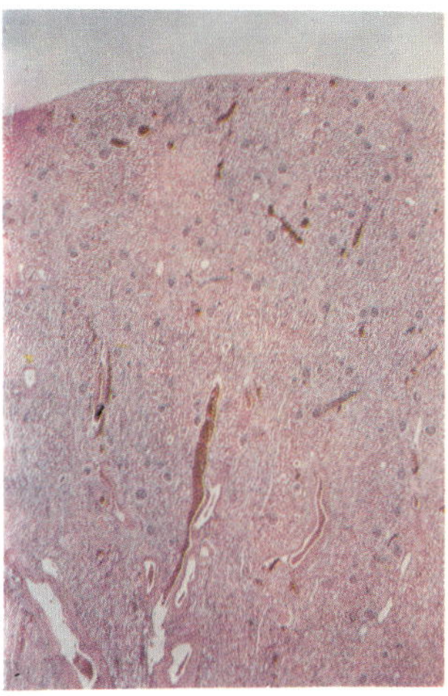

At scanning power two slight indentations of the cortex are visible, and subjacent to each there is a small focus of cortical fibrous connective tissue which has contracted slightly. Other than this, the tissue appears normal with abundant tubules and evenly spaced glomeruli of expected number. Arteries, small arteries, and arterioles are not unusual.

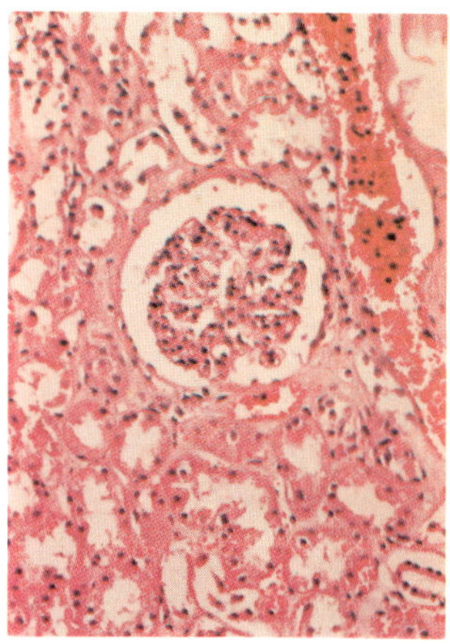

At higher power, a glomerulus reveals normal cellularity and delicate capillary buds. The space of Bowman is empty, and the glomerular membrane is uniformly thin. The adjacent tubules are not remarkable.

SHOCK KIDNEY

The capsules are stripped with ease to reveal large pale smooth kidneys.

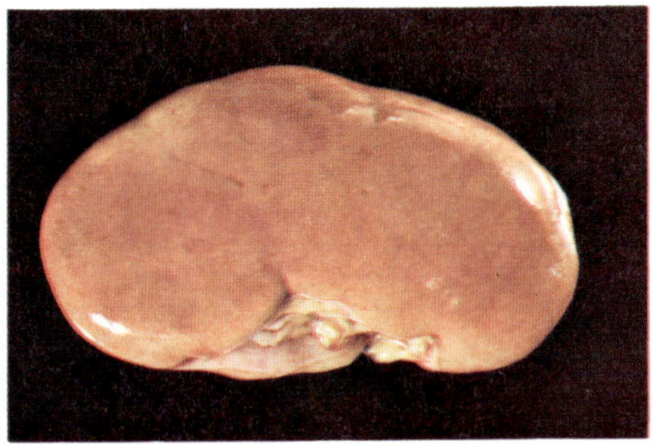

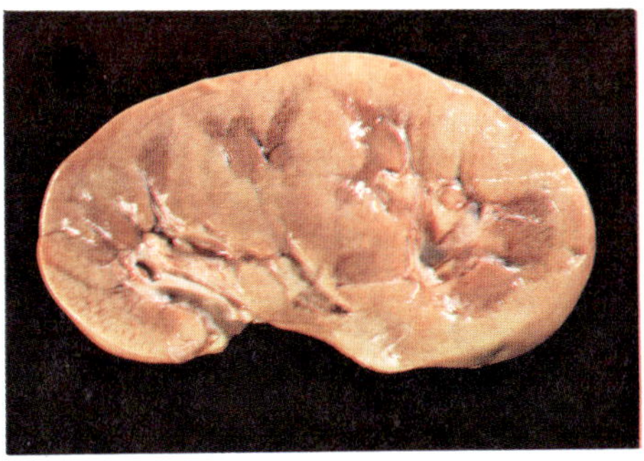

The cut surfaces disclose pallor and thickening of the cortex with cortical striations that are indistinct and a corticomedullary junction that is poorly delineated.

The microsection reveals glomeruli of normal appearance and tubules that display some casts. The interstitial tissue is edematous.

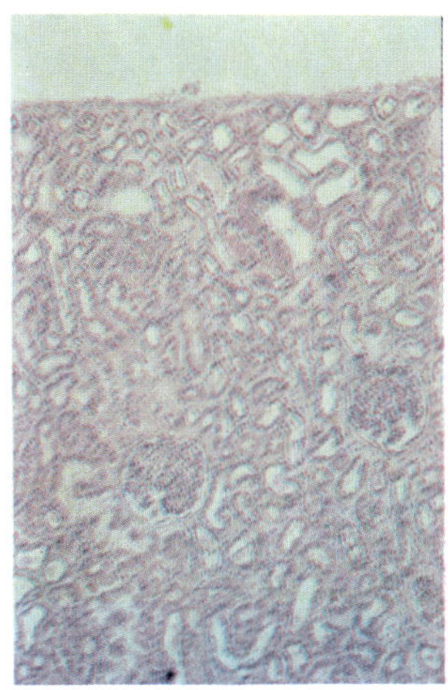

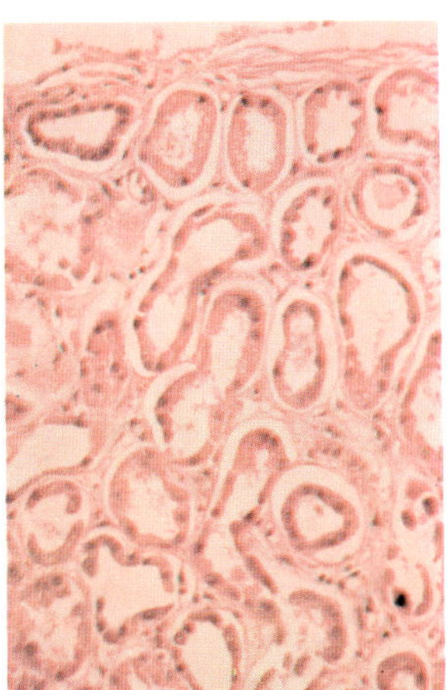

At higher power tubular cells display a loss of cytoplasm, some reveal a failure of nuclear staining, and the interstitial tissue between the tubules is abundant, loosely constructed, and edematous.

SHOCK KIDNEY

CLINICAL ACCOUNT 5915

The patient was a Negro woman 28 years old who took a steroid medication for two weeks because of swelling and tenderness of the thyroid. The symptoms subsided; the medication was continued. One week before admission her morning cough became worse, malaise was noted, and the temperature rose to 99.6 degrees F. On the day of admission she had a sharp pain in the right chest that was accentuated by deep breathing. She then became short of breath, the cough worsened, and abundant "dirty" sputum was raised.

The temperature was 102 degrees F., pulse 120, respirations 32, and blood pressure 120/70. Breath sounds were decreased, and coarse rales were heard. The urine disclosed 3 plus protein. The hemoglobin was 15.0 Gm., hematocrit 47, and leukocytes 11,000 with 66 neutrophils and 18 band cells. The serum glutamic transaminase and lactic dehydrogenase were elevated. During the hospital course an anemia developed. The leukocytes rose to 24,000 with 59 neutrophils and 22 band cells. A right thoracentesis yielded 300 ml. of bloody fluid. Dyspnea increased. A chest x-ray disclosed a widespread infiltration in both lung fields. Oliguria developed and peritoneal dialysis was performed. Respiratory distress increased, coma supervened, and death occurred on the fifteenth hospital day.

Autopsy examination revealed alveolar proteinosis of the right and left lungs. The lung weights were 950 and 755 Gms., respectively. There was also passive hyperemia of the liver. The right and left kidneys weighed 225 Gm. each.

THE ENTITY

The so-called shock kidney has certain anatomic, functional, and clinical features (1). The gross features are pallor and large size, i.e., in the range of 240 to 300 Gm. On section the cortex is wide, the cortical striations are indistinct, and the corticomedullary junctions are obscure. Under the microscope, the glomeruli appear normal, the interstitial tissue is edematous, and the tubules show a variety of changes that range from nearly normal appearance to widespread necrosis with or without protein or pigment (heme) casts.

Such kidneys are associated with acute renal failure. The clinical course begins with oliguria, i.e., less than 400 ml. per day, which is the least amount necessary to clear metabolites from the blood. This ordinarily lasts about two weeks. During this time the blood urea nitrogen and serum creatinine rise while the urine contains some protein and is of low specific gravity. Later, diuresis develops, i.e., more than 1,000 ml. per day. The specific gravity remains low. The diuretic period tends to last about as long as the oliguric period. Thereafter, the specific gravity rises and function improves until recovery is complete.

Most patients recover, although that is dependent on the cause. The main causes are shock, prolonged hypotension, pronounced hemorrhage, overwhelming infection, crush injuries, and tubular poisons.

1. Heptinstall, R.H. Pathology of the Kidney. Little, Brown, and Company, Boston, Mass., 1966.

ARTERIOLAR NEPHROSCLEROSIS

CLINICAL ACCOUNT 6369

The patient was a white male 47 years old who was admitted to the hospital because of chronic headaches, dyspnea on exertion, ankle edema, and, during the five days preceding admission, orthopnea and paroxysms of nocturnal dyspnea.

The blood pressure was 190/120 mm. Hg., and the pulse was 95 and irregular. Rales were heard over both posterior bases. The heart was enlarged to the left, and a systolic ejection murmur was audible at the apex. The hemoglobin was 8.7 Gm., hematocrit 26, and leukocytes 8,700 with a normal differential count. The blood urea nitrogen was 86 mg. per 100 ml. The urine revealed 3 plus protein, and the sediment disclosed hyaline and coarsely granular casts. A chest x-ray revealed cardiomegaly, pleural fluid at both bases, and a pulmonary infiltration suggestive of uremic pneumonitis. The patient's condition deteriorated; the blood urea nitrogen rose to 117 mg., and weakness, anorexia, and weight loss developed. Peritoneal dialysis was performed. Hypertension persisted, the blood urea nitrogen continued to rise and the patient became stuporous and then semicomatose. Death occurred after twenty-eight days in the hospital.

Autopsy examination revealed hypertrophy of the heart (675 Gm.), acute fibrinous pericarditis, and marked arteriosclerosis of the right and left coronary arteries. The lungs weighed 450 and 600 Gm., respectively and disclosed edema. The left lung was atelectatic. The peritoneum contained 750 ml. of ascitic fluid. The right and left kidneys weighed 100 and 90 Gm., respectively.

THE ENTITY

In arteriolar nephrosclerosis the kidneys are moderately reduced in size but rarely weigh less than 100 Gm. each. The external surface is finely and uniformly granular. The cut surfaces are firm, the cortical striations are indistinct, and the cortico-pelvic distance is decreased. Microscopically the main lesion is a thickening of the arterioles with a pale pink hyaline material that is most pronounced in the preglomerular segments. As the thickening increases, ischemia develops, the glomerulus atrophies, and the tubule disappears. The connective tissue that replaces these structures then contracts so that the surface is finely pitted and the parenchyma is focally fibrosed. The process is widespread but patchy in distribution so that intervening glomeruli and tubules appear normal. The same change is also seen in other arterioles, especially those of the adrenals, pancreas, and gut. The most common associated lesion is hypertrophy of the heart.

In such cases, so-called 'malignant' hypertension may develop. It is characterized clinically by a further elevation of blood pressure, progressive general deterioration, and rapidly advancing uremia. Anatomically there are, in addition to the arteriolar nephrosclerosis, fibrinoid necrosis of renal arterioles, necrosis of corresponding glomeruli, and necrotizing arteriolitis at other sites, especially gut, pancreas, and retinae (1). The cause of this abrupt clinical and morphologic change is not known.

1. Stoddard, L.D., and Puchtler, H. Human renal vascular lesions and hypertension. Pathology Annual, Vol. 4, p. 253. Appleton-Century-Crofts, New York, 1969.

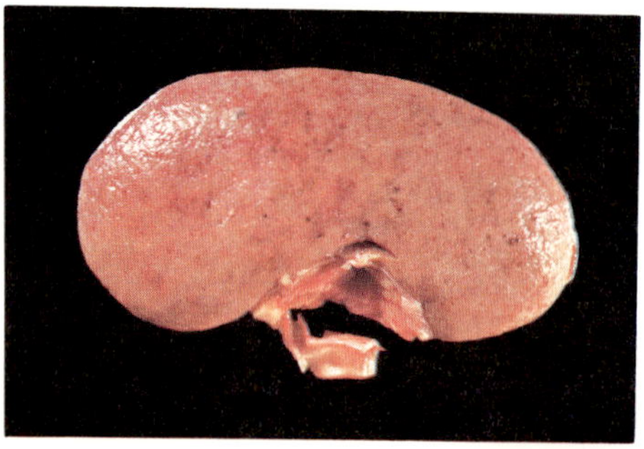

The external surface of the left kidney is pallid and finely granular, with a small number of minute petechiae scattered over the surface. The petechiae are the hallmark of necrotizing arteriolitis, which is the anatomic component of "malignant" hypertension.

The cut surface at a distance is not especially remarkable although the kidney is smaller than normal.

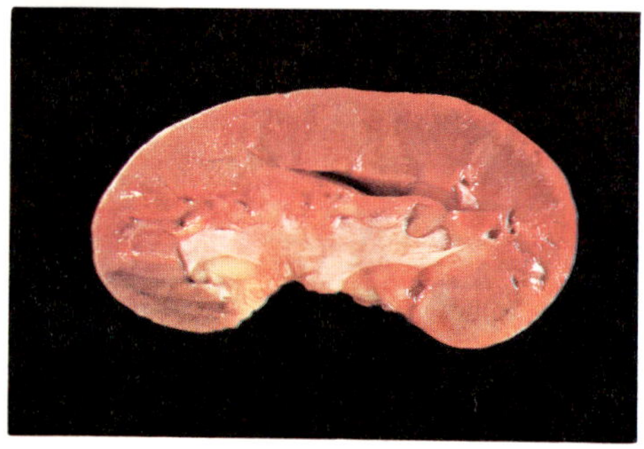

Left: A close-up view reveals that the cortical striations are indistinct and the cortico-medullary junction is obscure. Both of these changes are due to arteriolar narrowing with diffuse atrophy that develops gradually. **Right:** At high magnification three arterioles are seen. Two reveal smudgy pale red transmural alteration that is characteristic of fibrinoid necrosis. It is this vascular change that causes the glomerulus to undergo hemorrhagic necrosis, the tubule to succumb, the blood pressure to rise even further, and the uremia to advance.

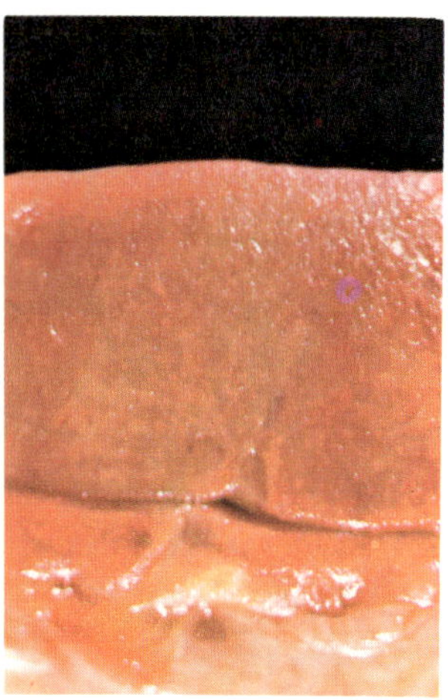

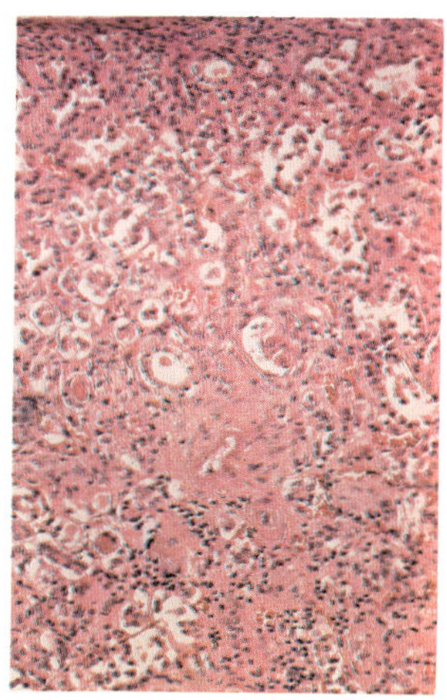

ACUTE PYELONEPHRITIS

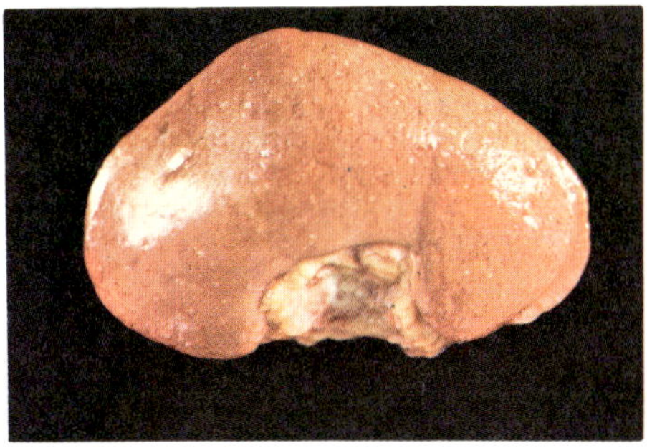

The external surface is smooth and pale red with scattered foci of pale yellowish gray. Foci are minute abscesses.

The cut surface is also pale red flecked with yellowish gray. The latter are due to exudate that fills the abscesses. The pelvic mucosa is hyperemic.

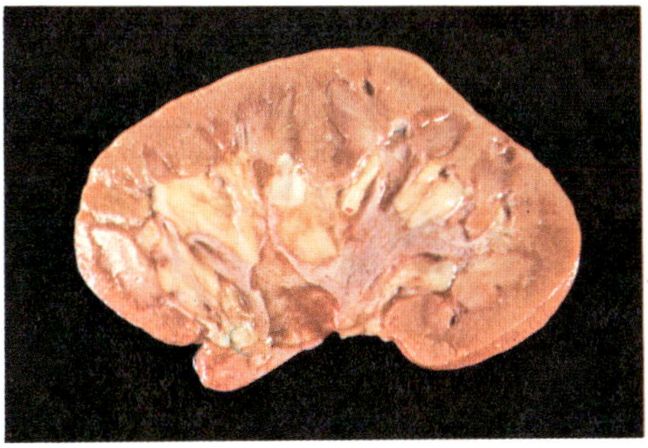

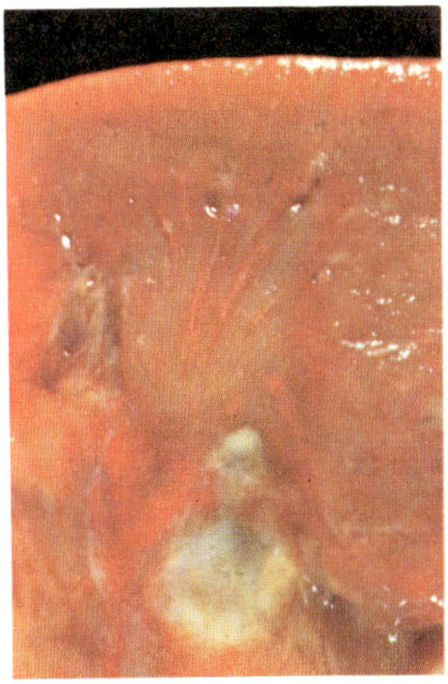

A close-up view reveals an abscess located in the medulla. It is filled with yellowish gray neutrophilic exudate.

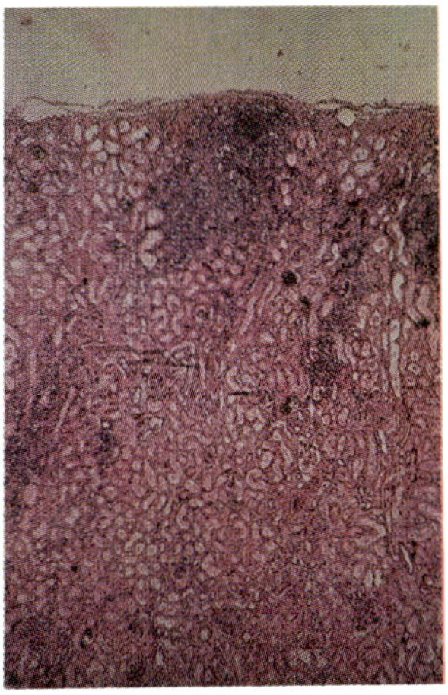

The tissue reveals more or less discrete collections of neutrophilic leukocytes that focally destroy the tissue and create minute abscesses.

ACUTE PYELONEPHRITIS

CLINICAL ACCOUNT 6387

The patient was a white male 85 years old who experienced a change of bowel habit of six weeks duration. He had two to three loose stools per day during this time and in the past month had noted the passage of a small amount of blood. Anorexia had also developed in the preceding two weeks. In addition, on the day before admission, the patient had developed chills, weakness, and chest pain.

The vital signs were normal. The positive physical findings included an enlarged thyroid, a systolic murmur over the entire precordium, a large right inguinal hernia, and a fungating mass on the posterior wall of the rectum 8 cm. above the anal sphincter. The blood and urine were normal. An abdomino-perineal resection was performed. The surgical specimen revealed adenocarcinoma of the rectum. The post-operative course was initially uneventful and thereafter stormy. The temperature rose, the blood pressure fell, and oliguria developed. There were signs of paralytic ileus. The patient died eighteen days after the operation.

Autopsy examination revealed acute suppurative peritonitis. The heart weighed 400 Gm. and disclosed calcific disease of the aortic valve with slight stenosis and calcification of the mitral annulus. The right and left lungs weighed 620 and 510 Gm., respectively, and both were focally atelectatic and moderately edematous. Pleural effusions were present; 400 ml., right, 500 ml., left. An unexpected finding was a small adenocarcinoma of the splenic flexure of the colon. Incidental diagnoses included hyperplasia of the prostate and a nodular colloid goiter that weighed 230 Gm. The kidneys revealed acute suppurative pyelonephritis with abscess formation; they weighed 155 and 150 Gm., respectively.

THE ENTITY

Acute pyelonephritis is a nonspecific bacterial infection of the renal tissue and the pelvic mucosa. It is often due to coliform bacteria (*Escherichia, Aerobacter, Paracolon bacilli*) that reach the kidney by filtration of circulating organisms (blood-borne or bacteremic), or by ascension from a lower urinary tract obstruction (ascending or obstructive) (1). The latter is more common than the former. Causes of obstruction include nodular hyperplasia of the prostate, renal or ureteral calculi, carcinoma of the bladder or uterine cervix, spinal cord injuries with atony of the bladder, pregnancy with compression of the ureters, and instrumentation with the placement of indwelling catheters.

The kidneys are swollen, the cut surfaces bulge, and the external and cut surfaces reveal scattered minute pale yellow abscesses over cortex and medulla. Microscopically there are collections of segmented granulocytes with and without abscess formation, and columns of leukocytes packing the lumens of renal tubules. The pelvic mucosa is hyperemic and acutely inflamed. Complications include perinephric abscess, especially with *Staphylococcus aureus,* and necrosis of the renal papillae, especially with diabetes mellitus.

Clinically there are chills, fever, loin pain, lumbar tenderness, urgency, dysuria, pyuria, bacteriuria, and pus casts in the centrifuged sediment.

1. Heptinstall, R.H. Pathology of the Kidney. Little, Brown and Company, Boston, 1966.

CHRONIC PYELONEPHRITIS

CLINICAL ACCOUNT 6259

The patient was a white male 72 years old who was admitted to the hospital because of chest pain of three days' duration. The pain was midsternal and subxiphoid and radiated to the arms and neck. The patient had experienced exertional angina in the recent past.

The vital signs were normal. The skin was pale. Physical examination otherwise revealed only a systolic ejection murmur along the left sternal border. The urine was normal. The hemoglobin was 14.6 Gm., hematocrit 43, and leukocytes 10,700 with a normal differential count. The serum glutamic transaminase was 205 units. A chest x-ray revealed clear lung fields. The electrocardiogram disclosed changes consistent with myocardial ischemia. On the sixth hospital day hypotension developed, the pain increased, and cyanosis developed. Later that day hypotension became extreme, resuscitative measures failed, and the patient died.

Autopsy examination revealed a recent infarct of the heart, a recent thrombus of the left coronary artery, and a mural thrombus of the left ventricle. The heart weighed 510 Gm. Incidental diagnoses included atherosclerotic stenosis of the left renal artery, arteriolar nephrosclerosis of the right kidney, and nodular hyperplasia of the prostate. The right and left kidneys weighed 125 and 120 Gm., respectively.

THE ENTITY

Chronic pyelonephritis evolves from acute pyelonephritis. It may be unilateral or bilateral. Grossly the external surfaces display broad, flat-based, finely granular, shallow scars of irregular outline that tend to be large and often occur on the "back" of the kidney in the form of a "saddle." Microscopically there are atrophy of nephrons, fibrosis of parenchyma, dilatation of tubules, pink protein-rich fluid resembling colloid within those tubules ("thyroidization"), thickening of arteries and arterioles, periglomerular fibrosis, and collections of lymphocytes and plasma cells throughout the cortex and medulla. The changes are patchy in distribution. If the process is widespread, the kidney may become extremely small.

Unless due to obstruction, the onset is often clinically silent and only such vague symptoms as lassitude, headache, loss of weight, nausea, and indigestion occur (1). The urine reveals frequent proteinuria, sporadic pyuria, and often bacteriuria with 100,000 organisms/ml. on culture. Intravenous pyelography may show reduction of renal size and focal dilatation of calyces. The lesion may heal, leaving only an incidental autopsy observation, may remain active with vague clinical signs, or may progress to renal atrophy with hypertension and cardiac failure or gradually progressive renal failure with uremia.

1. Heptinstall, R.H. Pathology of the Kidney. Little, Brown and Company, Boston, 1966.

CHRONIC PYELONEPHRITIS

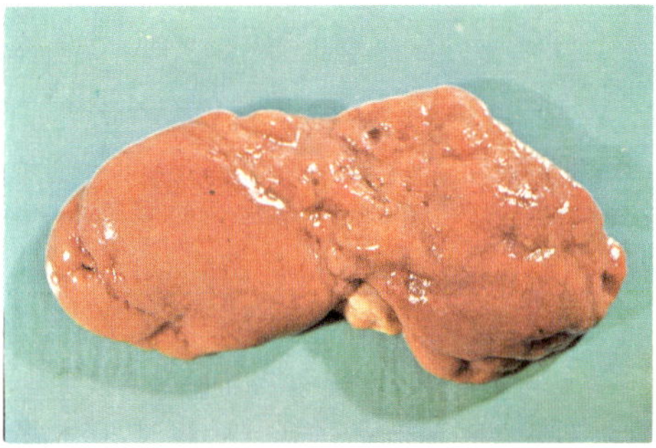

The external surface of the right kidney reveals the large flat scars of irregular outline that are characteristic of chronic pyelonephritis. The bases of such scars are finely granular.

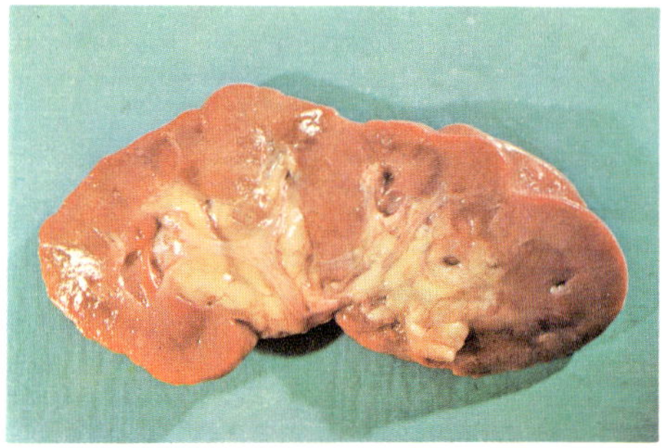

Section reveals focal cortical thinning due to atrophy from the vascular complications of inflammation. Cyst at upper pole is incidental.

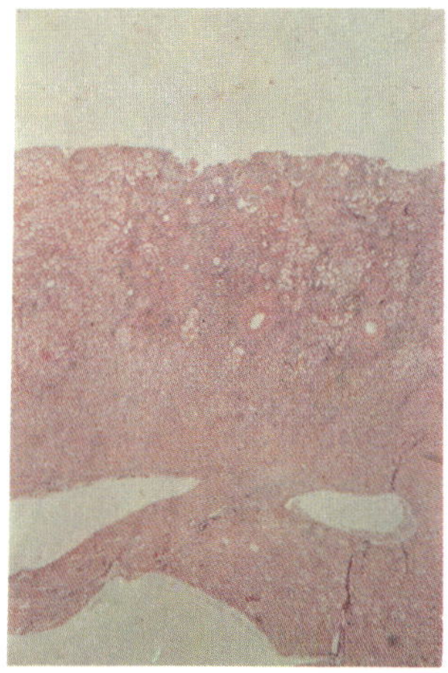

A close-up view discloses that the cortex and medulla are both thin at the sites of scar formation. With this change the pelvic adipose tissue tends to expand and become unusually prominent.

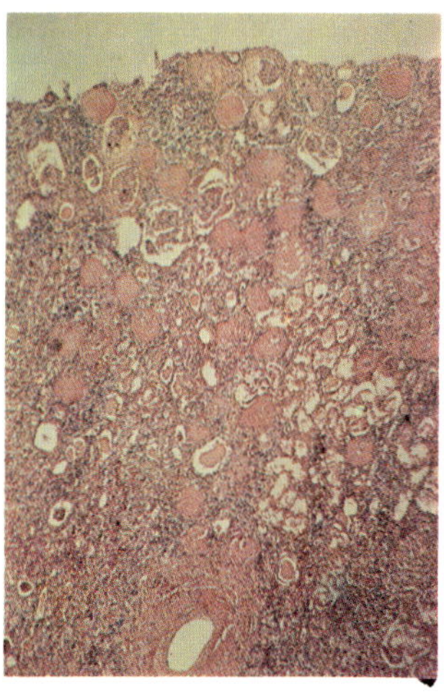

The magnified histologic view taken at the base of a scar reveals hyalinization of glomeruli, extensive interstitial fibrosis, and widespread lymphocytic infiltration. Not seen are three additional characteristics, i.e., dilated tubules filled with clear pale pink "colloid," concentric layers of periarterial fibrous connective tissue, and thick mantles of periglomerular fibrosis.

CHRONIC GLOMERULONEPHRITIS

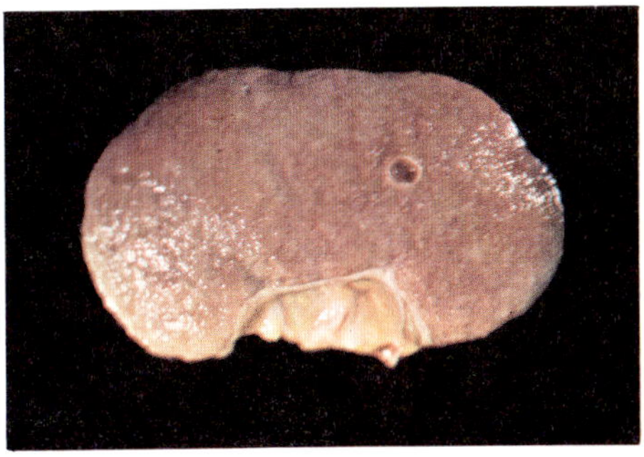

The capsules were stripped with difficulty to reveal a pale grayish pink external surface that is uniformly granular.

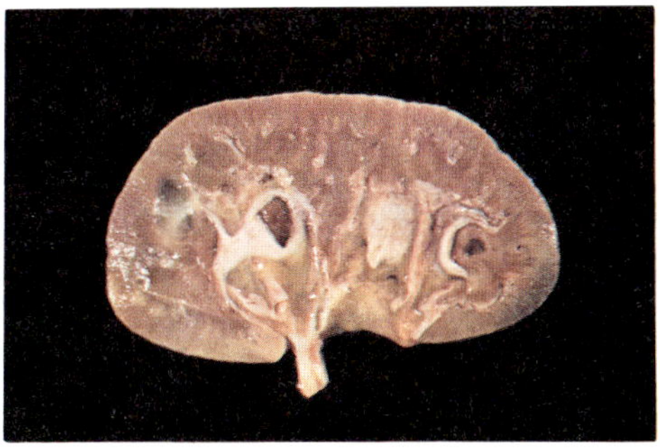

On section the cortex is thin, the cortical striations are indistinct, and the corticomedullary junction is ill-defined. In addition, the tissue is pale, the calyceal mucosa is normal, and two small medullary cysts are present.

Left: At scanning power nearly all of the glomeruli are hyalinized, nearly all of the tubules are atrophic, and nearly all of the interglomerular tissue is replaced with fibrous scar. As the glomeruli become fibrosed, the blood supply to the tubules is diminished, and as the tubules disappear the tissue shrinks and the glomeruli are brought closer together. Thus the concentration of glomeruli in a microscopic field is high. A light lymphocytic infiltration is present in the interstitium. **Right:** At higher power three glomeruli are shown. All are hyalinized. The Bowman's spaces and capillary lumens are obliterated. The periglomerular region is occupied by fibrous scar lightly infiltrated with lymphocytes. Only an occasional tubular remnant is seen. The most important histologic characteristic of chronic glomerulonephritis is the uniformity of the glomerular change.

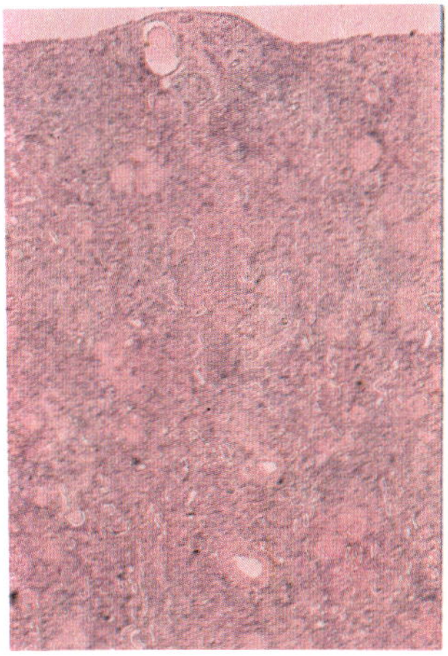

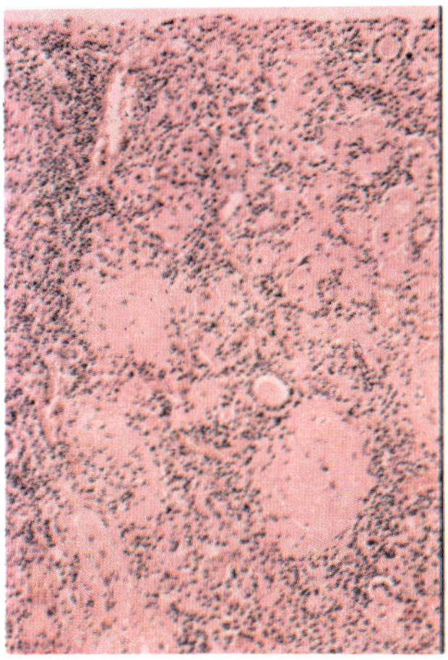

CHRONIC GLOMERULONEPHRITIS

CLINICAL ACCOUNT 5926

The patient was a Negro male 44 years old who was admitted to the hospital because of ankle swelling and shortness of breath of one week's duration. He had been in renal failure for many months and had undergone peritoneal dialysis several times. He was thought to have chronic membranous glomerulonephritis. A weight gain of 7 pounds had taken place during the week prior to admission.

The patient was emaciated and puffy-faced. The temperature was 98.2 degrees F., respirations 20, pulse 80, and blood pressure 160/110 mm. Hg. Physical findings included rales at both bases, enlargement of the heart, a reducible right inguinal hernia, and pronounced pitting edema of the extremities.

The urine was yellow, cloudy, and alkaline. There was a 2 plus proteinuria; the sediment revealed 10 leukocytes per high power field. The hemoglobin was 6.2 Gm., hematocrit 18 per cent, and leukocytes 11,900 with a slight neutrophilia. The blood urea nitrogen and serum creatinine were 99 and 10.6 mg. per 100 ml.

Peritoneal dialysis was performed. Paracentesis removed 1100 ml. of ascitic fluid. An ischiorectal abscess developed and was drained. Massive edema of the scrotum developed and the skin sloughed. He remained afebrile. His sensorium deteriorated and he died after two weeks in the hospital.

Autopsy examination revealed hypertrophy of the heart (560 Gm.), edema of the right and left lungs, empyema of the right pleural space, acute suppurative prostatitis, ischiorectal abscess, and chronic glomerulonephritis. The right and left kidneys weighed 75 Gm. each.

THE ENTITY

There are two kinds of glomerulonephritis: proliferative and membranous. The former affects children, begins abruptly about two weeks after a streptococcus (Beta hemolytic) infection, is manifested by hematuria and proteinuria, and gradually subsides so that about 80 per cent of cases recover completely. Membranous glomerulonephritis affects adults and children, begins gradually, is not preceded by infection, is manifested by subcutaneous edema, especially about the eyes, and is slowly progressive so that renal failure develops and recovery is unusual. Both proliferative and membranous types progress to a chronic state of renal failure in which functional and anatomic changes are similar. Despite these clinical distinctions, in most cases of chronic glomerulonephritis there is no awareness of the nature of the early stages of the condition. In about 20 per cent of cases, the first symptoms begin after the age of 50.

Regardless of initial events, the kidney of chronic glomerulonephritis is small, often weighing from 70 to 90 Gm. The external surface is granular, and on section the cortex is thin and the pelvic fat is increased. The cortical striations are indistinct, and the corticomedullary junction may be obliterated. Microscopically nearly all glomeruli are affected; they may be fibrosed, hyalinized, or hypercellular. Tubules are decreased in number, glomeruli are moved closer together on account of this, and interstitial fibrosis is widespread. Arterioles and small arteries tend to be thickened and hyalinized.

Chronic glomerulonephritis is often discovered in the course of routine urinalysis or in the investigation of periorbital edema or hypertension. The urine shows proteinuria, hematuria, casts, and fixation of the specific gravity at 1.010 to 1.012. The course progresses to uremia with nausea, vomiting, headache, fatigability, and anemia. Death usually occurs in several months to a few years from renal failure, CVA, or cardiac decompensation.

HYDRONEPHROSIS

CLINICAL ACCOUNT 5805

The patient was a white female 76 years old who was admitted to the hospital because of anorexia and orthopnea. The former had begun six weeks previously, and there had been a six-pound loss of weight. Orthopnea was of three weeks' duration and was progressive. The patient was hypertensive but had had no illness referable to the urinary tract.

The temperature was 98.2 degrees F., pulse 114, respirations 22, and blood pressure 200/90. Rales were heard over both lung bases. The heart was not remarkable. The physical examination was not otherwise revealing.

The urine disclosed 2 plus proteinuria. The hemoglobin was 8.8 Gm., the hematocrit was 28, and the leukocytes numbered 14,800 with a normal differential count. The blood urea nitrogen was 81 mg. The serum lactic dehydrogenase was 2160 units per 100 ml. During the hospital course the patient became oliguric. This progressed to anuria on the tenth day. Peritoneal dialysis was performed repeatedly. The blood urea nitrogen and serum creatinine climbed to 177 and 12 mg., respectively. On the fifteenth day a small specimen revealed 4 plus proteinuria. Pulmonary edema developed and the patient died on the seventeenth hospital day.

Autopsy examination revealed hypertrophy and dilatation of the heart, edema of the right and left lungs, pleural effusions of 500 ml. on each side, and bilateral renal cortical necrosis. The right and left kidneys weighed 225 and 175 Gm., respectively.

THE ENTITY

Hydronephrosis is a dilatation of the renal pelvis and calyceal system. It is due to obstruction to the outflow of urine. As the obstruction persists, the pressure increases and the parenchyma becomes atrophic. In extreme cases the cortex may be reduced to a thin rim. If the obstruction is on one side the process is unilateral. If the obstruction is in the ureter, the proximal segment dilates and hydroureter also develops. If the obstruction is at the bladder neck, the process is bilateral and hydronephrosis, hydroureter, and dilatation of the bladder are seen. Microscopically the principal change is dilatation of the distal tubules and collecting ducts with parenchymal atrophy. The process tends to be clinically silent unless atrophy is so extreme that function fails, or infection occurs and pyelonephritis is associated.

The causes of obstruction are organic and neuromuscular. Examples of the former are tumors, aberrant vessels compressing the ureteropelvic junction, and retroperitoneal fibrosis. Examples of the latter are paraplegia, multiple sclerosis, tabes dorsalis, and spina bifida.

HYDRONEPHROSIS

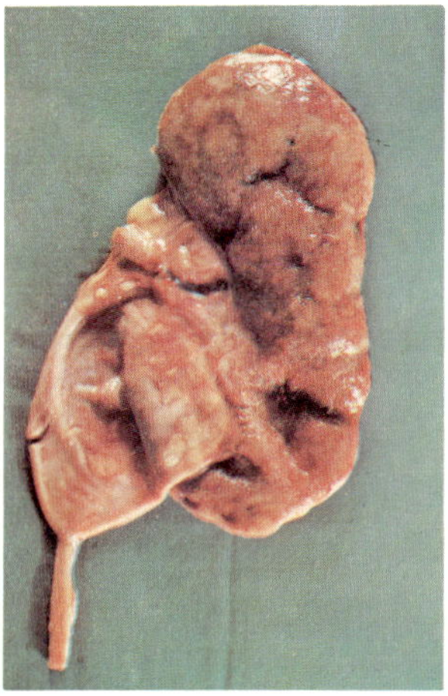

The capsule was stripped with slight difficulty to reveal granular surfaces that are focally deeply scarred. The granular portions are light red mottled with pale yellowish pink. The site of the obstruction is evident at the upper end of the ureter.

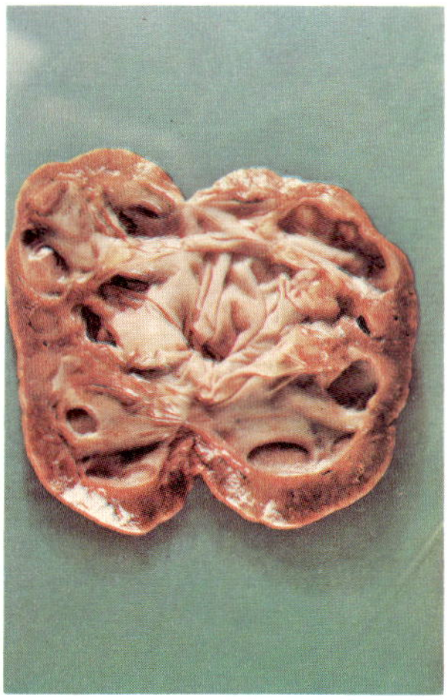

The cut surface discloses pronounced enlargement of the renal pelvis at the expense of the parapelvic adipose tissue and the renal parenchyma. At several sites the latter is reduced to a thin rim of tissue covering the dilated pelvic chamber.

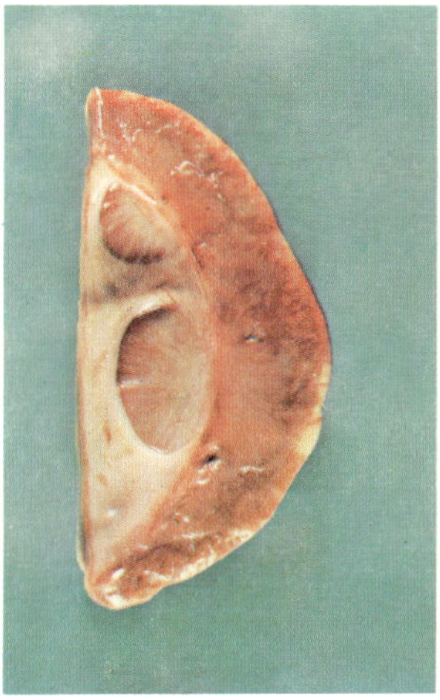

A close-up view shows the atrophy of the renal parenchyma, the enlargement of the calyces, and the smooth thin pale gray nature of the pelvic mucosa. The pale yellowish gray discolorations in the cortex are foci of cortical necrosis independent of the hydronephrosis.

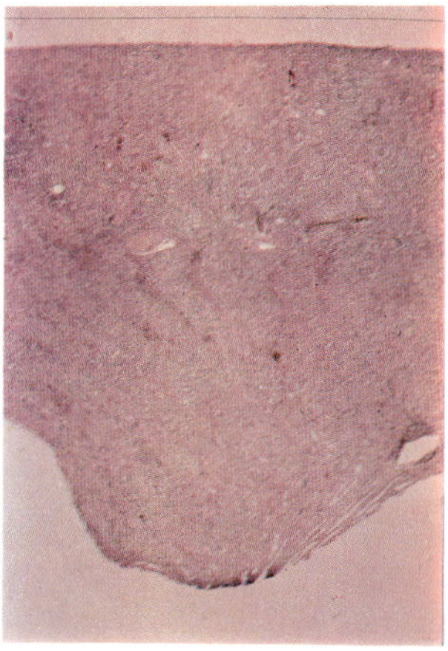

The entire thickness of the renal cut surface is shown with the papilla of a renal pyramid projecting downward in the center. Compression has taken place slowly so that the parenchyma is unscarred and reveals only atrophy.

CYST OF KIDNEY

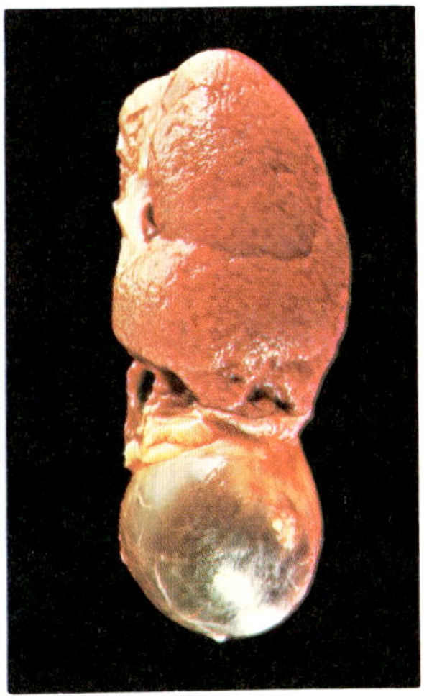

The cyst measures 4.5 cm. in diameter. It has a thin translucent wall and contains a clear pale yellow nonviscid fluid.

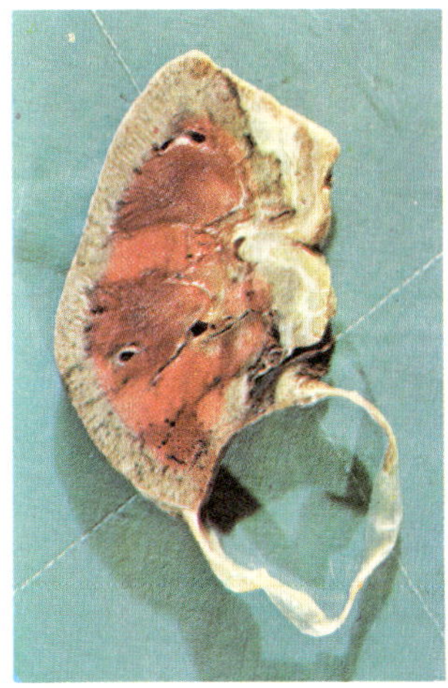

On section the thin wall is evident. The lining surface is smooth. The renal parenchyma and calyceal structure adjacent to the cyst is deformed so that a defect of outline would be expected on either retrograde or intravenous pyelography.

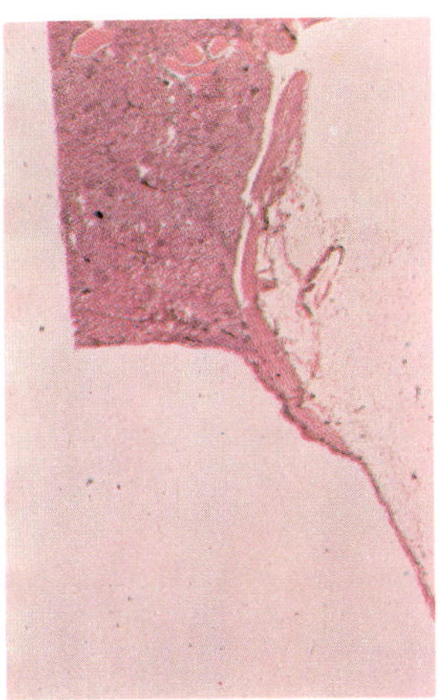

An unmagnified histologic section reveals that the wall of the cyst is composed of nothing more than a thin layer of fibrous connective tissue. The cyst lumen is in the right lower portion of the photo.

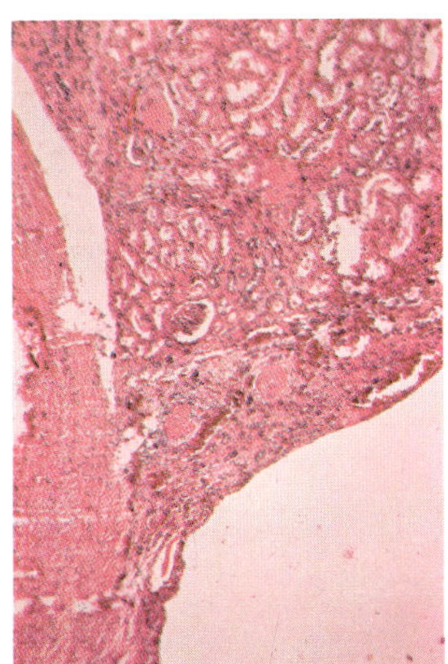

At higher power the juncture of the cyst wall with renal parenchyma is shown. The latter discloses slight compression, but neither inflammation nor significant atrophy is present.

CYST OF KIDNEY

CLINICAL ACCOUNT 6117

The patient was an obese white male 64 years old who had taken nitroglycerine for angina pectoris for several years. On the day of admission, after a big dinner, the patient suffered acute anterior chest pain, vomited, and collapsed. An electrocardiogram disclosed bradycardia, heart block and recent infarction. The blood pressure was 170/100. His skin was cool and moist. He was admitted to the emergency room where cyanosis and Cheyne-Stokes respirations were observed. The blood pressure fell to 60-70 systolic, and the heart rate increased to 130 per minute. Heart sounds were faint, and rales were audible over all lung fields. He was given Dilaudid, atropine, and Aramine. He died two hours after entering the hospital.

Autopsy examination revealed a recent infarct of the postero-medial papillary muscle of the left ventricle, an old infarct of the myocardium, marked arteriosclerosis of both coronary arteries, and edema of the right and left lungs. There were also focal chronic pyelonephritis, calculi of the left renal pelvis, and a cyst of the lower pole of the left kidney.

THE ENTITY

Renal cysts occur in three forms: small and multiple, single and large, and congenital and polycystic. At least half of all persons over 50 years of age have small multiple cysts in their kidneys. These cysts are of no clinical or functional significance. Since they are uncommon at birth, it is presumed that they are acquired, and it is likely that they are due to focal cortical obstructions of the nephrons. They tend to be associated with diffuse disease of the renal parenchyma (1).

Single large cysts likely arise by the same mechanism. The are less common, measure several centimeters in diameter, and are usually unilateral. The cyst wall is a thin layer of pale yellowish gray connective tissue that is translucent. The inner surface is smooth and glistening, and may be trabeculated. The lumen contains clear thin pale yellow fluid. The cysts are asymptomatic unless complicated by hemorrhage, infection or rupture. The larger cysts compress and indent the renal surface and may be discernible by abdominal palpation or radiographic examination. In these instances they must be distinguished from renal cell carcinoma. They are not associated with functional disturbance or abnormal excretion of enzymes in the urine.

1. Hepinstall, R.H. Pathology of the Kidney. Little, Brown and Company, Boston, 1966.

SCLERODERMA KIDNEY

CLINICAL ACCOUNT 6077

The patient was a white female 48 years old who entered the hospital because of headache and shortness of breath. She was last well eight months previously, when thrombophlebitis caused pain and swelling in the left arm. Later stiffness of the hands and feet developed, and this was associated with tightening of the skin, especially of the fingers. On exposure to cold the fingers blanched markedly and then turned purple. Dysphagia had been noted for the past two months. Three days before admission a persistent headache developed. There had also been recent blurring of vision in the right eye.

The blood pressure was 190/130 mm. Hg. The skin of the face was tight, shiny, and pale. The skin of the hands was similar, and the fingers could not be clenched. Laboratory examination revealed anemia and 3 plus proteinuria. There was restrictive impairment of pulmonary function; the vital capacity was 65 per cent of normal. Preparations for LE cells were negative. The blood urea nitrogen was 89 mg. per 100 ml. Renal failure developed and in four weeks the blood urea nitrogen rose to 300 mg. and the serum creatinine to 13 mg. per 100 ml. Anuria was treated by peritoneal dialysis. Lethargy was progressive, and the patient died in uremia on the thirtieth hospital day.

Autopsy examination revealed extensive fibrosis of both lungs, focal bronchopneumonia, and small foci of necrosis in the right and left adrenals. Collagen in the skin was excessive. Permission for examination of the brain was not given. The right and left kidneys weighed 160 Gm. each.

THE ENTITY

Scleroderma is a systemic disease of unknown cause that begins gradually, often between the ages of 20 and 50 years, and affects females more often than males. The skin, especially of the fingers, shows shiny atrophy, condensation of collagen, and flexure contractions with ulceration. Raynaud's phenomenon is frequently associated. Later, involvement of heart, lungs, and esophagus becomes evident. At these sites collagen replaces muscle, and function gradually fails. The course is slowly progressive.

Uncommonly the course is fulminant, and in these cases renal involvement is common. Medium and small arteries display subintimal fibrosis and fibrinoid necrosis with infarction of the renal cortex. Infarction occurred in five of thirty-one autopsied cases (1). The clinical indications of florid renal involvement include pronounced hypertension of sudden onset, cardiac failure, headache, visual disturbance, convulsions, and rapidly progressive renal failure (2).

1. Piper, W.N., and Helwig, E.B. Progressive systemic sclerosis. Arch. Derm. 72:535, 1955.
2. Rodnan, G.P., Schreiner, G.E., and Black, R.L. Renal involvement in progressive systemic sclerosis (generalized scleroderma). Am. J. Med. 23:445, 1957.

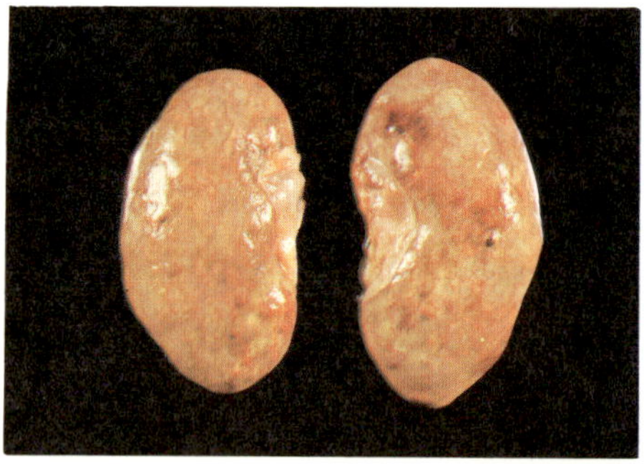

The renal capsules were stripped with ease, and the external surfaces are smooth and light red mottled with pale yellow.

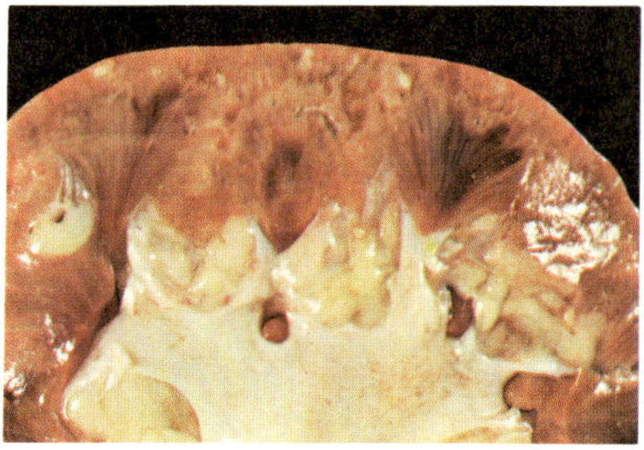

The cut surfaces on close examination reveal foci of cortical necrosis that are pale yellow and zones of recent hemorrhage that are dark red. The necrosis extends into the columns of Bertin, but not into the medulla or renal pyramids.

Left: The necrosis is coagulative in nature, and the junction of necrotic tissue (above) with viable tissue (below) is evident. **Right:** The reason for the cortical infarction is the fibrinoid necrosis of small arteries in the cortical tissue. This occurs elsewhere in the body but is especially common in the kidneys. It is the cause of the hypertension, oliguria, and progressive renal failure.

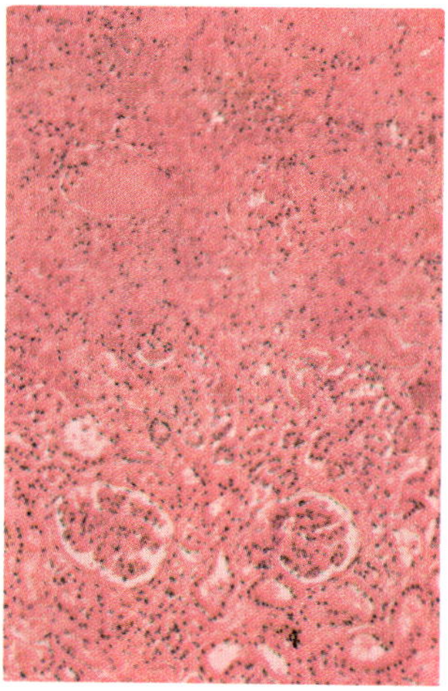

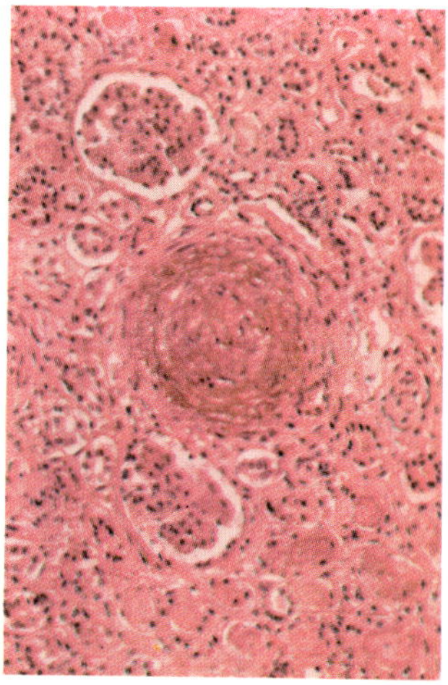

RENAL CORTICAL NECROSIS

The external surfaces are slightly granular and light red mottled with pale yellow. The foci of yellow discoloration are suggestive of cortical abscesses that are characteristic of acute suppurative pyelonephritis.

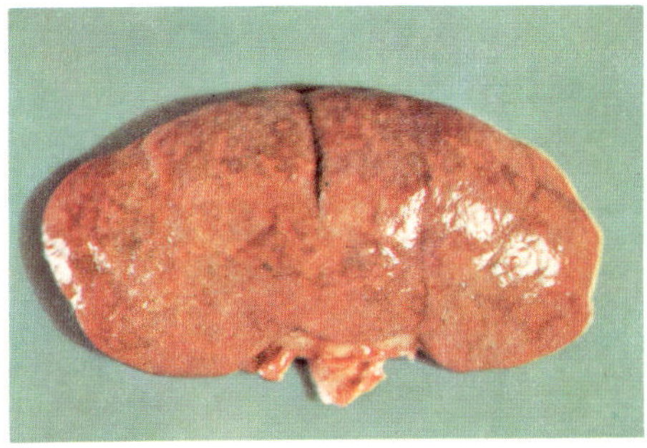

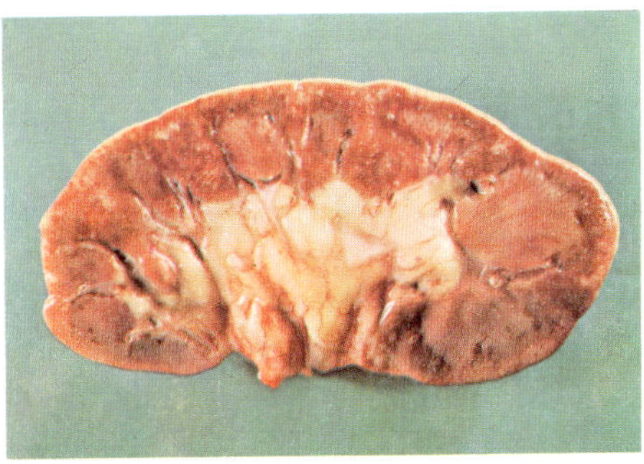

On section the yellow foci are limited to the cortex and instead of exuding pus from small abscesses, the lesions are solid and more or less dry. Sparing of the medullary pyramids is evident. Foci of hemorrhage in the cortex suggest new sites of more necrosis.

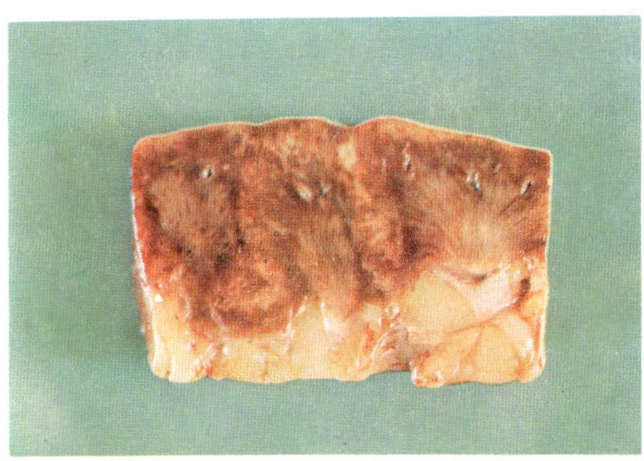

A closer view reveals extensive necrosis of the cortex that extends deeply into the columns of Bertin but spares the medullary tissue.

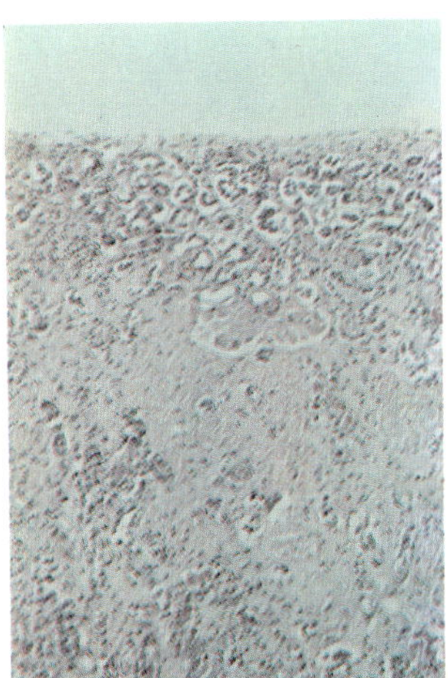

At scanning power the necrosis is evident. It usually extends just short of the surface so that a viable rim of tissue is left; this is seen in the picture. The coagulative nature of the necrosis due to ischemia is also apparent.

RENAL CORTICAL NECROSIS

CLINICAL ACCOUNT 5805

The patient was a white female 76 years old who was admitted to the hospital because of anorexia and orthopnea. The former had begun six weeks previously, and there had been a 6-pound loss of weight. Orthopnea was of three weeks' duration and was progressive. The patient was hypertensive but had had no illness referable to the urinary tract.

The temperature was 98.2 degrees F., pulse 114, respirations 22, and blood pressure 200/90. Rales were heard over both lung bases. The heart was not remarkable. The physical examination was not otherwise revealing.

The urine disclosed 2 plus proteinuria. The hemoglobin was 8.8 Gm., the hematocrit was 28, and the leukocytes numbered 14,800 with a normal differential count. The blood urea nitrogen was 81 mg. The serum lactic dehydrogenase was 2160 units per 100 ml. During the hospital course the patient became oliguric. This progressed to anuria on the tenth day. Peritoneal dialysis was performed repeatedly. The blood urea nitrogen and serum creatinine climbed to 177 and 12 mg., respectively. On the fifteenth day a small specimen revealed 4 plus proteinuria. Pulmonary edema developed, and the patient died on the seventeenth hospital day.

Autopsy examination revealed hypertrophy and dilatation of the heart, edema of the right and left lungs, pleural effusions of 500 ml. on each side, and bilateral renal cortical necrosis. The right and left kidneys weighed 225 and 175 Gm., respectively.

THE ENTITY

Renal cortical necrosis is an uncommon bilateral lesion that is characterized pathologically by ischemic necrosis of cortical tissue and thrombosis of interlobular arteries. The necrosis may be extensive and appear as a yellow cortical ribbon; it also may be patchy, appearing as foci of yellow cortical discoloration. The kidneys are large, the medullae and subcapsular portions are spared, and the tubules, arteries, veins, and glomeruli become necrotic. Necrosis may also occur in the adrenals, liver, pituitary, and gut (1).

The condition is almost always secondary to a serious illness, i.e., about ⅔ of the cases are associated with a complication of pregnancy, especially placenta previa and hemorrhage during delivery. Other cases are associated with septicemia and occasionally acute hemorrhagic pancreatitis. The condition affects males and females, adults and children. The clinical onset is characterized by flank pain, abnormal urine, and oliguria that rapidly progresses to anuria. The urine contains much protein, and many erythrocytes, leukocytes, and casts. When the lesion is widespread in both kidneys, the condition is irreversible. When patchy in distribution, however, recovery may occasionally follow the procedure of dialysis.

The reason for the arterial thrombosis is not known.

1. Hamburger, J. Nephrology II. W.B. Saunders Co., Philadelphia, 1968.

CARCINOMA OF KIDNEY

CLINICAL ACCOUNT 6074

The patient was a white man 57 years old who entered the hospital because of chills and fever of six weeks' duration. At age 41 proteinuria was discovered, at age 44 hypertension developed, and at age 54 back pain, fever and hematuria were noted. A cyst of the left kidney was diagnosed. Subsequently, there were episodes of prostatitis and urinary tract infections. At age 56 renal failure developed and peritoneal dialysis had been performed three times per week until admission. The patient was emaciated. The temperature was 98.4 degrees F., pulse rate 88, respiratory rate 18, and blood pressure 110/56 mm. Hg. Physical examination was not remarkable except for a slightly tender mass, thought to be spleen, in the left upper quadrant of the abdomen. The urine was hazy with 3 plus proteinuria and amorphous urates in the sediment. The hemoglobin was 6.2 Gm., the hematocrit 20 per cent, and the leukocytes numbered 3,300 with a normal differential count. The blood urea nitrogen was 51 mg. and the serum creatinine was 4.4 mg. The serum alkaline phosphatase was 60 units per 100 ml. X-rays disclosed normal bones and nodular densities in the lungs. The serum magnesium was 5 mg. Renal failure progressed and the patient became somnolent and died after five weeks in the hospital.

Autopsy examination revealed a carcinoma of the left kidney, marked chronic pyelonephritis of the right kidney, and metastatic carcinoma of the heart, lungs, pleura, and left adrenal. There were also hypertrophy of the heart (520 Gm.), acute fibrinous pericarditis, and pleural effusions (200 ml., right, 150 ml., left). Other findings were incidental. The left kidney weighed 150 Gm.

THE ENTITY

Renal cell carcinoma comprises 85 per cent of all malignant tumors of the kidney. It arises in tubular cells, is equally common in the two kidneys, occurs twice as often in males as females, and appears in the age interval of 50 and 75 years. The clinical features are hematuria, flank pain, and palpable mass. Less often there are fever, anorexia, and weight loss. Intravenous pyelography reveals a nonfunctional mass that is indistinguishable from a cyst. Urinary alkaline phosphatase and lactic dehydrogenase are elevated with carcinoma but not cyst and indicate the diagnosis (1). Uncommonly polycythemia is pronounced and is attributed to erythropoietin production by the tumor. The tumor is round, circumscribed, yellow mixed with red and gray, and tends to grow into the renal vein and embolize into the vena cava. Most tumors at operation measure 5 cm. in diameter, at which time about half extend into the renal vein. With that invasion, the 5-year survival is about 30 per cent; without that invasion, about 55 per cent. Metastases are especially common in lungs, liver, bone, and brain.

1. Amador, E., Zimmerman, T.S., and Wacker, W.E.C. Urinary Alkaline Phosphatase Activity. JAMA 185:769, 1963.

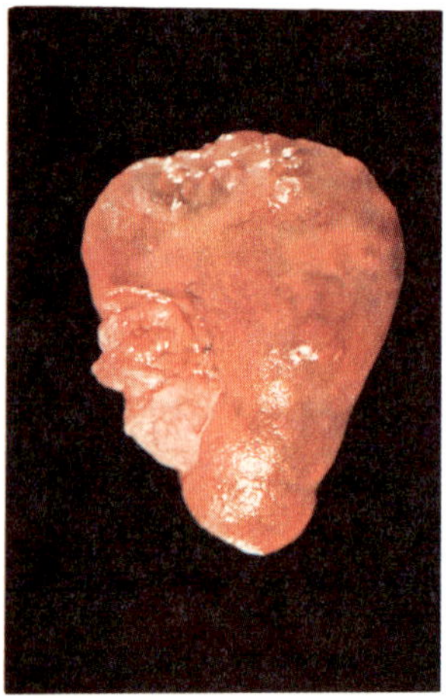

The upper pole is markedly enlarged and coarsely scarred; the lower pole is finely granular and light red.

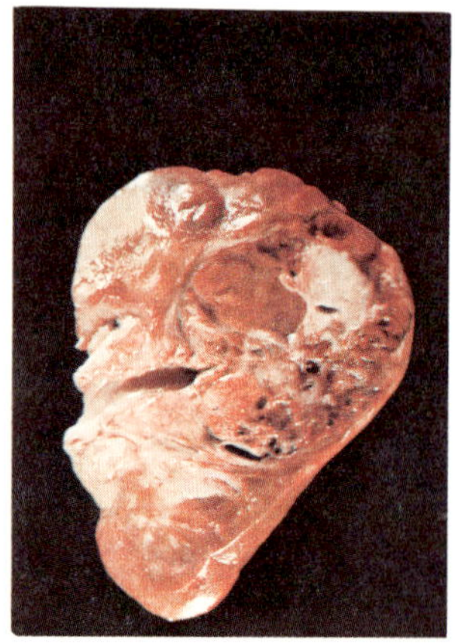

On section a sharply circumscribed approximately round tumor mass measuring 6 cm. in diameter is evident. The tumor tissue is red mottled with pale yellow. The renal parenchyma at the margin is thin and compressed. The renal vein is opened at the hilum and extension of tumor into it is not seen.

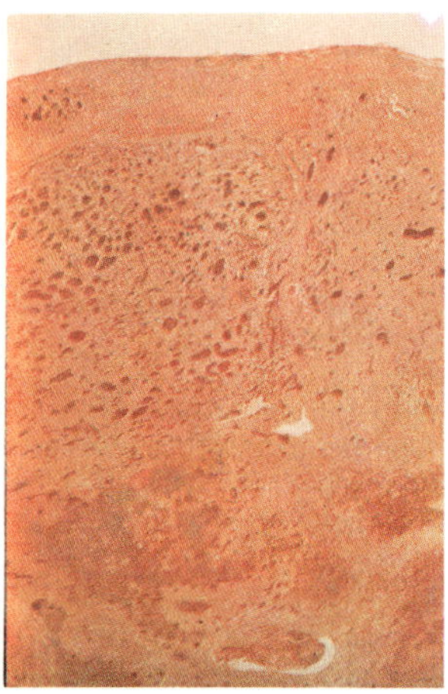

At scanning power the marginal cortex is thin and fibrosed, and the subjacent tumor mass is markedly vascular and hyperemic. Foci of necrosis are present in the lower portion of the picture.

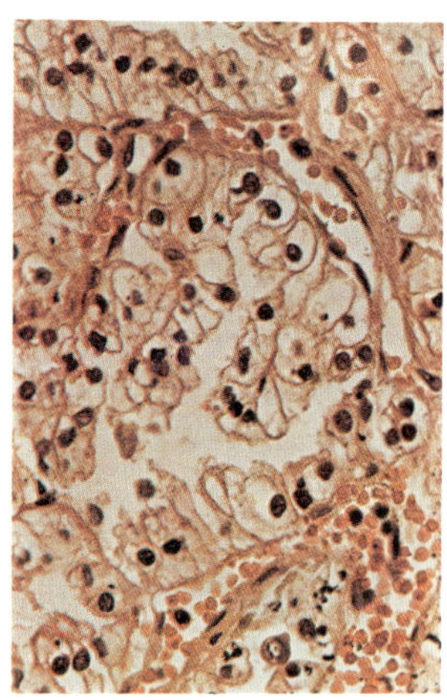

At high magnification, the "clear cells" characteristic of renal carcinoma are apparent. This is due to the dissolution of lipids in the cytoplasm of the tumor cells as the tissue is subjected to fat solvents in preparation for paraffin embedding. It is therefore artefact and is not a sound basis for the nomenclature of the tumor ("clear cell carcinoma"). An alveolated pattern is suggestive of tubule formation by the tumor cells. Mitotic figures are scarce.

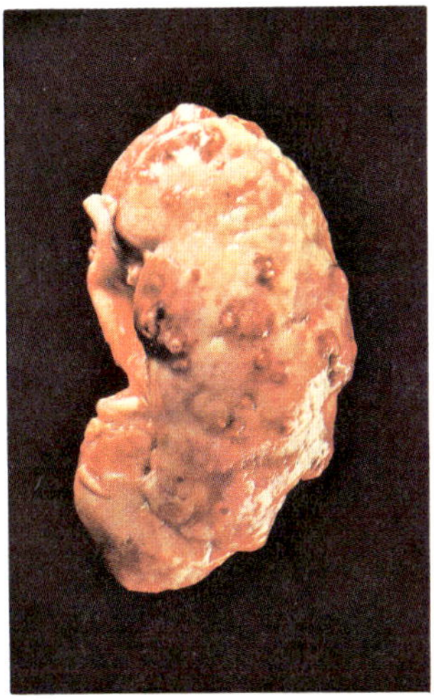

The right kidney was finely granular and displayed only arteriolarsclerosis; no tumor was identified. The left kidney is coarsely scarred and reveals large raised soft nodules that distort the surface.

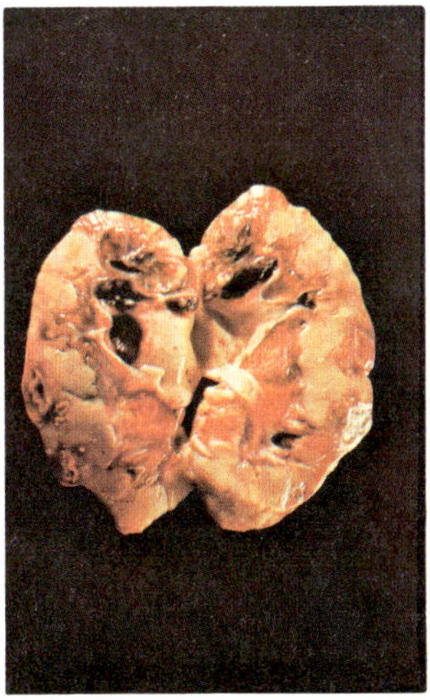

Section of the left kidney reveals large, raised, yellowish red tumor nodules that distort the cut surface. Recent hemorrhage occupies portions of the pelvis.

Left: At scanning power, the tumor nodules are seen to be composed of discrete leukemic cell infiltrations about which there are foci of recent hemorrhage, and within which there are zones of coagulative necrosis. **Right:** At higher magnification the leukocytic mass is seen to separate and destroy the renal tubules. The infiltration is myelocytic although cell type is not identifiable at this power, and is sometimes difficult with the hematoxylin and eosin stain which is designed for tissues rather than cellular elements of the blood.

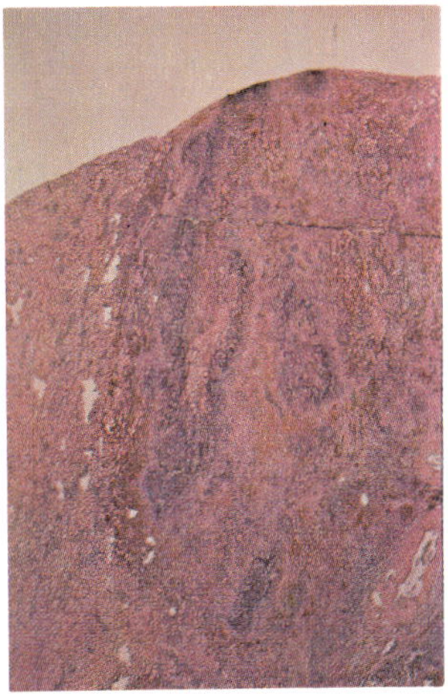

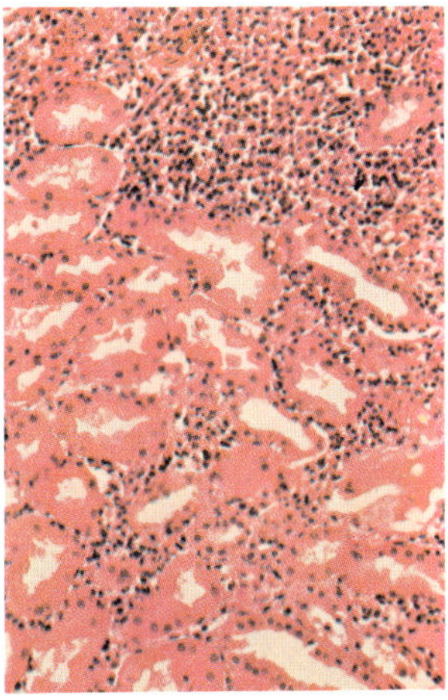

LEUKOSIS OF KIDNEY

CLINICAL ACCOUNT 6127

The patient was a white female 72 years old who entered the hospital because of slight vaginal bleeding of five weeks' duration. Prolapse of the uterus was discovered and a hysterectomy was performed. The hemoglobin was 12.5 Gm., the hematocrit was 39 per cent, and the leukocytes numbered 5,100 with a normal differential count. The patient recovered uneventfully.

Four months later she was readmitted because of headache, weakness, and poor appetite of several weeks' duration. There were also dizzy spells and calf pain on exercise. The skin was pallid. Liver, spleen, and lymph nodes were not palpable. The hemoglobin was 5.2 Gm., the hematocrit was 15 per cent, and the leukocytes numbered 3,300 with 47 segmented granulocytes, 36 lymphocytes, 14 band cells, and 3 monocytes. The bone marrow disclosed acute monocytic leukemia. The patient was given Purinethol and prednisone and was discharged after two weeks in the hospital.

One month later she was readmitted for transfusion. The physical findings were unchanged except for widespread ecchymoses. The urine was normal except for 2 plus proteinuria. The hemoglobin was 7.6 Gm., the hematocrit was 24 per cent, and the leukocytes numbered 6,500 with 63 neutrophils, 14 band cells, and 23 lymphocytes. The platelet count was 3,000 per cmm. Her condition regressed, and she died after six days in the hospital.

Autopsy examination revealed leukosis of the bone marrow and left kidney, recent hemorrhage in the stomach and intestine, and recent infarcts of the spleen. These findings confirmed the diagnosis of acute granulocytic leukemia. The right and left kidneys weighed 100 and 150 Gm., respectively.

THE ENTITY

The principal morphologic manifestation of leukemia is cellular infiltration of tissues. This process, called leukosis, regularly occurs in the hemopoietic organs, i.e., liver, spleen, bone marrow, and lymph nodes. The kidney is the most frequently involved extra-hemopoietic tissue; renal leukosis was seen in 78 of 123 cases in one series (1), and in 109 of 214 cases in another (2). The process occurs in two forms, nodular and diffuse. In the former the nodules arise especially in the cortex, elevate the surface, and display marginal hemorrhage. In the latter the infiltration is even and the kidney may be symmetrically enlarged.

The urine in cases of leukemia usually reveals proteinuria, erythrocytes, and leukocytes whether or not renal leukosis is present. Renal leukosis is therefore not a common cause of functional impairment, and neither azotemia nor hypertension can ordinarily be attributed to it. There is no predilection for any special type of leukemia with respect to renal involvement.

1. Kirshbaum, J.D., and Preuss, F.S. Leukemia. Arch. Int. Med. 71:777, 1943.
2. Norris, H.J., and Wiener, J. The renal lesions of leukemia. Am. J. Med. Sci. 241:512, 1961.

CARCINOMA OF RENAL PELVIS

CLINICAL ACCOUNT R3860

The patient was a white female 67 years old who developed a colicky pain in the left flank that radiated to the left labium. The pain began four months before admission to the hospital. It then subsided, and for the preceding three months there had been painless hematuria. During the latter part of this time, small blood clots had also appeared in the urine.

The blood pressure was 174/100 mm. Hg. The only positive physical finding was a mass in the right breast. The hemoglobin was 9.7 Gm., hematocrit 29, and leukocytes 7,500 with a normal differential count. The urine revealed 4 plus protein and 6 to 8 leukocytes and 8 to 10 erythrocytes per high power field of centrifuged sediment. A chest x-ray disclosed cardiac enlargement and clear lung fields. Retrograde pyelograms revealed incomplete filling of the lower pole on the left, and cystoscopic examination disclosed a normal urinary bladder and patent ureteral orifices. On the fifth hospital day a left nephro-ureterectomy was performed. The patient recovered uneventfully. Although bilateral mammograms were normal, biopsy of the right breast disclosed a carcinoma. The patient was discharged after twenty days in the hospital.

THE ENTITY

Carcinoma of the renal pelvis comprises about 8 per cent of all renal cancers, occurs equally in the two kidneys, and arises from transitional mucosa of the pelvic or calyceal surface (1). The tumor tends to be flat and sessile with a papillary surface and an invasive base. The chief biologic characteristic is spread by contiguous surface extension in the renal pelvis and by separate implantations down the ureter and occasionally into the urinary bladder, especially about the ureteral orifice. The invasive bases at these sites eventually penetrate the ureteral lymphatics so that spread occurs to the para-aortic lymph nodes adjacent to the renal hilum.

The tumor occurs more often in men than women (4:1), usually after the age of 40. The outstanding clinical characteristic is hematuria that is first intermittent, then becomes constant, and later progresses to the passage of blood clots and minute bits of tissue. Pain is infrequent unless the uretero-pelvic junction becomes obstructed. In that event hydronephrosis develops and there is a dull ache in the loin. The diagnosis is indicated by pyelography which discloses an irregular filling defect of the pelvis or calyx, and by cytology of the urine which may reveal papillary fronds of transitional mucosa. Metastases are first clinically evident in the supraclavicular region and are neither massive in lung ("cannonball"), nor common in bone. The tumor does not respond to radiation or chemotherapy; treatment consists of nephro-ureterectomy.

1. Campbell, M.F., and Harrison, J.H. Urology, Vol. 2, p. 930. W.B. Saunders Co., Philadelphia, 1970.

CARCINOMA OF RENAL PELVIS

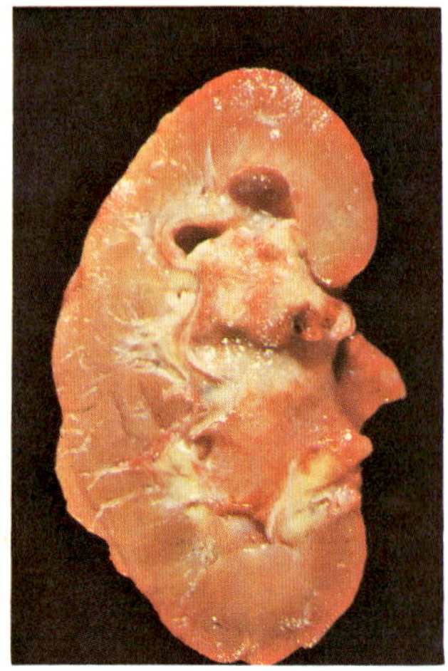

The kidney is of normal size and weight. The cut surface reveals the flat broad scars of chronic pyelonephritis. Also, the pelvic mucosa of the lower pole reveals a sessile pale gray granular tumor that projects into the calyx and extends outward as far as the uretero-pelvic junction. The mucosa of the calyx behind the tumor is unusually thick.

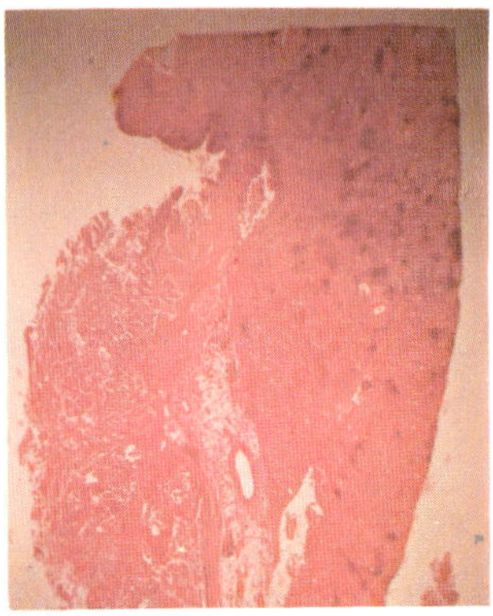

The unmagnified histologic section reveals that the tumor is papillary, the tissue subjacent to the sessile base is only slightly invaded, and pyelonephritis extensively involves the renal parenchyma.

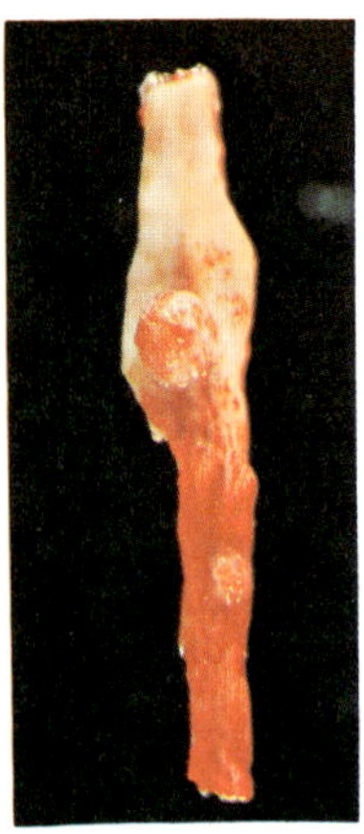

The attached ureter reveals two separate tumors, the upper large and pedunculated, the lower small and sessile. On histologic examination, both were found to be papillary. The upper tumor caused obstruction of the ureter proximal to it. Infection of that stagnant urine likely contributed to the pyelonephritis of the kidney. The obstruction may also have been the cause of the flank pain experienced by the patient.

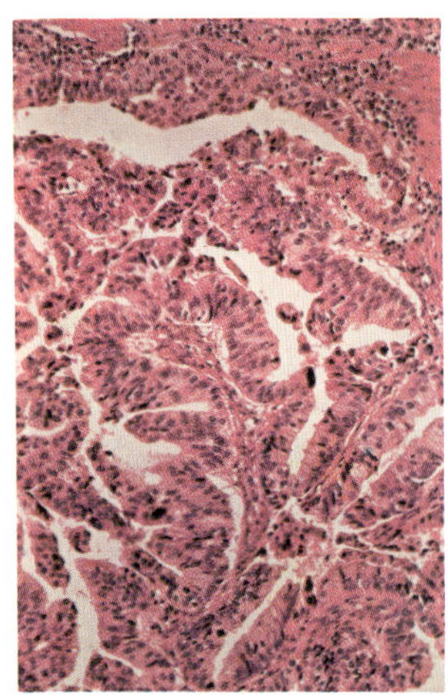

The magnified section shows that the renal pelvic tumor is papillary in nature with scant stroma, moderate anaplasia, and a light leukocytic infiltration. Nuclear size, shape, and staining are irregular, and occasional mitotic figures are present. Although occasional cells are columnar, the tumor is transitional, and the diagnosis is papillary transitional cell carcinoma of the renal pelvis.

LUPUS KIDNEY

The external surface is finely granular. There is no gross feature that is characteristic of lupus erythematosus.

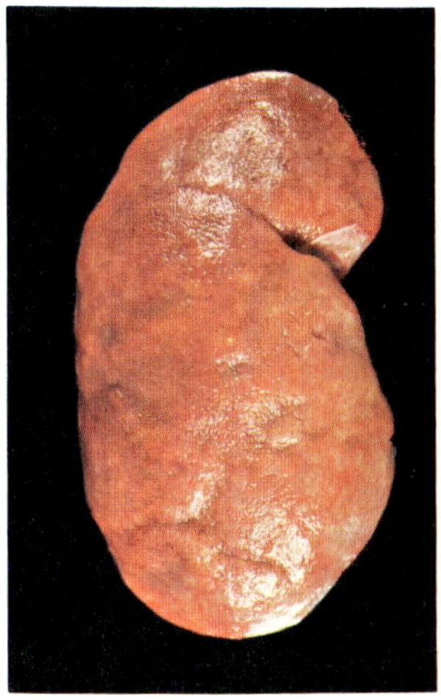

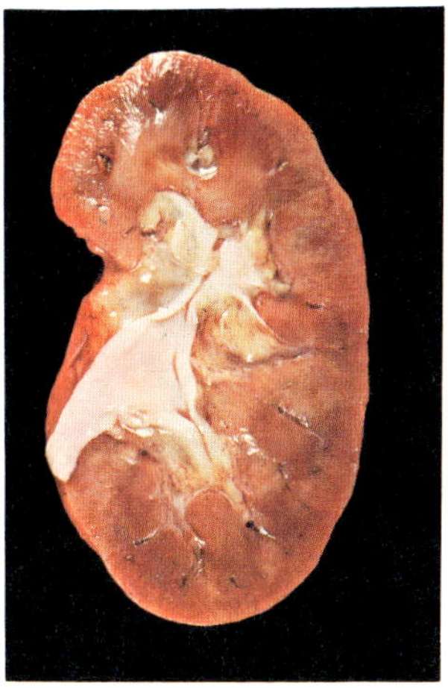

The renal cut surface is not distinctive; a gross diagnosis of lupus is not warranted.

The glomerulus shows hyalinization of the capillary loops so that they are thick, structureless, pale pink, and decreased in number. It is this process that resembles a "wire loop" when extreme.

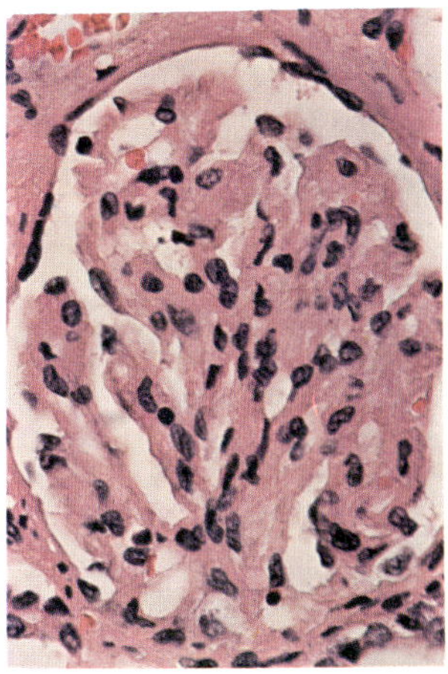

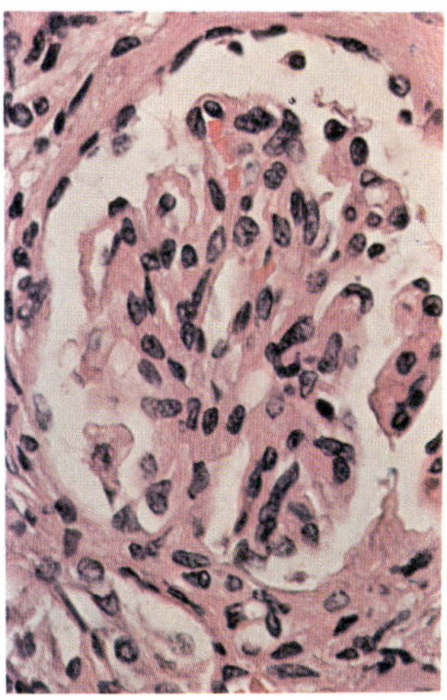

A second glomerulus is similar; no hematoxylin bodies are evident.

LUPUS KIDNEY

CLINICAL ACCOUNT 7374

The patient was a black female 33 years old who was admitted to the hospital for treatment of renal failure. She had been well until four years previously, when she developed arthralgia, transient photosensitive face rash, fever, and widespread subcutaneous edema. Associated with this were a pleural effusion, lymphadenopathy, leukopenia, elevated sedimentation rate, and a positive LE cell test. She had been treated with adrenal cortical steroids, and her condition had improved except for the gradual onset of hypertension and renal failure.

The temperature was 97.9 degrees F., pulse 86, respirations 28, and blood pressure 160/120 mm. Hg. Physical examination revealed enlargement of the heart and widespread subcutaneous edema.

The urine disclosed 3 plus protein and 2 to 3 leukocytes, 12 to 15 erythrocytes, and a few finely granular casts per high power field. The hemoglobin was 7.7 gm., hematocrit 23, and the leukocyte count 2500 with a slight neutrophilia. The LE cell preparation was positive and the blood urea nitrogen rose from 32 to 93 mgs. over a hospital course of two weeks. She was discharged from the hospital but returned two months later and died of renal failure.

The autopsy examination revealed chronic glomerular disease, acute pancreatitis, hypertrophy of the heart (425 gm.), and arteritis of the spleen consistent with lupus erythematosus.

THE ENTITY

Systemic lupus erythematosus occurs especially in the second, third, and fourth decades and is more frequent in women than men. Several anatomic systems are affected, and there is predilection for the skin, serous membranes, joints, kidneys, heart, and hemopoietic organs. Diagnosis is aided by the identification of LE cells in the blood and the demonstration of an antinuclear factor in the serum. The Coomb's test is often positive, and serologic tests for syphilis may be falsely positive. The disease waxes and wanes, often lasts many years, and causes death by renal failure, or, more often, bacterial infection of the lungs.

Renal involvement is manifested by proteinuria, slight hematuria, and abnormal sediment which contains leukocytes, red cell casts, fatty casts, and oval fat bodies (1). The proteinuria may be massive and cause the nephrotic syndrome; hypercholesterolemia, however, is usually absent. Renal failure may be due to progressive glomerular disease or to unrelated tubular degeneration or pyelonephritis.

There is no unique gross lesion. The characteristic microscopic finding is a uniform thickening of the glomerular basement membrane so that a "wire loop" configuration is formed. The specific finding is the hematoxylin body which usually occupies a glomerulus. There may also be glomerular fibrosis, focal cell proliferation, intracapillary hyaline thrombi, and crescent formation. The outlook is poorest when biopsy reveals widespread glomerular disease.

1. Heptinstall, R.H. Pathology of the Kidney. Little, Brown and Company, Boston, 1966.

URETERITIS CYSTICA

CLINICAL ACCOUNT 7235

The patient was a black female 72 years old who had been well until ten months before admission to the hospital. At that time she noted bloody vaginal spotting. This persisted for the ensuing four months, when she consulted a physician; a curettage was performed, and an adenocarcinoma of the endometrium was identified. The patient was in congestive heart failure and was extremely obese, so she was deemed unsuitable for surgical treatment. Four months before admission intracavitary and external irradiation were given in 20 treatments over 37 days; the midplane tissue dose was estimated to be 4,000 rads. Thereafter, the patient experienced temporary diarrhea and pelvic discomfort; the vaginal bleeding stopped.

She was admitted because of cough, shortness of breath, and ankle edema. She was 5 feet in height and weighed 217 pounds. The temperature was 98.6 degrees F., the pulse was 110, and the blood pressure was 130/80 mm. Hg. Breath sounds were decreased in the right chest, the liver was enlarged to the umbilicus, and no other masses were palpated. The blood revealed a moderate anemia. A chest x-ray disclosed elevated diaphragms, basilar atelectasis, and a pleural effusion on the right. No metastases of bone were seen. An intravenous pyelogram indicated dilatation of the right ureter and renal pelvis. Pleural fluid was aspirated and cytologic examination disclosed malignant tumor cells. Swelling of the legs became pronounced, and the patient died after nine days in the hospital.

Autopsy examination revealed carcinoma of the endometrium, metastatic carcinoma of the lungs, liver, and right pleura, a recent thrombus of the inferior vena cava, fibromyomas of the myometrium, bilateral ureteritis cystica, and slight dilatation of both ureters.

THE ENTITY

The term "ureteritis cystica" designates submucosal cysts that bulge into the ureter and distort the lumen. They measure up to 2 cm. in diameter and are usually widely scattered but may be clustered in small groups. They are most common in the upper third of the ureter and occasionally extend into the adjacent renal pelvis. They may be unilateral or bilateral. The cysts are most common in adults over the age of 50, they usually cause no symptoms, and they are sometimes found on excretory urograms which display a characteristic scalloping of the margins. Complications are uncommon and neoplastic transformation is rare.

Ureteritis cystica was first described by Morgagni in 1761, the first detailed microscopic description was given by von Brunn in 1893, and the first clinical diagnosis was made by Jacoby in 1929 (1). The popular concept of pathogenesis is that inflammation stimulates the ureteral mucosa to undergo hyperplasia, the epithelium focally projects downward beneath the mucosa to form discrete crypts, the crypts become disconnected from the surface, and fluid transudates into the centers of these cell nests to form cysts that bulge into the lumen. The urographic differential diagnosis includes tuberculous ureteritis in which the ulcerated margins are fuzzy and strictures are common, and tumors of the ureteral mucosa in which the lesion is single, the base is broad, and the surface is irregular in contour.

1. Loitman, B.S., and Chiat, H. Ureteritis cystica and pyelitis cystica. Radiology 68:345-351, 1957.

URETERITIS CYSTICA

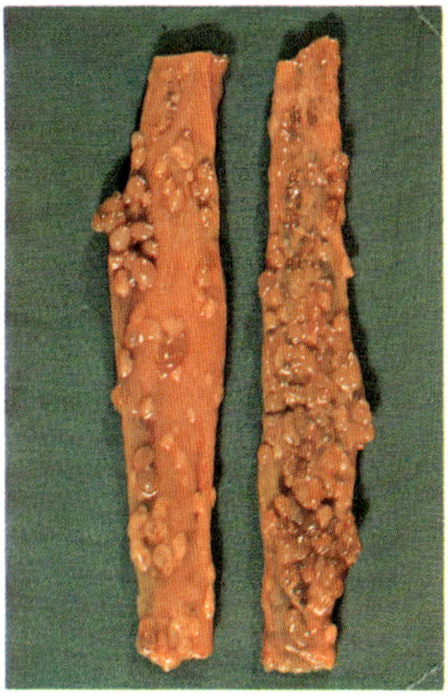

The photograph reveals the mucosal surfaces of the right and left ureters. The cysts are both scattered and in localized clusters.

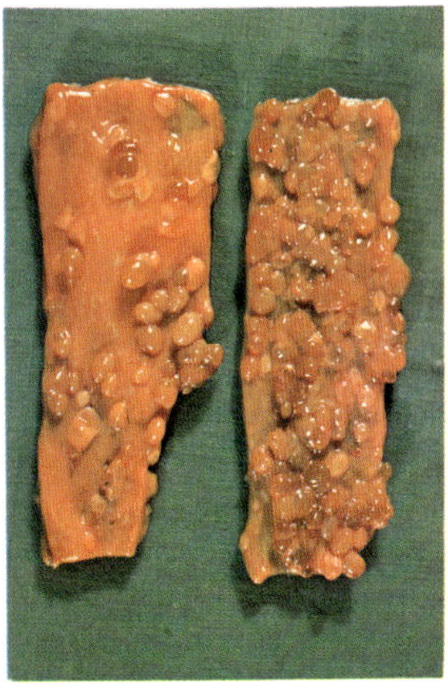

A closer view displays the clear nature of the cysts and the apparently normal adjacent mucosa.

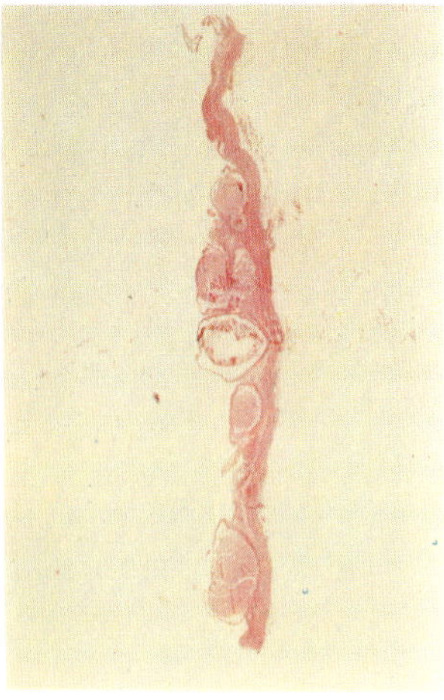

Projection of the cysts onto the luminal surface is evident in the unmagnified photograph.

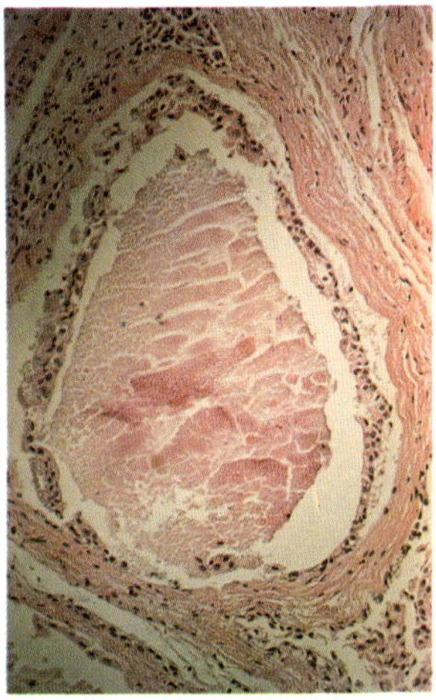

At higher power a single cyst reveals a thin wall, a peripheral margin of transitional epithelium, and a central accumulation of eosinophilic fluid.

CARCINOMA OF URINARY BLADDER

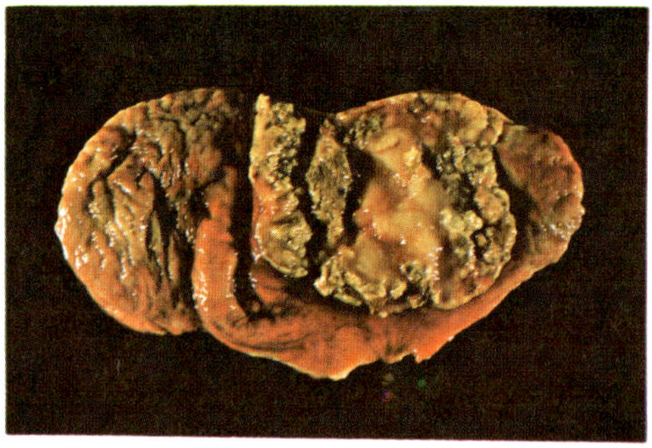

The opened urinary bladder reveals massive replacement of the mucosa with a thick raised greenish-gray mass of tumor that presents a coarsely corrugated necrotic surface.

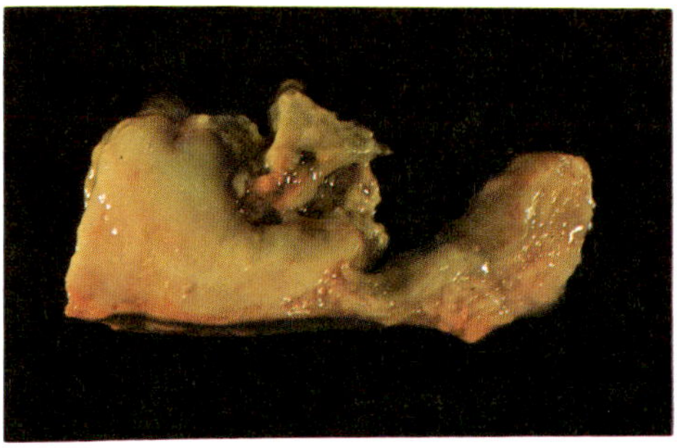

Section displays intact bladder wall on the right and massive tumor infiltration on the left.

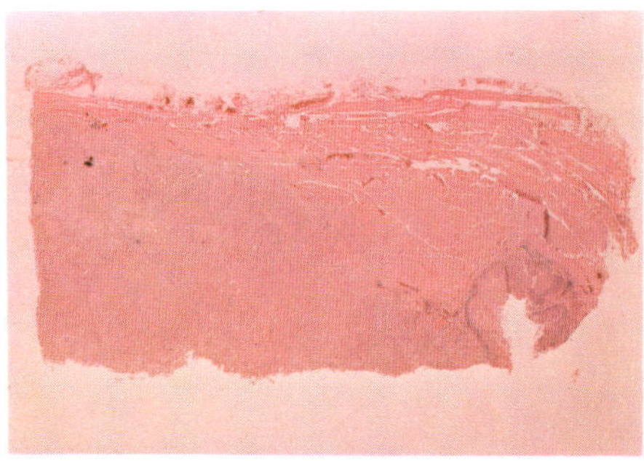

The unmagnified histologic section reveals a short segment of intact mucosa on the left and extensive infiltration of the wall by tumor.

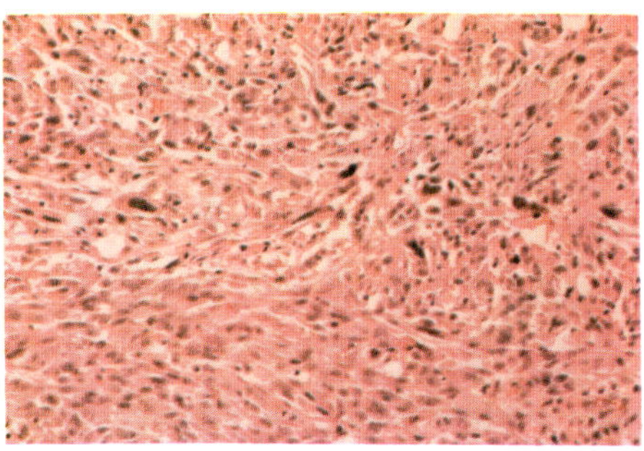

The magnified histologic section discloses a solid mass of epithelial tumor in which the cells and nuclei display pronounced variation in size, contour, and staining characteristics. Moderate numbers of mitoses are present.

CARCINOMA OF URINARY BLADDER

CLINICAL ACCOUNT 469

The patient was a Ugandan female 45 years old who had been well until six months before coming to the hospital. At that time she developed dysuria and pain in the lower abdomen. The pain spread to the rectum and vagina, and the dysuria worsened. More recently there had been headache, anorexia, vomiting, and loss of weight.

Physical examination revealed emaciation, dehydration, and pallor of the mucous membranes. The head, neck, and chest were not remarkable. Palpation of the abdomen disclosed a dilated urinary bladder with a mass on the right side. Pelvic examination revealed a mass in the region of the fornix. The patient's extremities were not remarkable.

The hemoglobin was 11.5 Gms. per 100 ml., and the leukocyte count was 30,000 per cmm. The urine revealed masses of leukocytes and a trace of protein. Culture disclosed colonies of E. coli. The blood urea nitrogen was 103 mg. per 100 ml. The stool was not remarkable except for hookworms. The patient lapsed into coma and died.

Autopsy examination revealed a carcinoma of the urinary bladder with acute and chronic cystitis, hydronephrosis, and acute pyelonephritis. Death was attributed to these lesions with associated uremia.

THE ENTITY

Carcinoma of the urinary bladder occurs especially in middle aged adults and affects males more often than females. The tumors arise on a wall or in the region of the trigone and spread eventually to involve the entire mucosa. The surface of the tumor is ulcerated, infected, necrotic, shaggy, and friable. The histologic type in Uganda is most often squamous; in Western nations it is usually transitional. Adenocarcinomas form a small third group. Squamous metaplasia is often seen in the mucosa adjacent to the tumor; carcinoma-in-situ is less frequent. The tumor penetrates deeply into the wall of the bladder and spreads to pelvic lymph nodes and soft tissues but does not often metastasize to extrapelvic sites. Ureteral obstruction with hydronephrosis, pyelonephritis, and uremia is the usual terminal event. In advanced cases, vesicovaginal and vesicorectal fistulae may form.

While the cause of vesical cancer is not known, environmental factors seem to be of special importance. For example, urbanites are affected more often than suburban dwellers, and especially those in the dye, rubber, or cable industries in some step of which there is exposure to 2-naphthylamine. Schistosomiasis of the hematobium species, which is frequent in the Arab countries, is associated with an increased incidence of the tumor. Presumably the urine contains a carcinogenic substance so that related practices, including cigarette smoking and possibly an unusual diet, together with conditions that cause the urine to be retained in the bladder, such as urethral stricture, may predispose to the onset of the cancer. In Ugandan males stricture of the prostatic urethra, probably post-gonococcal, is common. Cigarette smoking has been variously estimated to increase the liability of developing vesical carcinoma by a factor of 2 to 5 (1). Hereditary, genetic, or racial factors seem unimportant.

1. Anthony, P.P. Malignant tumors of the kidney, bladder, and urethra. Unpublished observations. Dept. of Pathology, Makerere University, Kampala, Uganda.

HYPERPLASIA OF PROSTATE

CLINICAL ACCOUNT 6323

The patient was a white male 69 years old who was admitted to the hospital from a nursing home because of fever, cough, and failure to take food and fluids. He suffered from chronic alcoholism and cerebral atrophy and had been treated for arteriosclerotic heart disease with atrial fibrillation.

The blood pressure was 110/80 mm. Hg.; the pulse was 80 and irregular. The patient was thin, the pharynx was dry, and the outstanding physical findings were a Parkinson's tremor and absence of the dorsalis pedis and posterior tibial pulses.

The urine was normal except for a trace of albumin. The hemoglobin was 11.2 Gm., hematocrit 33, and leukocyte count 8,300 with a normal distribution. The spinal fluid contained 1500 erythrocytes per cmm., and the remainder of the laboratory data was within normal limits. A chest x-ray was suggestive of pneumonitis. On the second hospital day the temperature rose to 101 degrees F., and the patient died.

Autopsy examination revealed bronchopneumonia of the right and left lungs with multiple abscess formation. The lungs weighed 790 and 660 Gm., respectively. The heart weighed 340 Gm. and disclosed only atherosclerosis of the right and left coronary arteries. Incidental diagnoses included cholangiomatosis of the liver, focal chronic pyelonephritis of both kidneys, hyalinization of the splenic capsule, and a healed infarct of the brain.

THE ENTITY

Hyperplasia of the prostate is characterized by peri-urethral nodules that cause the gland to be enlarged two to three times normal size (1). The nodules are round, of various diameters, and are composed of dilated glands and fibromuscular stroma. The former are often large and well circumscribed; the latter are usually small and poorly defined. On histologic examination both reveal non-anaplastic tissue in which mitotic figures are scarce. Infarcts of the nodules are common; they are initially hemorrhagic and later undergo metaplasia to leave oval masses of squamous epithelium.

Nodular hyperplasia is clinically evident because of its secondary changes. The nodules compress the urethra and bulge into the trigone. The obstruction causes difficulty in starting urination, pain during urination, and dribbling after urination from interference with the function of the vesical sphincter. The bladder hypertrophies, false diverticula develop, and the ureters dilate. Residual urine then becomes infected and there are cystitis, vesical calculi, ureteritis, and eventually pyelonephritis with abscess formation and terminal uremia.

Nodular hyperplasia is rare before age 50 but common in the elderly. It has been attributed to the imbalance of sex hormones with predominance of estrogen that takes place in males after middle-life. It is not related to the development of carcinoma of the prostate.

1. Moore, R.A. A Textbook of Pathology, W.B Saunders Company, Philadelphia, 1944.

HYPERPLASIA OF PROSTATE

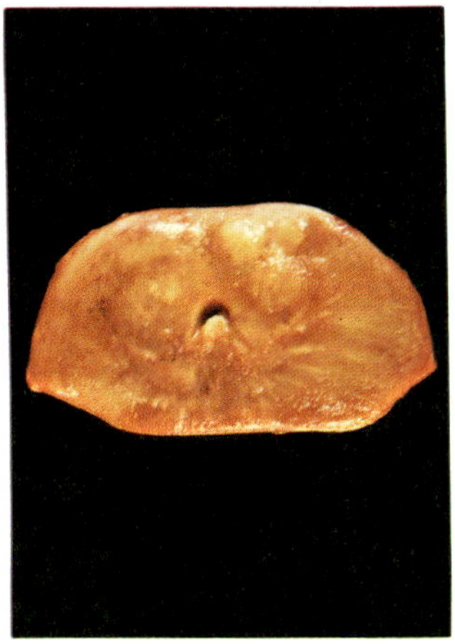

The prostate is only slightly enlarged. The photograph reveals the transverse cut surface with the prostatic urethra in the center. Slightly bulging oval nodules are present in the lateral lobes adjacent to the urethra. The posterior lobes are uninvolved; they lie at the lower portion of the picture and are the usual sites of cancer formation.

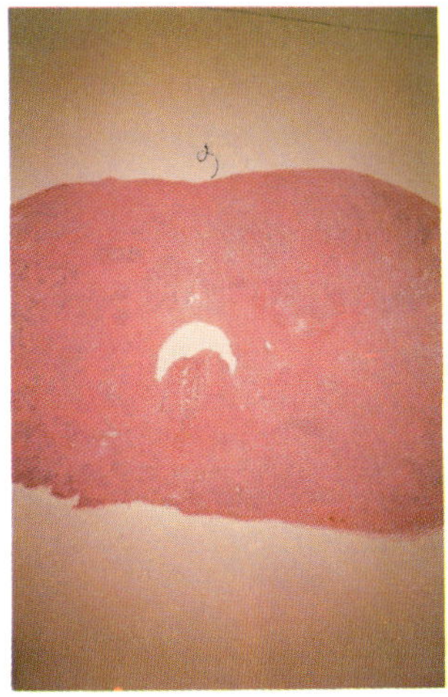

The histologic section shows the same orientation with the urethra in the center and the posterior lobes on either side of the lower margin. Three nodules of glandular tissue are present in the right upper portion of the picture. When such nodules become large, and are present on both sides, the urethra is compressed and urinary obstruction results. All of the consequences of prostatic hyperplasia are due to such obstruction.

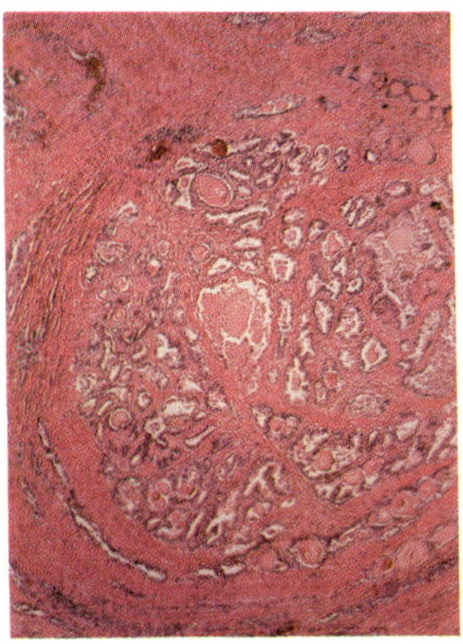

At higher power a hyperplastic nodule of glandular tissue is seen. The outline is round and the margin is distinct. The glands are often dilated in such nodules so that clear pink proteinaceous material within them becomes inspissated to form solid masses known as corpora amylaceae.

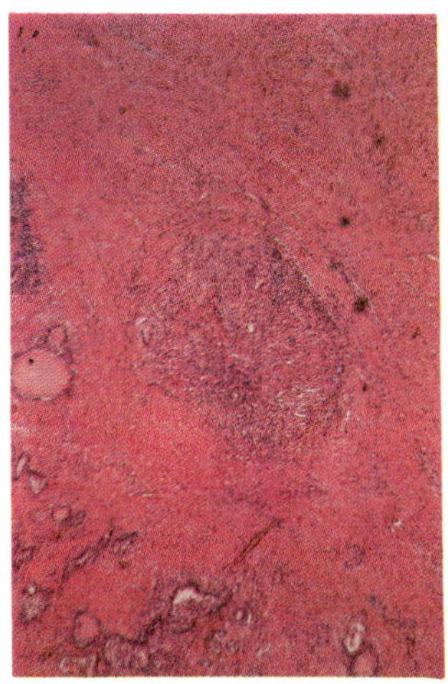

Stromal nodules often accompany the glandular nodules so that the precise diagnosis is "glandular and stromal hyperplasia of prostate." Since the condition is not neoplastic and does not increase the function of the gland, the words "benign" and "hypertrophy" are inappropriate in the terminology of this condition.

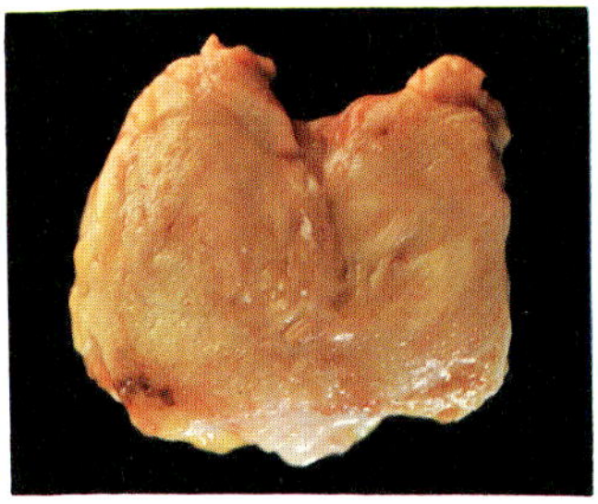

The cut surface of prostate reveals poorly defined glandular hyperplasia in the lateral lobes and a granular focus of firm pale gray tissue in the lower part of the cut surface on the viewer's left. The latter is the cancer.

A close-up view gives the nature of the cut surface; it is pale gray and firm whereas the adjacent hyperplastic tissue is light red and resilient. As most are, the tumor is located in the posterior lobe on one side.

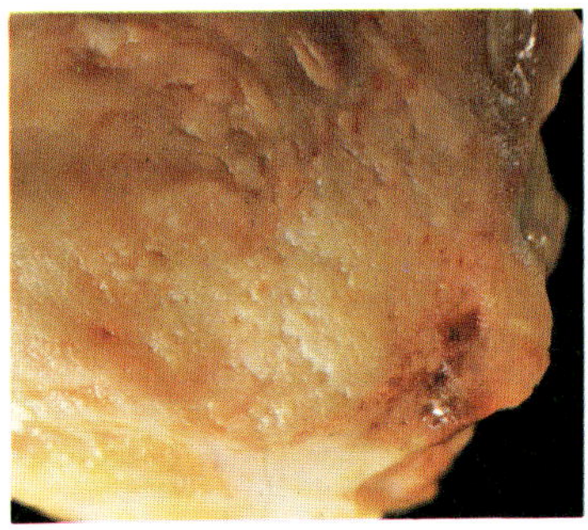

The tumor cells are irregularly distributed throughout the fibromuscular stroma. The tumor cells are in solid clusters in which central necrosis is conspicuous. The undifferentiated nature of this tumor differs from most other tumors which are well differentiated adenocarcinomas.

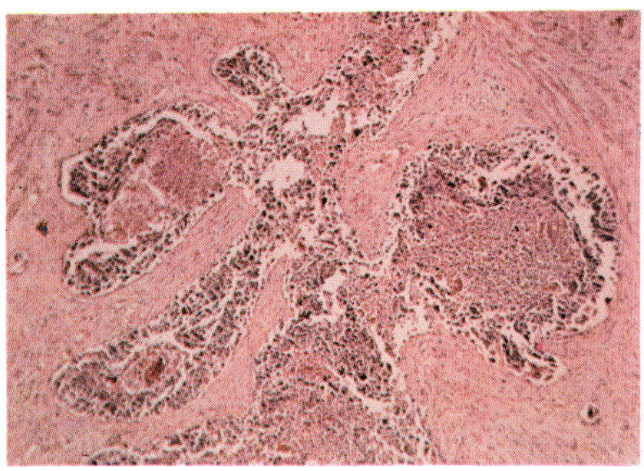

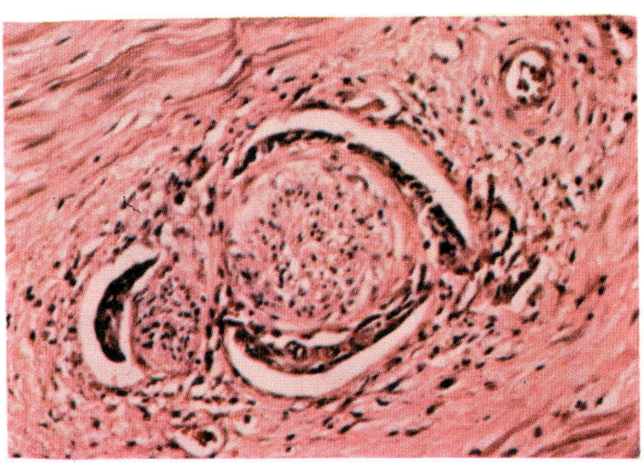

Nerve fibers are abundant in the posterior capsule, and cancers of the prostate infiltrate the perineural lymph sheaths at an early stage in the evolution of the tumor. This finding establishes the diagnosis of malignancy.

CARCINOMA OF PROSTATE

CLINICAL ACCOUNT 6134

The patient was a white male 75 years old who was chronically ill and confused. One year previously a diagnosis of cancer of the prostate had been made, he was presently in chronic renal failure, and he had recently had two episodes of melena. For the past year he had been treated with estrogens.

Physical examination revealed gynecomastia, a palpable spleen, and a hard prostate. The urine revealed 30-50 leukocytes per high power field. The hemoglobin was 5.2 Gm., the hematocrit was 14, and the leukocytes numbered 3,500 with a normal differential count. The blood urea nitrogen was 115 mg. The total serum protein was 4.5 Gm. with 1.9 Gm. albumin and 2.6 Gm. globulin. The alkaline phosphatase was 650 units per 100 ml. An x-ray of the pelvis revealed radiolucent foci suggestive of metastatic disease.

Transfusions were given and the patient was discharged on the fourth hospital day. He was readmitted one month later for dialysis. He died three hours after admission to the hospital.

Autopsy examination revealed a dissecting aneurysm of the aorta, a recent subarachnoid hemorrhage, pulmonary edema, splenomegaly, and a carcinoma of the prostate. The dissecting aneurysm was large, with a saccular component in the thoracic portion and a distal defect so that blood coursed in part through a false channel and then re-entered the true lumen of the aorta. The prostate was large from hyperplasia, the prostatic urethra was compressed, and the urinary bladder was dilated and hypertrophic with marked trabeculation of the wall.

THE ENTITY

Carcinoma of the prostate is the most common cancer in men. It is rare in persons less than fifty years old but increases thereafter so that approximately every third man over 70 has the tumor. About four-fifths of these are small and clinically silent. The rest are invasive and cause symptoms. The former are called latent; the latter are called overt. These two biologic forms are histologically indistinguishable.

Most cancers of the prostate arise in the posterior lobes, and most are adenocarcinomas. The tumor invades the capsule first and then the seminal vesicles, but not the rectum, which is protected by a fascial layer. Later the tumor spreads upward into the prostate to the urethra and undersurface of the bladder. In the posterior capsule invasion of perineural lymph sheaths takes place, and spread into the vertebral veins is common. Metastases therefore arise first in the spine and pelvis and later in the internal iliac and peri-aortic lymph nodes. Lungs and liver may eventually be affected. The tumor is endocrine dependent so that regressive changes, although temporary, follow castration or the administration of estrogens.

Symptoms are late and are due to urethral obstruction. The earliest physical sign is a firm nodular asymmetric prostate as felt by rectal examination. The epithelial cells normally produce acid phosphatase; when tumor cells invade blood or lymph vessels this enzyme increases in the serum and indicates the diagnosis, especially in the presence of metastatic disease. Metastases to bone often stimulate bone growth, and in this event, alkaline phosphatase also rises.

CARCINOMA OF UTERINE CERVIX

CLINICAL ACCOUNT 451

The patient was a black female 30 years old who was diabetic. She reported to a clinic and was controlled with tolbutamide. One week before admission widespread subcutaneous edema and a circumferential ischemic ulcer of the right lower leg developed. Her pulse was 104, and blood pressure 110/70 mm. Hg. Physical examination revealed diabetic cataracts in both eyes, anasarca, an ulcerated uterine cervix, and an ischemic ulcer of the right lower leg. The patient unexpectedly died on the second hospital day. No laboratory investigations were completed.

Autopsy examination disclosed ascites of 1,000 ml., a right pleural effusion of 1,000 ml., marked arteriosclerosis of the coronary arteries and aorta, a recent thrombus of the left internal iliac artery, and ischemic necrosis of the right lower leg. The kidneys were not grossly remarkable. The uterine cervix disclosed an ulcerated carcinoma, and metastatic tumor was thought grossly to be present in the pelvic lymph nodes.

THE ENTITY

Carcinoma of the uterine cervix occurs half as frequently as cancer of the breast and accounts for 10 per cent of cancer deaths in women. The lesion arises at the external os and presents an irregularly papillated surface that ulcerates. The tumor may extend into the subjacent tissue to form a large excavation or into the vagina to form a bulky friable mass. Most are squamous in histologic type although adenocarcinomas, presumably arising from endocervical mucosa, do occur. The tumors may be graded according to their degree of histological differentiation, the more anaplastic tumors showing the more aggressive behavior. The tumor spreads upward to the endometrium, downward to the vagina, and outward to the round ligament. Iliac, hypogastric, presacral, and para-aortic nodes are sooner or later affected. In advanced cases the tumor may spread anteriorly to the bladder to form a vesicovaginal fistula, or posteriorly to the rectum to form a recto-vaginal fistula. The patients are "staged" according to the distribution of the tumor as judged by clinical examination. Different classifications are used; the stages usually progress from I to IV, and while the practice is not especially accurate, it is presumed to be helpful in judging the effectiveness of treatment. The more localized the tumor, the better the result. The carcinoma tends to remain in the pelvis so that although distant metastases may form, death is usually due to uremia from obstruction of the ureters or urethra. The cause is not known although smegma and certain viruses may be carcinogenic when the exposure is repeated or prolonged.

Carcinoma-in-situ precedes invasive carcinoma by about 10 years, i.e., 35 versus 45. It arises at the external os and consists of transmural anaplasia without invasion through the basement membrane of the mucosa. It is clinically silent and is usually discovered by cytologic examination of a cervical smear. Over a period of years the lesion may progress to invasive carcinoma or regress to normal mucosa. The cause is unknown.

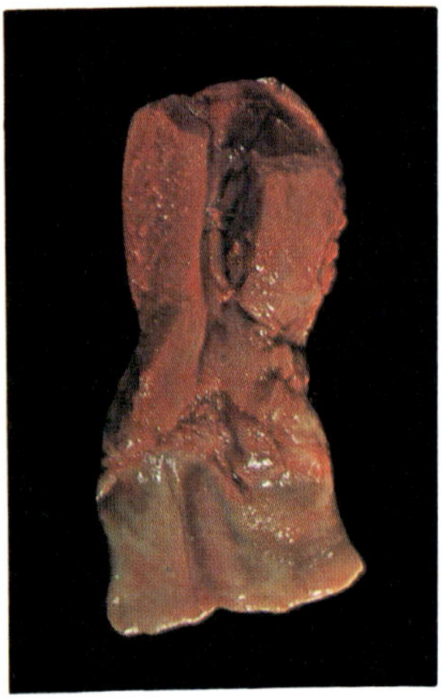

The uterine fundus is at the top, the cervix in the middle, and the vagina below. Irregularity of the cervical surface is evident.

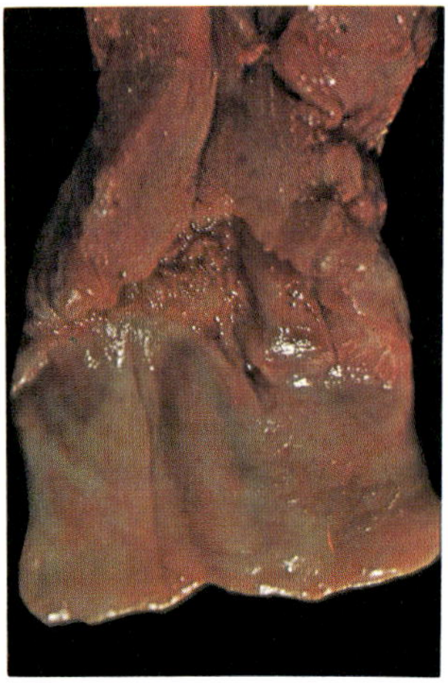

Closer examination reveals ulceration and coarse granularity of the cervix in the region of the external os.

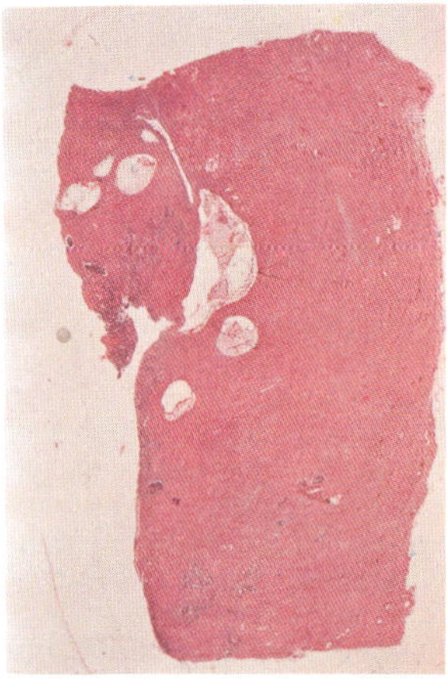

The unmagnified histologic section discloses the mucosal surface on the left with the ulcerated portion in the upper part and the vaginal surface subjacent to it. The tumor infiltrated the overhanging projection of cervical tissue. In the lower part of the section minute nodules of tumor may be seen in vascular spaces deep within the stroma.

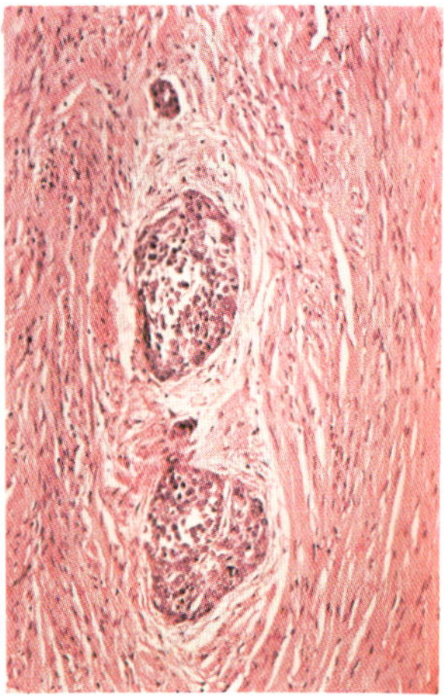

The photograph shows nodules of squamous cell carcinoma in vascular spaces deep within the wall of the vagina.

The opened uterus reveals a fibromyoma in the upper portion of the fundus and a smooth vaginal mucosa at the lower margin of the specimen. In between, the endometrium displays a carcinoma that extends from nearly the uterine cervix to the midportion of the cavity.

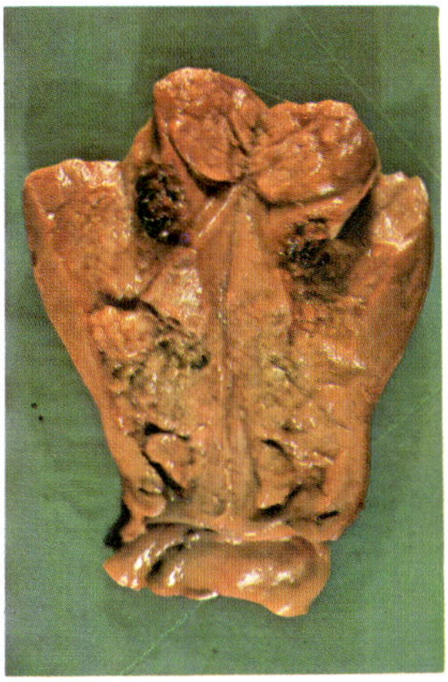

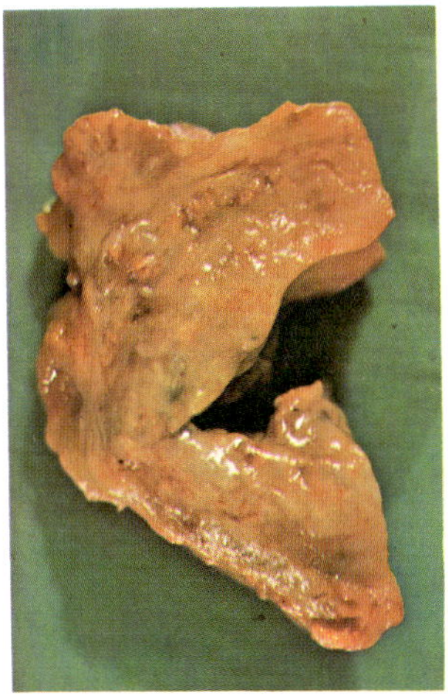

On cross section of the fundus, a yellowish gray tumor may be seen extending through the entire thickness of the muscle wall.

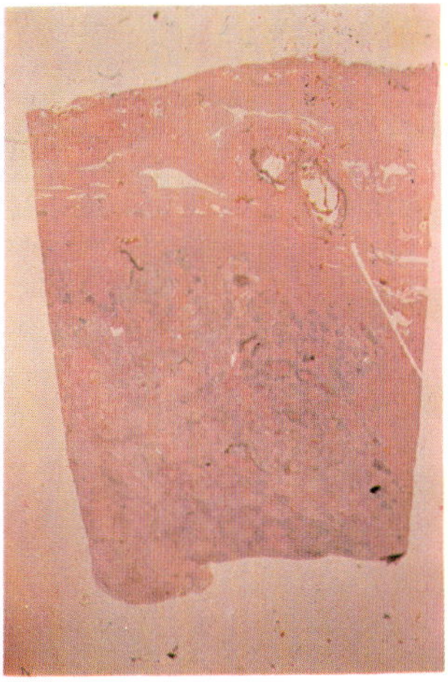

In the unmagnified section, solid masses of basophilic and focally necrotic tumor extend slightly more than half way through the myometrium.

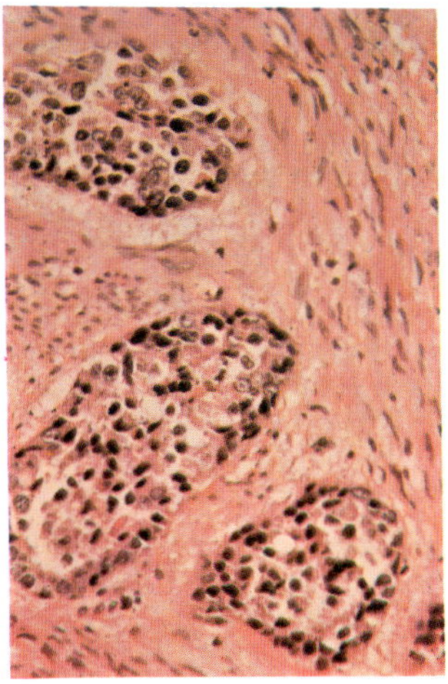

Sections of deep muscle, however, reveal tumor emboli in vascular spaces of the uterine wall.

CARCINOMA OF ENDOMETRIUM

CLINICAL ACCOUNT 7235

The patient was a white female 27 years old who had delivered a normal baby three months before admission to the hospital. Three weeks before hospital entry she noted a right inguinal lump that was red and painful. Fever then developed and antibiotic therapy was given. The temperature rose to 103 degrees F., and chills and nausea and vomiting began. Swelling and tenderness in the inguinal region persisted.

The temperature was 102.2 degrees F., pulse 112, respirations 12, and blood pressure 100/70 mm. Hg. Physical examination revealed warm dry skin, no lymphadenopathy except in the right inguinal region, slight enlargement of the liver, and a negative pelvic examination.

The urine was normal except for 4 to 6 leukocytes per high power field of centrifuged sediment. The hemoglobin was 9.7 Gm., the hematocrit was 30.2 per cent, and the leukocytes numbered 60,700 per cmm. with a neutrophilia that included 26 band cells. Subsequently the leukocyte count decreased to 20,000 per cmm. The spinal fluid was normal. An electrocardiogram was normal. A chest x-ray was normal. The first of two bone marrow examinations was normal. On the seventh hospital day a biopsy of the tender right inguinal lymph node revealed undifferentiated malignant tumor. The patient's condition progressively deteriorated, and death occurred after the tenth day of hospitalization.

THE ENTITY

Carcinoma of the endometrium is a postmenopausal disease. It arises most often between the ages of 50 and 60 years, especially in women with obesity, hypertension, diabetes, and nulliparity in combination. The cause of the cancer is not known, although hyperestrinism is thought to be involved. Adenomatous hyperplasia often precedes the development of the carcinoma. The presenting signs are leukorrhea and irregular vaginal bleeding. Diagnosis is established by histologic examination of curetted endometrium.

The cancer arises in any part of the chamber, projects bulkily into the cavity, infiltrates widely into the myometrium, and ulcerates extensively to produce a soft, shaggy, necrotic tumor mass that fills the uterine vault. Infection and pyometrium often develop. Extension into the cervical canal is common. Progressive penetration of the muscle wall allows tumor cells to invade blood and lymphatic vessels and eventually reach the peritoneal surface. Transperitoneal spread then occurs to the broad ligaments, uterine tubes, ovaries, and pelvic peritoneum. Lymph vessels of the myometrium carry tumor emboli to the pelvic, inguinal, and para-aortic lymph nodes. In advanced cases, metastases form in the liver and lungs. Histologic examination reveals that all are adenocarcinomas although in some, squamous metaplasia of the glandular pattern is focal and distinct (adenoacanthoma).

Treatment consists of surgical removal often preceded by intracavitary or external irradiation. The principal measure, however, is the excisional procedure (1). Five-year survival rates range from 60 to 80 per cent depending on the extent of the tumor spread at the time therapy is applied.

1. Smith, J.C. The superiority of surgical treatment of endometrial carcinoma. J.A.M.A. 160:1460, 1956.

NORMAL SPLEEN

CLINICAL ACCOUNT 6196

The patient was a white female 75 years old who had been hypertensive for the past ten years and had experienced angina pectoris for the past five years. For some months she had also had shortness of breath, dyspnea on exertion, 2-pillow orthopnea, nocturia, and ankle edema which disappeared in the morning. On the night before admission she had a severe pain in the left anterior chest that radiated to both shoulders and was not relieved by nitroglycerine.

The temperature was 98.6 degrees F., pulse 150, respirations 32, and blood pressure 92/60 mm. Hg. Rales were audible over the lower posterior lung fields. The heart was enlarged to the left, the rhythm was regular, and no murmurs were heard. The abdomen was protuberant; no masses were palpated. There was no fluid wave. There was no ankle edema.

The urine was not remarkable except for 15 leukocytes and many epithelial cells and hyaline casts in the sediment. The hemoglobin was 12.9 Gm., hematocrit 41, and leukocyte 9,000 with a normal differential count. An electrocardiogram disclosed atrial fibrillation. The patient was digitalized, the heart rate decreased, and a harsh systolic murmur radiating to the neck and axilla was then heard. The blood urea nitrogen was 42 mg. per 100 ml. A chest x-ray indicated pulmonary hyperemia, pleural effusions, and cardiac enlargement. On the fourteenth hospital day dyspnea became pronounced and the patient died.

Autopsy examination revealed hypertrophy of the heart (475 Gm.), rheumatic disease of the aortic valve with stenosis, arteriolar nephrosclerosis, carcinoma of the thyroid, and carcinoma of the right breast. The spleen weighed 130 Gms.

THE ENTITY

The capsule and trabeculae of the spleen are elastic so that pronounced distension is possible. After death the elastic fibers contract, blood flows from the hilar vessels, and in this state the normal adult organ weighs about 150 Gm. The cut surface is red flecked with gray. The former is the red pulp, the latter is the lymphoid tissue evenly dispersed as minute follicles. Blood enters at the hilum through the splenic artery. The artery immediately divides into small vessels that pass through the white pulp, i.e., are surrounded by lymphoid collars that expand into follicles with germinal centers. Thereafter the arterial blood enters the sinusoids of the red pulp, through which it moves slowly past the lining cells that are phagocytic. In this passage particles are engulfed and erythrocytes are sequestered, phagocytized, and disassembled so that the unusable parts (pyrroles) are sent to the bile and the usable parts (iron, globin) are returned to the circulation. The splenic vein emerges at the hilum, follows the splenic artery, and joins with the superior mesenteric vein to form the portal vein.

The spleen produces erythrocytes for the first six months of fetal life; after this, hemopoiesis is a function of the bone marrow (1). In adulthood, the spleen filters the blood, disposes of old erythrocytes, generates new lymphocytes, and produces serum antibodies. It also provides blood to the circulation in emergencies by contraction and resumes hemopoiesis when the bone marrow loses this capability, i.e., by fibrosis or tumor cell replacement. While not essential to life, removal causes a transient anemia, leukocytosis, and thrombocythemia.

1. Miale, J.B. Laboratory Medicine—Hematology. The C.V. Mosby Co., St. Louis, 1962.

NORMAL SPLEEN

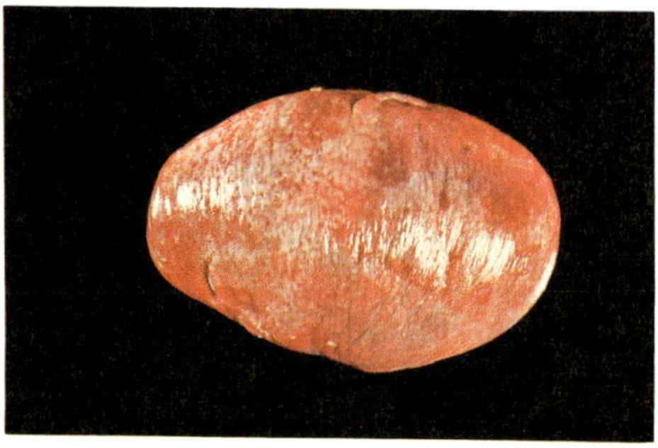

The spleen is normal in weight, size, and contour. The capsule is red mottled with pale gray. In this instance the pale gray discoloration is due to slight capsular thickening; it is normally smooth, glistening, and uniformly dark red.

The cut surface is normally dark red and uniform except for short pale gray fibrous septae.

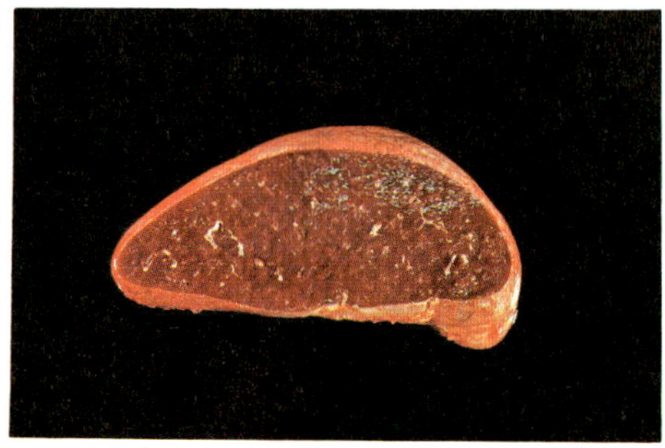

At low power, several normal structures are visible, i.e., a thin smooth capsule, an abundant subjacent red pulp, a small mass of white pulp (lymphoid cells forming a lymph follicle), a small central artery in the lymphoid follicle, and a fibrous septum.

At higher power lymphoid cells of the white pulp with minute arterioles may be seen. The periphery is composed of red pulp traversed by splenic sinusoids.

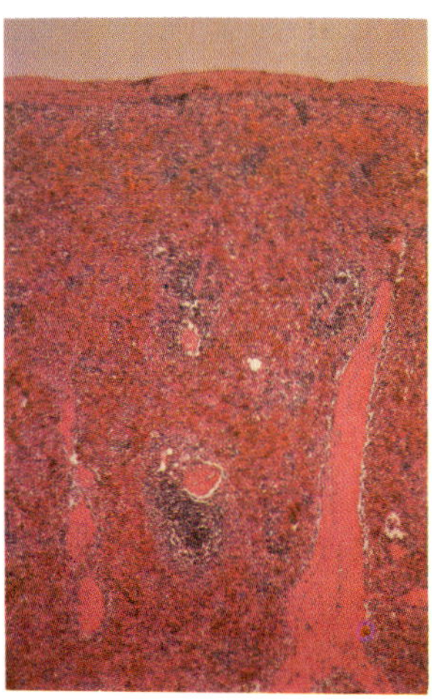

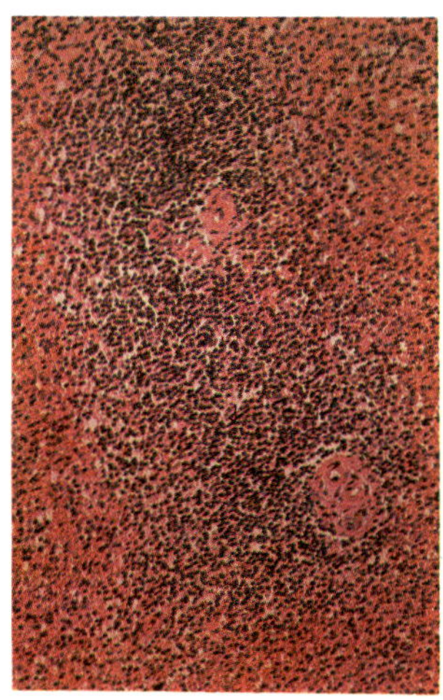

ACUTE HYPERPLASIA OF SPLEEN

The capsule is smooth and tense; the texture is extremely soft.

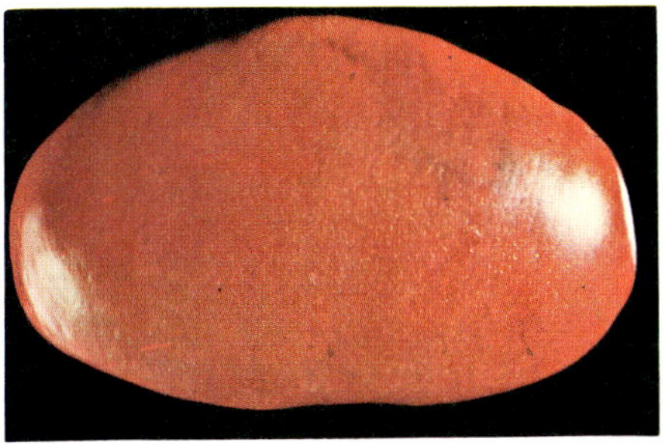

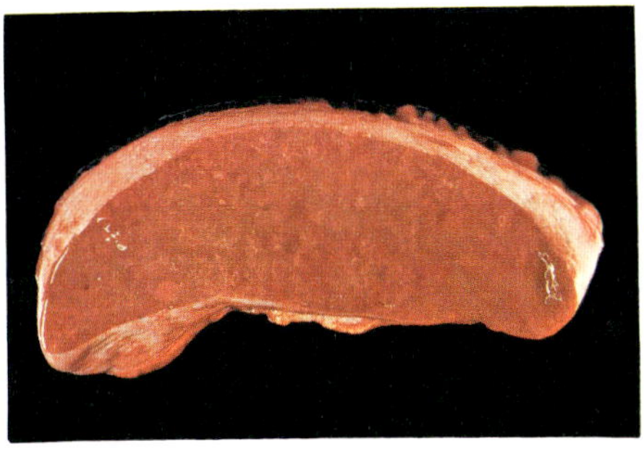

Sections release a thick dark red semifluid that flows freely from the cut surface. The semiliquid pulp flowing onto the black background may be seen over the convex surface. The capsule is not thickened.

Close up examination reveals structural details obscured by the semiliquid red pulp that issues over the surface.

Histological examination reveals leukocytic infiltration, endothelial hyperplasia, extreme hyperemia, and recent hemorrhage. A small central hemorrhagic focus appears to be undergoing necrosis.

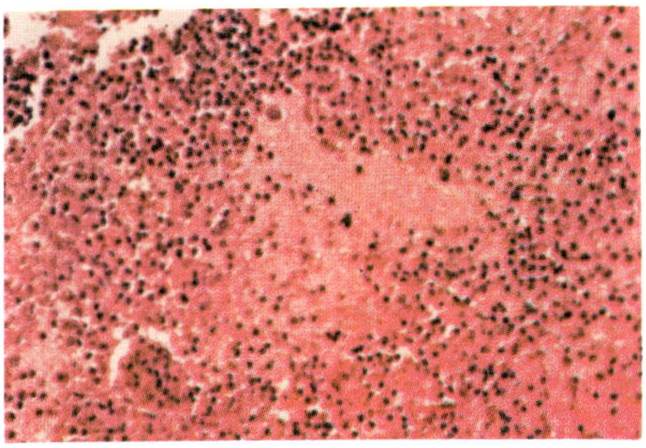

ACUTE HYPERPLASIA OF SPLEEN

CLINICAL ACCOUNT 6157

The patient was a white male 62 years old who was admitted to the hospital because of low back pain of three months' duration that radiated to the perineum, suprapubic region, and left testicle. A transurethral prostatectomy had been performed and a prostatic abscess was drained. Over the past two months there had been a weight loss of 10 pounds. Recently the patient had noted a sensation of bowel obstruction. Past history revealed that a myocardial infarction had occurred nine years earlier and that the patient was presently under treatment for angina pectoris.

Physical examination was not remarkable except for nodularity over the right side of the prostate. The deep tendon reflexes were normal, and there were no neurologic complaints.

The urine was normal. The hemoglobin was 11.6 Gm., hematocrit 36.5, and leukocytes 57,400 with 76 segmented granulocytes, 17 band cells, 3 lymphocytes, 3 monocytes, and 1 eosinophile. The serum alkaline phosphatase was 8.0 units per 100 ml. On the fifth hospital day a pelvic abscess was drained through a suprapubic incision. Tissue removed at that time revealed a malignant tumor of uncertain type. On the twelfth hospital day the patient felt weak, and later that day he unexpectedly died.

Autopsy examination revealed a sarcoma of the lower ileum that had metastasized to the mesenteric lymph nodes. The tumor had spread through the bowel wall and a pelvic abscess had formed. The urinary bladder, prostate, and colon were not remarkable. There were also a recent infarct of the myocardium, edema of the right and left lungs, and hyperemia of the liver. The spleen weighed 425 Gm.

THE ENTITY

Acute hyperplasia is the most common cause of splenic enlargement. It is caused by infectious disease, perhaps because the spleen acts as a sieve for the blood. Inciting examples include septicemia, typhoid fever, lobar pneumonia, acute bacterial endocarditis, and acute meningococcemia. In the past the condition has been referred to as "acute splenic tumor" or "acute hyperplastic splenitis."

Grossly the spleen is big and soft; it may weigh as much as 500 to 600 Gm. The capsule is smooth and tense, and the cut surface is soft, pultaceous, and usually dark bluish red. A thick dark red semifluid oozes from the cut section. Microscopically the follicles are of usual size and the intervening pulp is abundant and rich with blood. Lymphocytes are numerous, and endothelial cells proliferate. Segmented granulocytes may also be present in substantial numbers depending on the nature of the infectious disease. Many cells undergo degeneration, and foci of necrosis are often present. Both contribute to the soft texture of the tissue.

Clinically the spleen is too soft to be felt. As the infectious disease subsides, the spleen returns to its normal size and state so that no residual change is left.

RECENT INFARCT OF SPLEEN

CLINICAL ACCOUNT 6127

The patient was a white female 72 years old who entered the hospital because of slight vaginal bleeding of five weeks' duration. Prolapse of the uterus was discovered and a hysterectomy was performed. The hemoglobin was 12.5 Gm., the hematocrit was 39 per cent, and the leukocytes numbered 5,100 with a normal differential count. The patient recovered uneventfully.

Four months later she was readmitted because of headache, weakness, and poor appetite of several weeks' duration. There were also dizzy spells and calf pain on exercise. The skin was pallid. Liver, spleen, and lymph nodes were not palpable. The hemoglobin was 5.2 Gm., the hematocrit was 15 per cent, and the leukocytes numbered 3,300 with 47 segmented granulocytes, 36 lymphocytes, 14 band cells, and 3 monocytes. The bone marrow disclosed acute monocytic leukemia. The patient was given Purinethol and prednisone and was discharged after two weeks in the hospital.

One month later she was readmitted for transfusion. The physical findings were unchanged except for widespread ecchymoses. The urine was normal except for 2 plus proteinuria. The hemoglobin was 7.6 Gm., the hematocrit was 24 per cent, and the leukocytes numbered 6,500 with 63 neutrophils, 14 band cells, and 23 lymphocytes. The platelet count was 3,000 per cmm. Her condition regressed, and she died after six days in the hospital.

Autopsy examination revealed acute granulocytic leukemia with leukosis of the bone marrow and left kidney. There were also an acute hemorrhagic gastritis, a recent hemorrhage in the gastrointestinal tract, acute ulcers of the colon, and a recent hemorrhage of the subarachnoid space. The spleen weighed 150 Gms.

THE ENTITY

Infarcts of the spleen are comparatively common and are due to occlusion of the splenic artery or its branches. One cause is embolism from the valves of the left side of the heart. In that instance the embolus may be infected, the infarct is septic, and an abscess forms. Another cause is local thrombosis which is usually associated with a hematologic disorder such as leukemia, polycythemia, sickle cell disease, or lymphoma. In this instance the thrombus is sterile, the infarct is bland, and the healing proceeds without abscess formation. Most infarcts of the spleen are bland.

As the artery is blocked and necrosis takes place, fluid seeps in, hemorrhage occurs, and the tissue swells. The capsule bulges and fibrin appears on the surface. The hemoglobin then breaks down, macrophages carry it away, and the early hemorrhagic lesion decolorizes and becomes pale yellowish gray. Finally, fibroblasts grow toward the center from the viable margin and the necrotic zone is replaced with fibrous tissue. As the connective tissue contracts a depressed scar is left.

Infarction of the spleen causes sharp pain in the left abdomen that may radiate to the left shoulder and cause splinting of the left diaphragm and abdominal muscles. The destruction of splenic tissue is not functionally significant, the infarcts do not tend to rupture, and bed rest with sedation is sufficient treatment. It is important that more serious conditions not be mistaken for infarcts, i.e., rupture of the spleen or perforation of the gut or stomach. Infarction of the left kidney is distinguished by blood in the urine.

RECENT INFARCT OF SPLEEN

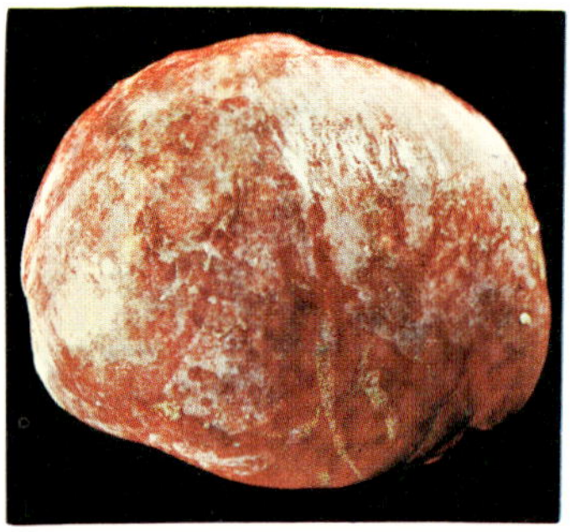

The spleen is of normal size. The capsule is roughened by fibrous adhesions and displays scattered foci of slight hyalinization.

Section reveals the usual dark red surface with pale gray fibrous septae at the hilum. The convex surface discloses a roughly triangular focus of pale yellowish gray discoloration that extends to the splenic capsule. This is a recent infarct. Although the word "recent" is used, the lesion has lasted long enough for the margins to become sharply delineated and the hemoglobin in the necrotic tissue to be broken down and carried away by the macrophages. Several days are required for this change.

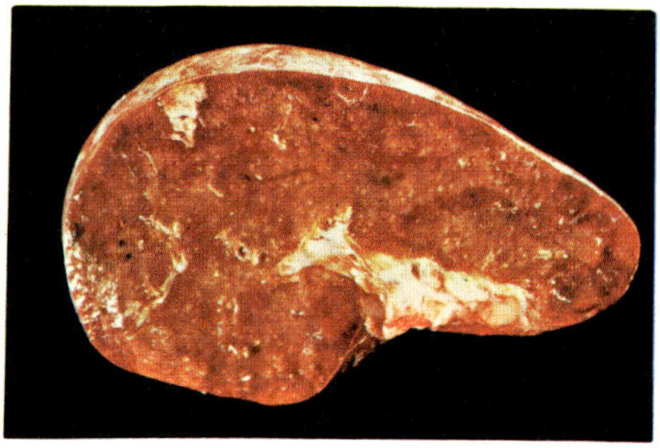

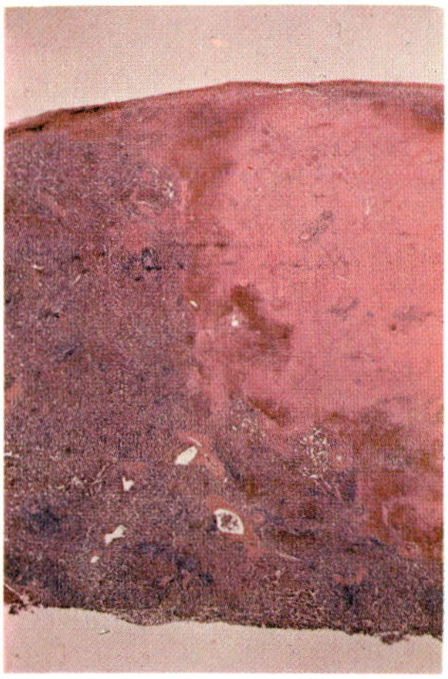

At scanning power the necrotic region extending to the capsule is seen. The necrosis is sharply delineated from the adjacent pulp, and a conspicuous zone of hemorrhage delineates this margin. Follicles can be discerned in the uninvolved tissue.

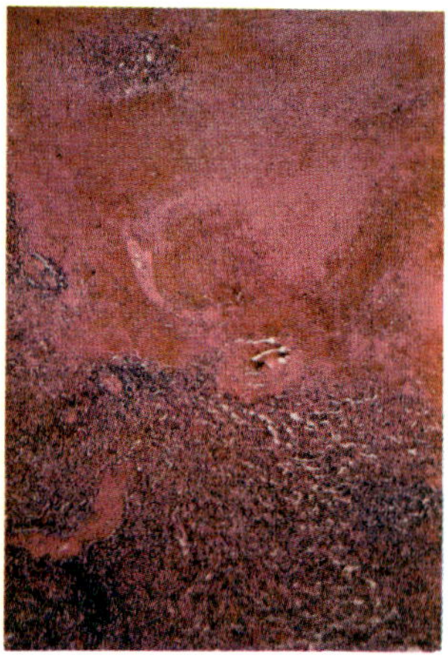

At higher power the marginal zone is again seen with necrosis above and viable tissue below. Most of the cells remaining in the necrotic region fail to stain; those that do disclose pyknotic nuclei.

AMYLOIDOSIS OF SPLEEN

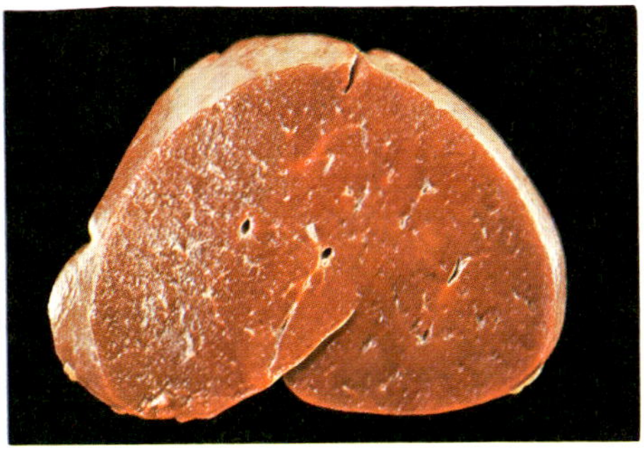

The organ is slightly enlarged and the capsule thin and smooth; the cut surface is firm, pale red, and somewhat lardaceous.

At low power the tissue is evenly infiltrated with a pale pink structureless material that obliterates the lymphoid follicles. The tissue is scarcely recognizable as spleen.

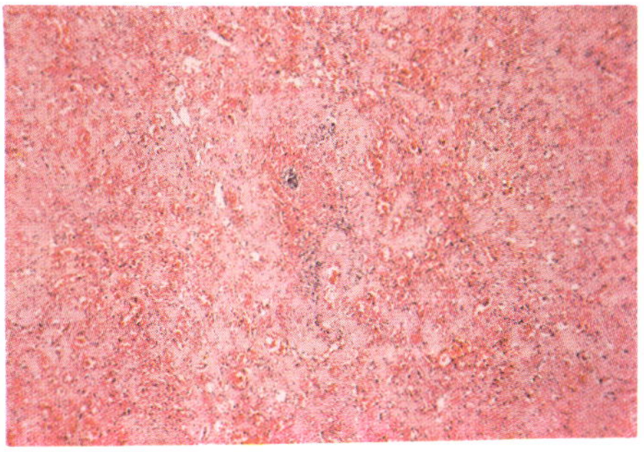

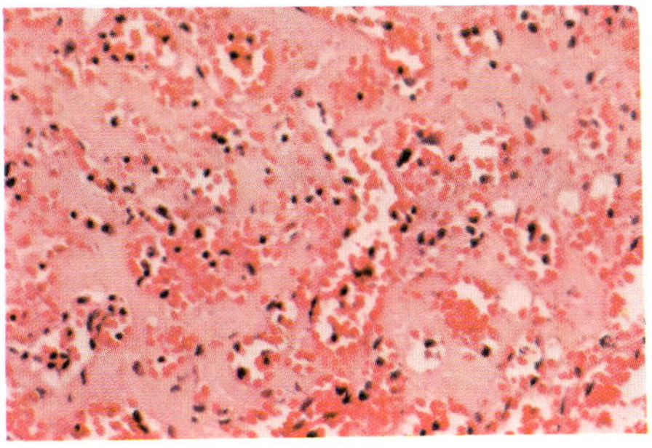

A closer view reveals the pale pink material replacing the red and white pulp and leaving only the vascular sinusoids winding through the tissue.

At higher magnification the pale pink hyaline material (amyloid) may be seen in the walls of small arteries as well as throughout the pulp. Occasional lymphocytes are present but no follicle has resisted the infiltration.

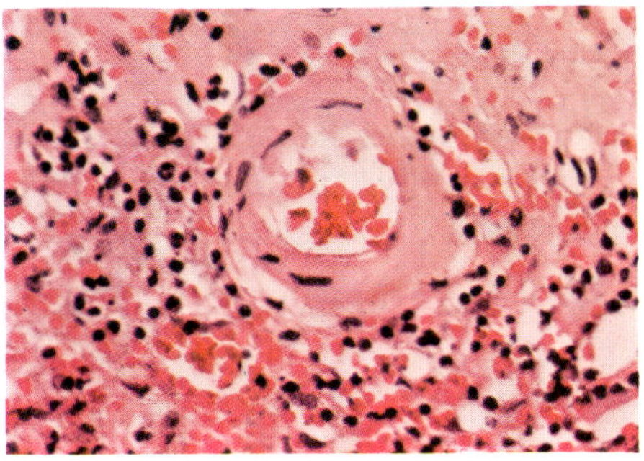

AMYLOIDOSIS OF SPLEEN

CLINICAL ACCOUNT 6002

The patient was a white male 63 years old who developed hepatomegaly four years before the last hospital admission. Biopsy disclosed amyloidosis. Since then his condition had steadily worsened; weight decreased and weakness developed. Diarrhea began three years before admission and seemed to follow the ingestion of meat, green vegetables, and citrus fruits. Renal disease developed eighteen months before admission and was manifested by nocturia and intermittent swelling of the lower extremities.

The temperature was 98.2 degrees F., pulse 96, respirations 18, and blood pressure 110/70 mm. Hg. The patient was weak and emaciated. The heart and lungs were normal. The liver margin was hard, nontender, and 7 fingerbreadths below the right costal margin. There was a 3 plus pitting edema of the ankles.

The urine revealed 4 plus proteinuria, a few coarsely and finely granular casts, and a small number of leukocytes. The hemoglobin was 16.7 Gm., hematocrit 51, and leukocytes 10,800 with a slight neutrophilia. The blood urea nitrogen and serum creatinine were 115 and 6.9 mg. per 100 ml., respectively. The total protein was 5 Gm. with 2 Gm. albumin and 3 Gm. globulin. The alkaline phosphatase was 200 units (normal 30-85).

On the day after admission bright red blood was passed per rectum, the blood pressure fell to 50/50 mm. Hg., and the patient died.

Autopsy examination revealed amyloidosis of the heart, liver (4,000 Gm.), pancreas, kidneys (300 Gm., 250 Gm.), spleen, lymph nodes, bone marrow, adrenals, parathyroids, spleen, and tongue. The lungs were edematous and weighed 900 and 875 Gm., respectively. There were also an acute fibrinous enterocolitis that was attributed to uremia, and a slight plasmacytosis of the vertebral bone marrow. The spleen weighed 200 Gm.

THE ENTITY

Amyloid, originally misnamed because of a presumed starch composition, is a translucent protein material of uncertain structure that grossly transmits the color of the underlying tissue and microscopically accumulates between parenchymal cells and within connective tissues. Primary amyloidosis is uncommon, occurs in the absence of known predisposing conditions, and affects especially the muscles of the tongue (macroglossia), heart (failure), and gastrointestinal tract. Secondary amyloidosis is more common, occurs with diseases that cause extensive tissue destruction, and affects especially the spleen, liver, kidneys, and adrenals. Predisposing diseases include tuberculosis, osteomyelitis, bronchiectasis, and rheumatoid arthritis. Amyloidosis also occurs with some cases of multiple myeloma, and least commonly in a localized form in the larynx or upper respiratory tract. Lugol's solution (10% iodine) applied to fresh tissue selectively stains the amyloid deposits dark brown.

In the spleen, amyloidosis occurs in two forms, follicular and diffuse. In the former the spleen is firm and slightly enlarged, and the capsule is normal. The cut surface reveals small glassy round hyaline deposits that correspond to enlarged lymphoid follicles which are replaced with amyloid. In the diffuse form the spleen is larger but does not exceed 500 to 600 Gm. (1). The cut surface is firm, tumid, red, and waxy. Microscopically the red pulp is affected and often the follicles too. Iodine shows the distribution of the deposit in each instance.

1. Karsner, H.T. Human Pathology, 7th Edition, J.B. Lippincott Co., Philadelphia, 1949.

HODGKIN'S DISEASE OF SPLEEN

CLINICAL ACCOUNT 6191

The patient was a white female 66 years old whose illness began twenty years previously with biopsy of a lymph node in the neck. That revealed Hodgkin's disease. She was subsequently treated with irradiation and had a partial gastrectomy because of a peptic ulcer. She was currently taking cyclophosphamide and an adrenal corticosteroid. One week before admission she developed an acute urinary tract infection with chills, fever, dysuria, and low back pain relieved by micturition.

The temperature was 101 degrees F., respirations 18, pulse 96, and blood pressure 90/65 mm. Hg. The patient was emaciated. The lung fields revealed rales and rhonchi. The abdomen was not remarkable. There was slight pretibial pitting edema. Neurologic function was normal.

The hemoglobin was 9.2 Gm., hematocrit 31, and leukocytes 3,150 with a slight neutrophilia. The urine was yellow, cloudy, and acid with a specific gravity of 1.006. The sediment disclosed 5 leukocytes per high power field. The serum protein was 5.8 Gm. with 2.3 Gm. albumin and 3.5 Gm. globulin. Anorexia developed, weakness was progressive, and the patient died after thirty days in the hospital.

Autopsy examination revealed nonbacterial thrombotic endocarditis of the mitral valve, acute laryngotracheobronchitis, acute fibrinous pleuritis of the lower lobe of the right lung, bronchopneumonia of both lungs, acute pyelonephritis of the right kidney, and Hodgkin's disease of the liver, spleen, ovaries, and thoracic and abdominal lymph nodes. The spleen weighed 190 Gms.

THE ENTITY

Hodgkin's disease is regarded as a form of lymphoma that usually begins in lymph nodes, often of the neck, and gradually progresses to widespread involvement with a fatal outcome. The lesions are nodular, discrete, and composed of an intermingling of reticulum cells, lymphocytes, plasma cells, fibroblasts, often neutrophils, and usually a scattering of eosinophils. Sternberg-Reed cells with large bizarre irregular or multiple deeply basophilic nuclei are a histologic feature. The nodules display a striking tendency to undergo fibrosis.

The condition arises in the 20-to-40-year age group and occurs twice as often in males as females. Enlargement of lymph nodes on one side of the neck is usually the first sign. Onset may begin, however, by splenomegaly, recurring (Pel-Ebstein) fever, anemia, or widened mediastinal shadow on x-ray examination. Spread occurs to other groups of lymph nodes and to spleen, liver, bone marrow, and lungs. The spleen commonly weighs 500 to 600 Gm., and involvement ranges from microscopic lesions to massive nodules with extensive fibrosis. Infarcts may result for vascular effects.

The disease progresses irregularly, often with long periods of inactivity, and eventually recurs. Progressive debility leads to emaciation, infection, and death. Two uncommon forms include an indolent type that progresses slowly and tends to lack Sternberg-Reed cells, and a rapidly progressive form in which anaplasia is pronounced. Prognosis is best indicated, however, by clinical stage; i.e., whether involvement is limited to a single site or to multiple sites. Prospects decline in the latter instance. The overall 5, 10, and 20 year survival rates are approximately 30, 15, and 5 to 10 per cent (1).

1. Aisenberg, A.C. Hodgkin's disease—prognosis, treatment, and etiologic and immunologic considerations. New Eng. J. Med. 270:508, 1964.

HODGKIN'S DISEASE OF SPLEEN

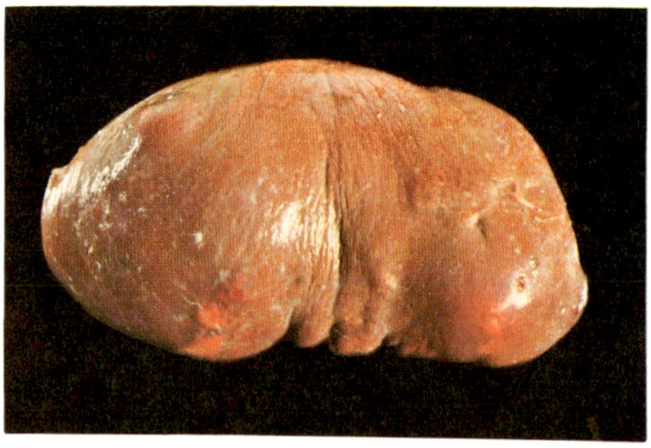

The capsule is roughened by fibrous adhesions, and the contour is distorted by firm nodules within the tissue.

The cut surface reveals two of the nodules. Both are firm, sharply circumscribed, and pale yellowish gray.

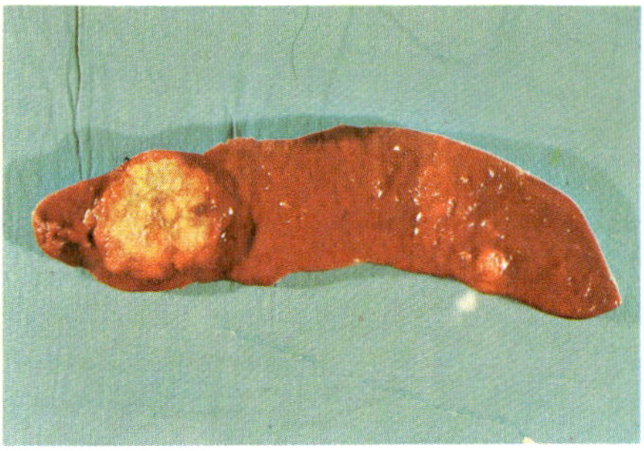

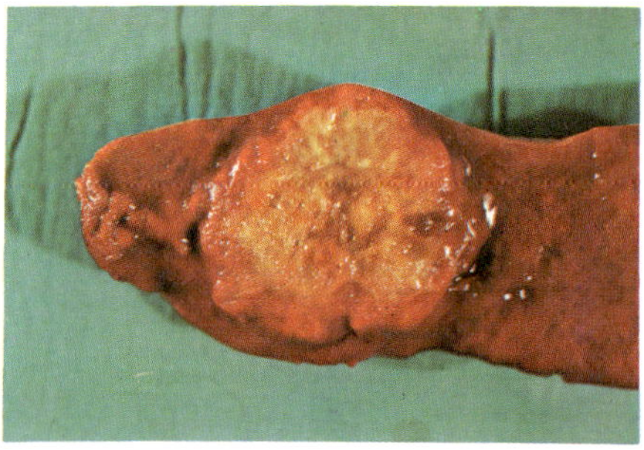

A closer view of the larger nodule discloses the cut surface in which central necrosis may be seen. Necrosis is not an especially conspicuous feature of the disease process, however.

Histologic examination reveals the polymorphous nature of the neoplastic process with neutrophils, lymphocytes, plasma cells, eosinophils, and reticulum cells in the same field. In the center a Sternberg-Reed cell is present; it is a giant cell with an irregular outline and tripolar nucleus. Such cells are regularly large and bizarre, but not necessarily trinucleated.

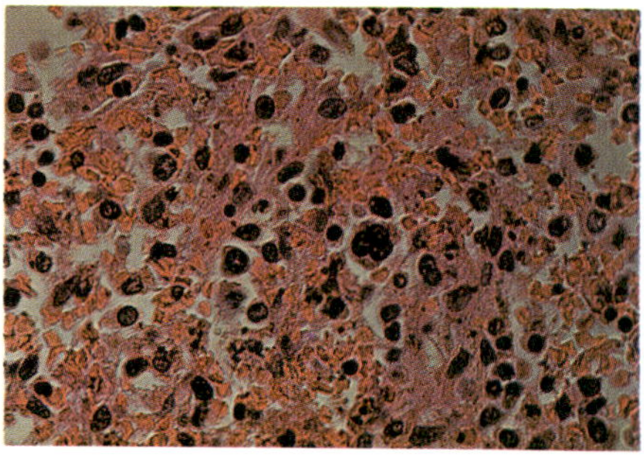

BURKITT'S LYMPHOMA

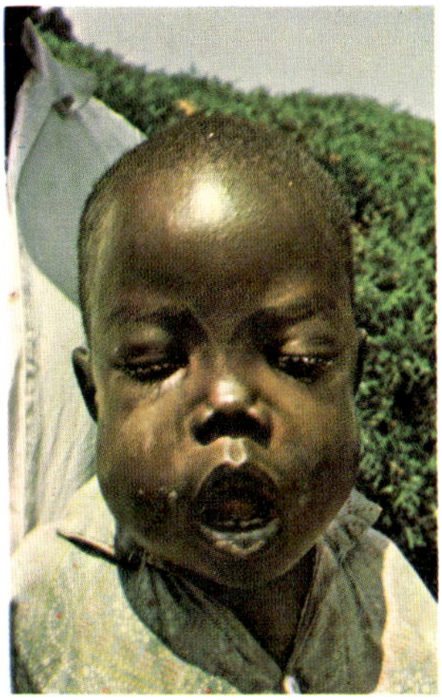

The patient presents distortion of the face due to tumor involvement of the upper jaws. A clinical characteristic is that facial disfigurement may become pronounced while symptomatic distress remains only slight.

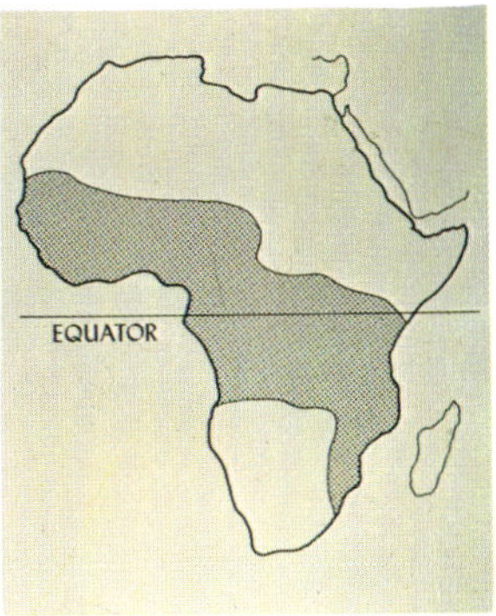

The "lymphoma belt" of Africa. The climate in this region is warm and damp so that arthropod vectors (mosquitoes) are abundant.

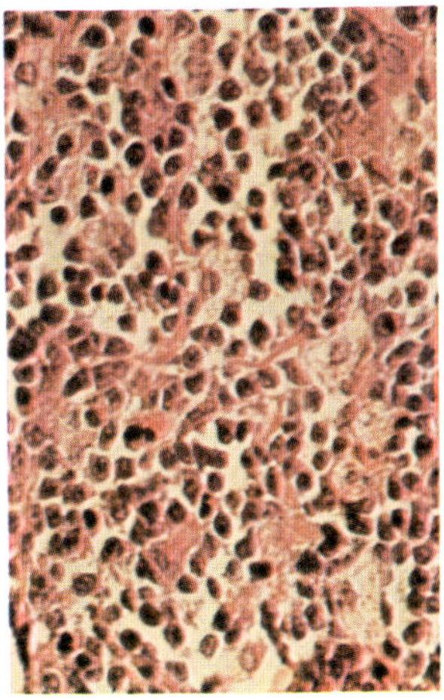

The histologic pattern is monocellular and uniform except for interspersed macrophages containing cellular debris.

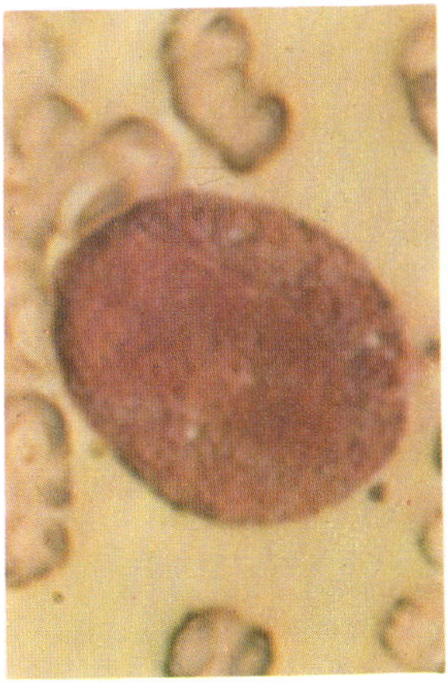

The uniformly immature tumor cells contain large nuclei with nucleoli and finely stippled chromatin; the cytoplasm is uniquely rich in ribonuclease and often displays minute lipid vacuoles.

BURKITT'S LYMPHOMA

CLINICAL ACCOUNT 7394

The patient was a 3½-year-old Ugandan male child who was well until one month before hospital admission. At that time, swelling of the upper jaws was noticed. Associated with this was pain in the teeth. There had been no loss of weight, and the child had felt well. Except for the face, physical examination was not remarkable. The blood and urine were normal.

THE ENTITY

Burkitt's lymphoma was first satisfactorily described in 1958 (1). It accounts for more than half of the childhood neoplasms in East Africa, it is the least differentiated of the malignant lymphomas, and it occurs in children of both sexes principally in the age group of 3 to 12 years. The illnesses are short, i.e., two weeks to three months, the tumors grow rapidly, and the most frequent presentation is a painless enlargement of the mandible and maxilla. Next most common is a swelling of the abdomen due to tumor arising in the ovaries, retroperitoneal lymph nodes, and abdominal viscera including the liver, spleen, and intestine. Nearly one-third of the cases have central nervous system involvement manifested by paraplegia and ocular palsies, and due to blood-borne meningeal spread or direct extension through the orbits. Isolated sites of origin include breasts, testes, thyroid, and long bones. Peripheral lymph nodes tend not to be affected.

The tumor is lacking in stroma, the monomorphic cells resemble lymphoblasts, and the pattern is uniform with dispersed macrophages containing cellular debris that gives a "starry-sky" appearance. The tumor cells measure 10 to 12 microns in diameter, the nuclei are large and round, and the cytoplasm consists of a thin basophilic rim often containing lipid-laden vacuoles. The chromatin is finely stippled, and there are 2 to 5 large nucleoli. The cytoplasm is uniquely rich in ribonuclease as disclosed by the methyl-green-pyronine-Y stain (2). Mitotic figures are abundant and all cells are equally immature.

The tumors respond dramatically to cyclophosphamide therapy and "melt away" rapidly with complete restoration of normal features. The frequency of multiple organ involvement precludes radiation therapy, although the tumor is extremely radiosensitive. Treatment of localized disease achieves long remission and possibly cure. The outlook is much less favorable when the tumor is widespread. Without treatment the tumor is rapidly fatal, and life seldom lasts more than six months after onset.

Burkitt's lymphoma occurs world-wide but is endemic in equatorial Africa and eastern New Guinea. At these sites the yearly temperature exceeds 60 degrees F., and the yearly rainfall exceeds 20 inches. This climatic combination corresponds to the distribution of arthropods, including mosquitoes, that could act as vectors. The tumor cells contain a virus of the Herpes group (Ebstein-Barr). While the relationship of these factors is not clear, it has been suggested that the EB virus, which is ubiquitous and lymphoproliferative, acts as an initiating factor, and malaria, which is localized to vector-borne regions, acts as a climate-controlled cofactor in the development of the malignant process (2).

1. Burkitt, D. A sarcoma involving the jaws in American children. Brit. J. Surg. 46:218-223, 1958.
2. Burkitt, D.P., and Wright, D.H. Burkitt's Lymphoma. E & S Livingstone, London, 1970.

SICKLE AUTOSPLENECTOMY

CLINICAL ACCOUNT 6765

The patient was a black female 65 years old who experienced vomiting and syncopal episodes four days before admission to the hospital. Seventeen months previously she had had a "heart attack" that was associated with congestive failure and pulmonary thrombo-emboli. At that time she was told that she had sickle cell anemia.

The vital signs were normal. The patient was obese. The physical examination was not remarkable except for a slight enlargement of the liver and a systolic ejection murmur heard over the left sternal border.

The urine disclosed three plus albumin, moderate bacteriuria, and 16 to 20 leukocytes per high power field. The hemoglobin was 10.6 gm., hematocrit 31 per cent, and leukocytes 19,600 per cmm. There was a reticulocytosis of 18.5 per cent, the sickle cell test was positive, and hemoglobin electrophoresis revealed SC hemoglobin. Two days after admission the patient complained of chest pains and died.

Autopsy examination revealed recent and organizing pulmonary thrombo-emboli, pelvic phlebothrombosis, cardiac hypertrophy (560 gm.), acute pyelonephritis, and marked atrophy and fibrosis of the spleen (10 gm.).

THE ENTITY

Sickle cell disease began in Africa from a mutation that causes an amino acid substitution in the structure of otherwise normal hemoglobin, i.e., valine for glutamic acid. Hemoglobin of this structure crystallizes to form sharp spicules in red cells that later hemolyze or fail to pass through small vessels. The mechanism of the disease is therefore hemolysis with anemia or vascular obstruction with infarction. The condition is restricted to blacks, and the individual may be homozygous or heterozygous. The former are ill from infancy, and most die in late childhood. The latter are asymptomatic and immune from falciparum malaria, perhaps because the hemoglobin is not suitable to the parasite. Before modern times, therefore, normal blacks often died of malaria, homozygous sicklers died of that condition, and heterozygous sicklers were protected from both. This selective advantage explains the wide distribution and high frequency of the mutation. In American Negroes, 7 to 13 per cent are sicklers, and about 3 per cent of these are homozygous (1).

The condition is manifested by recurring hemolytic crises causing acute pain in the abdomen and joints associated with jaundice, fever, and leukocytosis. A vigorous reticulocytosis persists between crises, i.e., 5 to 10 per cent. Erythrocytes sickle from oxygen consumption under a sealed cover glass, or from the addition of a reducing agent such as sodium metabisulfite. The spleen is enlarged only in infancy; infarcts and fibrosis reduce it to a vestige later. Pigment stones may obstruct the bile channels and increase the jaundice. The bone marrow shows erythroid hyperplasia, and the skull thickens as the tables atrophy and the medullary space widens. Bone cortex undergoes aseptic necrosis. Painful priapism results from sludged blood in the corpora cavernosa. Ulcers of the ankles are frequent from impeded circulation, and neurologic damage is due to micro-vessel ischemia.

1. Miale, J.B. Laboratory Medicine—Hematology, Third Edition, The C.V. Mosby Co., 1967, p. 787.

The spleen weighs only 10 gm. The surface is markedly irregular from the resolution of many infarcts. The process that eventuates in this nonfunctioning vestige is called "autosplenectomy."

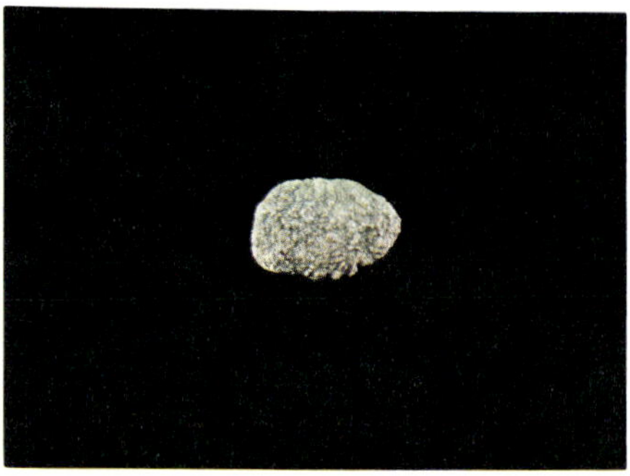

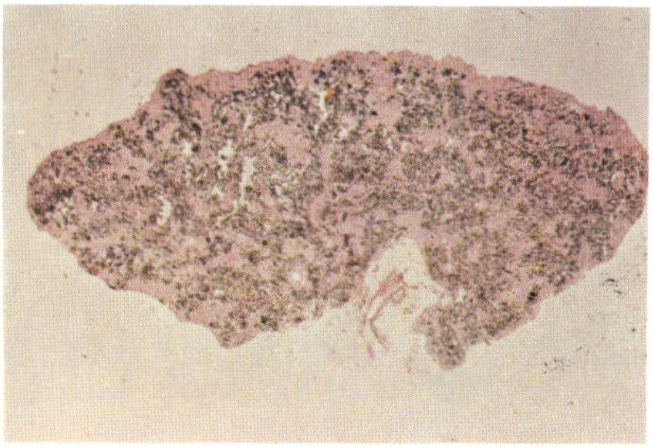

The cut surface of the entire spleen is displayed in this unmagnified cross section. The organ is reduced to a mass of dense fibrous connective tissue that is abundantly calcified.

At low magnification the large accumulations of calcium and hemosiderin are seen; these accumulations are called Gamna-Gandy bodies.

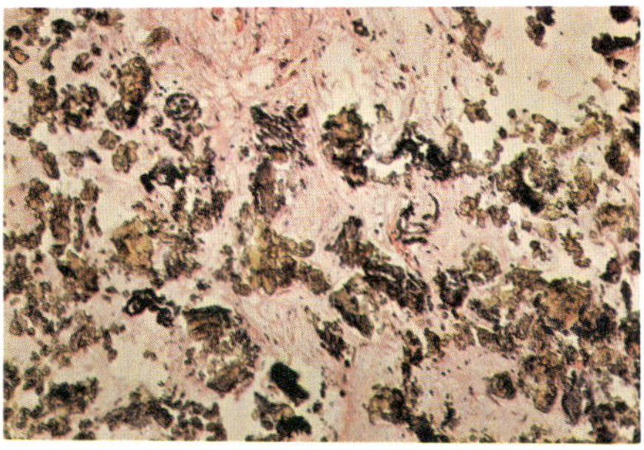

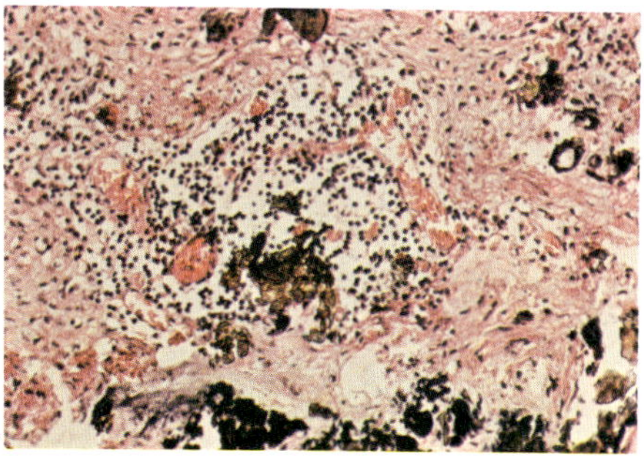

At slightly higher power the siderotic nodules (Gamna-Gandy bodies) are again seen. The amount of calcium in such spleens may be sufficient to be seen on an x-ray film of the abdomen.

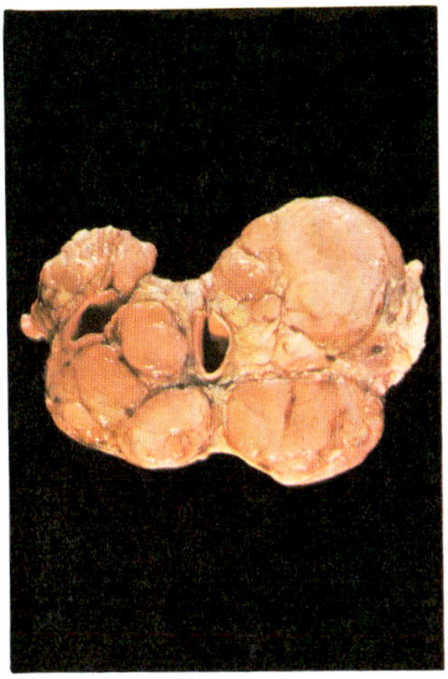

The cut surface of markedly enlarged lymph nodes at iliac bifurcation reveals beginning fusion of adjacent nodes and a uniform pinkish gray pallor that is characteristic.

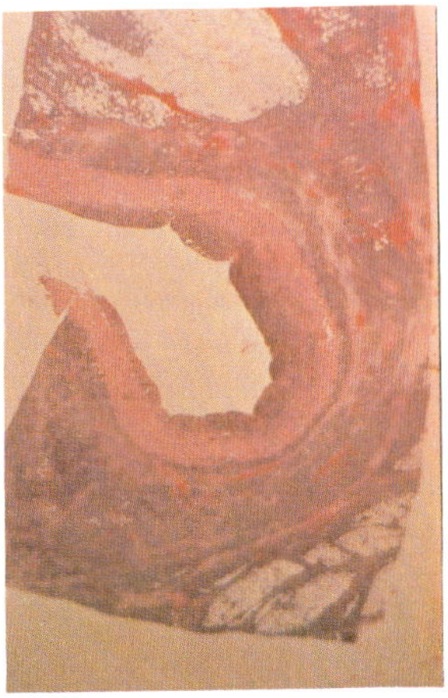

An unmagnified histologic section of abdominal nodes adjacent to the inferior vena cava discloses infiltration of the vein and extension into the retroperitoneal adipose tissue.

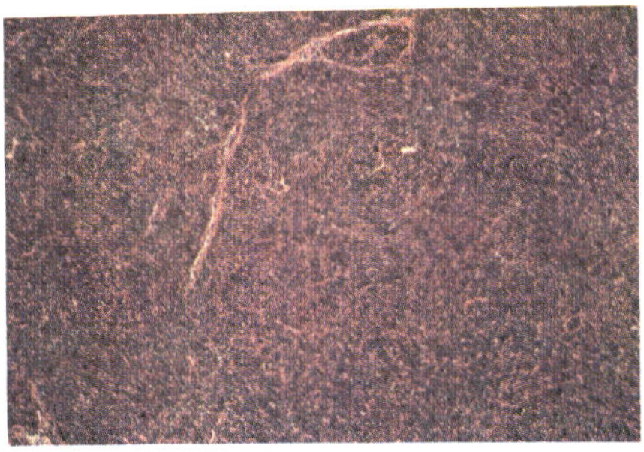

At low scanning power the nodal tissue displays uniform tumor cell infiltration that obliterates the germinal centers and normal follicular pattern.

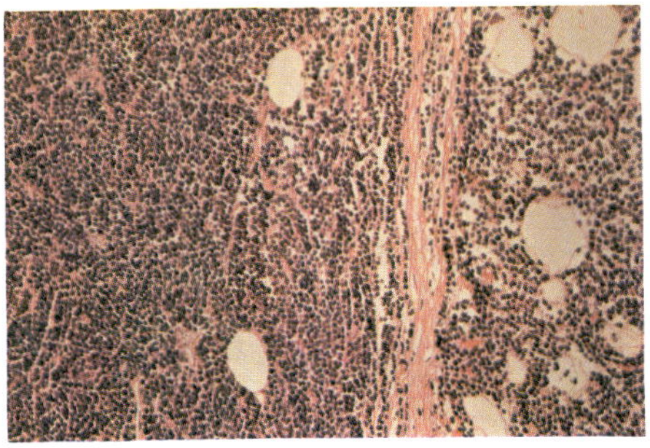

At higher power the extension of tumor cells through the capsule of the lymph node and into the perinodal adipose tissue is evident.

LYMPHOMA OF NODES

CLINICAL ACCOUNT 6419

The patient was a white female 52 years old who was well until two months before hospital admission, when she noted vaginal spotting. Physical examination revealed a vaginal mass that on biopsy disclosed a lymphoma of lymphoblastic type. An intravenous pyelogram displayed dilatation of the left renal pelvis. Irradiation treatment was given. Diarrhea, weakness, and weight loss ensued and the hospital admission was for these complaints.

The vital signs were normal. A 1 cm. movable lymph node was palpated in the left axilla. The liver was slightly enlarged. The spleen was not palpable. The remainder of the examination was not remarkable.

The urine was normal except for a few erythrocytes and leukocytes per high power field. The hemoglobin was 7.6 gm., hematocrit 22 per cent, and leukocytes 2,800 per cmm. with 51 segmented granulocytes, 7 band cells, 23 lymphocytes, and 19 monocytes. The blood urea nitrogen was 98 mg. per 100 ml. and the blood uric acid was 14.5 mg. per 100 ml.

The patient was treated with alkylating agents and steroids. A terminal pancytopenia developed, and there was gastro-intestinal hemorrhage. A staphylococcus septicemia contributed to the cause of death after twenty-nine days in the hospital.

The autopsy examination revealed pancytopenia of the bone marrow, hemorrhage of the gastro-intestinal tract, and lymphomatous invasion of the heart, stomach, liver, colon, spleen, pancreas, kidneys, pelvic organs, lymph nodes, bone marrow, and dura mater.

THE ENTITY

Malignant disease of the reticuloendothelial system, i.e., the liver, spleen, lymph nodes, and bone marrow principally, consists of the leukemias and lymphomas. The leukemias are named according to the dominant proliferating cell, i.e., granulocytic or lymphocytic, and are characterized by excessive numbers of immature cells in the circulating blood. The lymphomas arise in the reticuloendothelial tissues, especially the lymph nodes, later spread widely throughout the body, and do not extend into the blood in excessive numbers.

There are four types of lymphoma, i.e., lymphocytic, mixed cell type, reticulum cell, and Hodgkin's. All are either diffuse or nodular as seen microscopically under low magnification, and the first is further classified according to the developmental stage of the cells as poorly, moderately, or well differentiated (1).

Grossly the lymph nodes are enlarged in clusters, the cut surfaces are uniformly pale gray, and the adjacent margins are often fused. Microscopically the normal follicular pattern is fully effaced, the capsule is infiltrated, and the tumor cells frequently extend into the perinodal adipose tissue. Within the node the cell population tends to be immature and mitotic figures are abundant. Infiltration of vessel walls is often seen. The disease is progressive, and the rate of tissue infiltration increases with the immaturity of the cells. Intercurrent infection, especially of the lungs, is a frequent terminating event.

1. Rappaport, H. Tumors of the Hematopoietic System. Fascicle 8, Atlas of Tumor Pathology, Armed Forces Institute of Pathology, Washington, D.C., 1966.

LEUKEMOID REACTION

CLINICAL ACCOUNT 6699

The patient was a white female 53 years old who was well until four years before admission, when she developed a nodule in her right breast. Examination revealed carcinoma, a radical mastectomy was performed, and metastatic tumor was found in the axillary lymph nodes. Two years later abdominal pain was attributed to metastatic disease. One month before admission the abdominal pain recurred and was associated with confusion and a tendency to fall.

Positive findings included nodules in the skin of the chest, tenderness of the abdomen, a mass in the left upper quadrant, and a liver edge 10 cm. below the right costal margin. There were also an expressive aphasia, hyperactive tendon reflexes, and a positive Babinski sign on both sides.

The hemoglobin was 13.6 gm., and the leukocytes numbered 25,100 with 46 segmented granulocytes, 11 band cells, 3 juvenile cells, 3 myelocytes, 3 progranulocytes, 16 blast cells, 15 lymphocytes, and 3 monocytes. The blood uric acid, serum glutamic transaminase, and lactic dehydrogenase were 16.6 mgs., 163 units, and 3,840 units respectively. A bone survey indicated metastatic disease of the skull and pelvis, and a brain scan suggested metastatic carcinoma of the cerebrum. The patient's condition steadily worsened. On the twelfth hospital day the leukocyte count was 27,200, of which 43 per cent were blast cells. Bleeding developed, coma supervened, and the patient died after fifteen days in the hospital.

Autopsy examination revealed extensive widespread carcinomatosis that included the liver, spleen, lymph nodes, and bone marrow. The liver weighed 2400 gm., the spleen 800 gm. The latter was massively filled with metastatic carcinoma cells. The bone marrow was also diffusely infiltrated with metastatic tumor. Myeloid and erythroid cells were also widely spread throughout the hematopoietic organs.

THE ENTITY

The leukemoid reaction is a pronounced leukocytosis with immature cells in the circulating blood so that the differential count is suggestive of leukemia. The condition is self-limited and nonneoplastic. The principal causes are metastatic carcinoma, Gram negative bacteremia, trauma with bone marrow embolism, necrotizing liver disease, and disseminated granulomatous disease, especially miliary tuberculosis. Metastatic carcinoma of the breast is an especially common cause of the leukemoid reaction in women. In adults there is virtually no cytologic or morphologic distinction between acute myeloblastic leukemia and the leukemoid reaction; i.e., Auer bodies, histocytology, electron microscopy, and chromosomal karyotypes fail to demarcate one from the other (1). The hyperuricemia and elevation of the serum glutamic acid and especially the lactic dehydrogenase are evidence of increased cell synthesis and destruction, but it is not clear whether these signs are due to the metastatic carcinoma cells or the hemopoietic cells. Alkaline phosphatase is normally present in the cytoplasm of mature neutrophils and is increased in the leukemoid reaction. Moreover, this enzyme is decreased or absent in leukemia. The reaction, however, is unreliable when most of the leukocytes are immature. A final distinction is that of leukoblastic invasion of parenchymatous structures which is unique to leukemia. This was not seen in the present case, although it may have been obscured by the extensive metastatic tumor. Thus in some cases the distinction cannot be made.

1. Smith, J.C. Leukemia or leukemoid reaction? A clinico-pathologic conference. Med. Ann. Dist. Columbia 40:706-709, 1971.

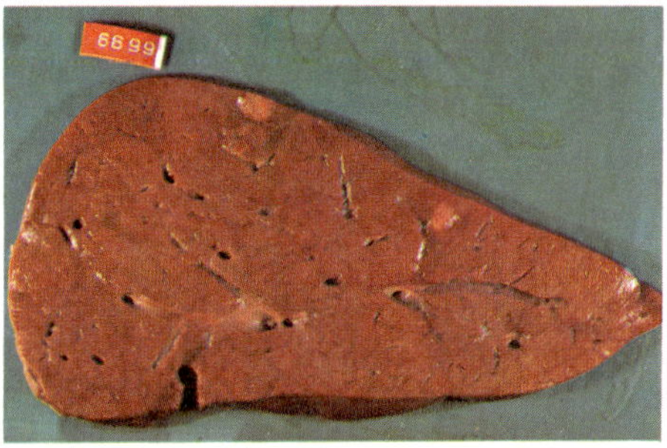

The cut surface of the liver reveals two nodules of metastatic carcinoma. Elsewhere the cut surface displays pallor suggestive of leukosis.

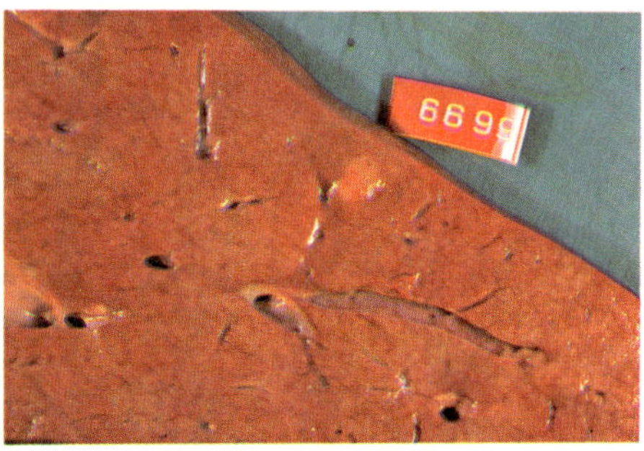

A close-up photograph gives a better view of both findings.

The microsection reveals the junction of the metastatic nodule with the adjacent parenchyma. Myeloid cells are numerous in the sinusoids of the latter.

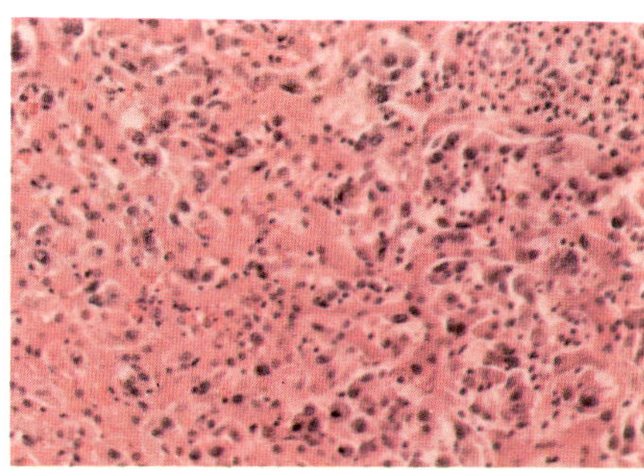

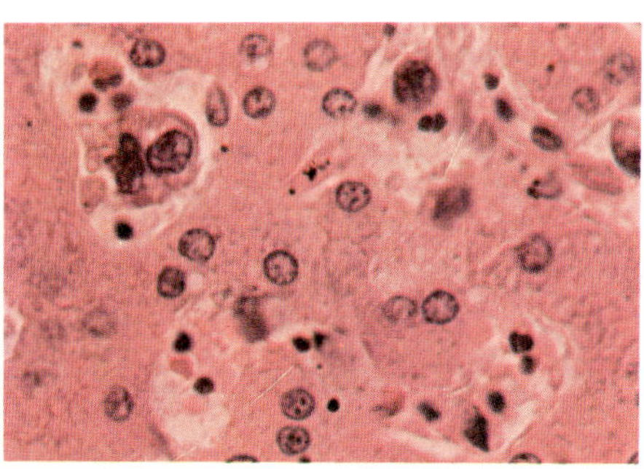

At higher power carcinoma cells with large nuclei and myeloid cells with small nuclei may be seen in the hepatic sinusoids.

KAPOSI'S SARCOMA OF LEG

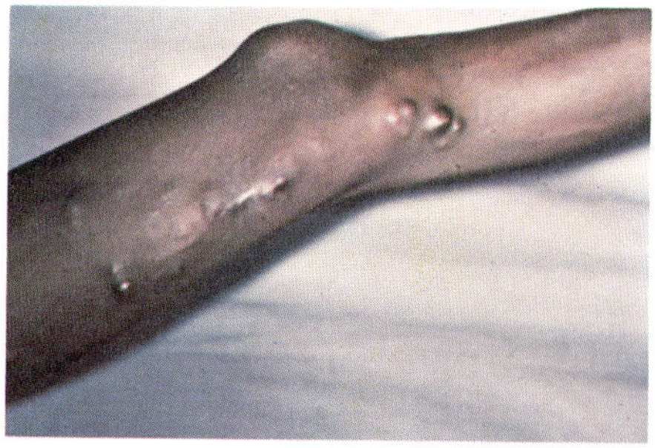

The medial aspect of the left leg reveals firm subcutaneous nodules that arose approximately 18 months before the patient was admitted to the hospital.

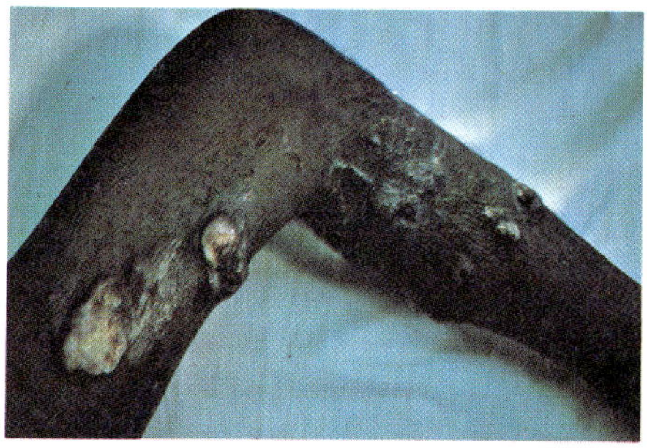

The same nodules showing ulceration that began two months before the patient was hospitalized.

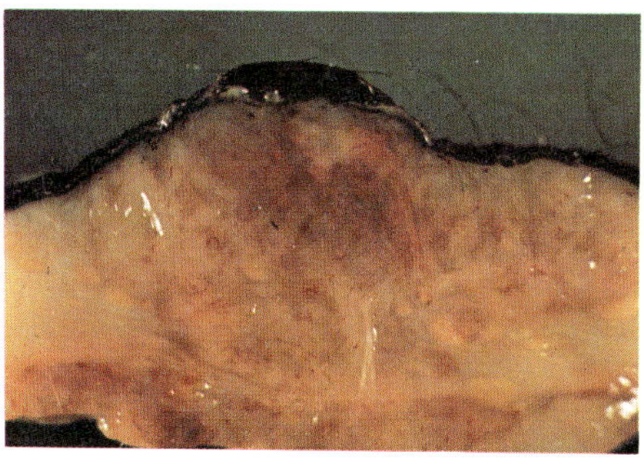

The cut surface of one of the nodules reveals a firm, poorly demarcated tumor mass that extends deeply into the subcutaneous tissue. Near the skin surface a yellow focus of necrosis is present. Capillaries and small vascular channels cause the red discoloration.

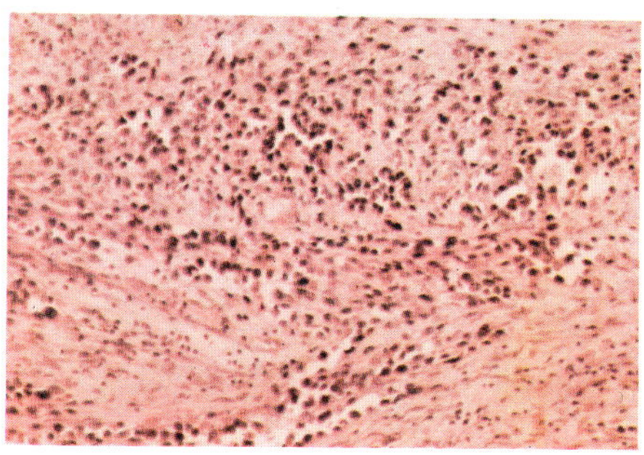

Large cells, presumably endothelial, compose the tumor and form small irregular channels so that vascularity is a feature of the lesion.

KAPOSI'S SARCOMA OF LEG

CLINICAL ACCOUNT U-439

The patient was a black male 22 years old who was well until 3½ years before entering the hospital. At that time the dorsum and medial aspect of his left foot began to itch. Scratching relieved the itching and was continued until six months later, when the skin of the foot became thick and nodular, and portions of the medial aspect sloughed. Two years before hospital entry a nodule was noted on the medial aspect of the right forearm. Eighteen months before admission additional nodules were discovered in the hypochondrium and over the lateral aspect of the right hip. During the past eighteen months the ulceration spread to involve most of the left foot, and multiple firm subcutaneous nodules appeared over the medial aspect of the left leg, extending to the groin. In the last two months the groin and a nodule of the left lower leg became ulcerated. Nitrogen mustard was given, but the spreading ulceration of the groin was not slowed. The patient became febrile, respiratory distress with coughing developed, and death occurred in respiratory failure.

THE ENTITY

Kaposi's sarcoma is a vascular tumor of the skin and subcutaneous tissue that occurs most often in African Negroes, especially in the equatorial countries of Nigeria, Zaire, Uganda, and Kenya. It was first described by the Hungarian dermatologist Moritz Kaposi in 1872. The condition affects mainly adults and occurs much more often in males than females, i.e. circa 12:1. The tumors tend to arise on the extremities, the feet more often than the hands, and appear as firm subcutaneous nodules measuring up to 2 cm. in diameter or as deeply pigmented dermal plaques that are markedly indurated. The simultaneous development of several nodules suggests multicentric sites of origin. While the tumors may be agressive from the onset and pursue a fulminant course, most are indolent for long periods, occasionally more than a decade, before invasion of the deeper tissues takes place. Concurrent with this aggressive course, one or more of the subcutaneous nodules enlarge, ulcerate, and weep a clear serum. Approximately 5 per cent of the cases occur in children under the age of 11 years, and in these patients the tumors tend to arise in and remain restricted to lymph nodes. Also, in these cases the condition is markedly aggressive from the onset, and death within a few months is due to compression of adjacent structures. Visceral tumors without skin involvement have been seen.

The cut surface of a subcutaneous nodule is firm and pinkish gray or red and hemorrhagic. The nodule is traversed by coarse bands of dense fibrous connective tissue, and the margins are poorly demarcated. Histologic examination reveals interweaving bundles of connective tissue that form capillaries lined by endothelial cells or slit-like spaces containing erythrocytes lined by spindle cells. Mixed forms are common, and either form may undergo anaplastic change. There is no histologic difference, however, between the clinically aggressive and indolent forms of the disease (1). The tumor is presumed to arise from primitive mesenchymal cells. The cause is unknown, although environmental factors are suspect because of the unusual ethnic and geographical distribution of the disease.

1. Slavin, G., Cameron, H. McD., and Singh, H. Kaposi's sarcoma in mainland Tanzania: A report of 117 cases. Brit. J. Cancer 23: 349-357, 1969.

NORMAL THYROID

CLINICAL ACCOUNT 6188

The patient was a white female 63 years old who felt well until noon of the day of admission to the hospital. At that time she developed neck pain and a headache. These promptly became severe. About one hour later she lay down and shortly thereafter became unresponsive.

The temperature was 98.6 degrees F., pulse 76, respirations 16, and blood pressure 160/90 mm. Hg. The patient was unconscious. The lung fields were clear. The heart was not enlarged, the rhythm was regular, and no murmurs were heard. The abdomen was soft and not remarkable. The spinal reflexes were exaggerated and the left pupil was dilated and fixed.

The urine revealed glucose and 6 erythrocytes per high power field. The hemoglobin was 13.4 Gm., hematocrit 40, and leukocytes 19,300 with a slight neutrophilia. The blood sugar was 164 mg. An arteriogram indicated bleeding, and a left craniotomy evacuated a large subdural hematoma. Continued bleeding necessitated clipping of the left common carotid artery. The bleeding did not stop, the blood pressure became difficult to maintain, and the patient died on the morning of the following day.

Autopsy examination revealed atelectasis of the right and left lungs, pneumatosis of the ileum and colon, and a subdural hematoma on the left. The thyroid weighed 20 Gms.

THE ENTITY

The thyroid is a symmetrical bilobed gland that normally weighs about 20 Gm. It consists of acini filled with colloid that are lined by a single layer of cuboidal epithelial cells. The cells extract iodine from the blood, incorporate it into thyroxine, and secrete the thyroxine into the capillaries that course between the acini. What is not secreted is stored in the gland.

Thyroxine stimulates metabolism so that an excess causes excitability, restlessness, and intolerance to heat, while a reduced amount causes a slowing of mental and physical processes and an intolerance to cold. Two tests are especially useful in measuring thyroid function; the protein-bound iodine and the uptake of radioactive iodine. About 95 per cent of the serum iodine is attached to protein in the form of thyroxine (1). From serum the protein may be precipitated and the iodine measured. The normal protein-bound iodine (PBI) is 4-8 mcgm. per 100 ml. In hypothyroidism (myxedema, cretinism) the blood level is about 2 mcgm., while in hyperthyroidism (Graves' disease) the circulating level is often 15 mcgm. Since the thyroid concentrates iodine and stores it, the avidity of the gland for this substance is indicated by the uptake of radioactive iodine. The normal uptake is 15 to 40 per cent in 24 hours.

1. Ravel, R. Clinical Laboratory Medicine, Year Book Medical Publishers, Inc., Chicago, 1969.

NORMAL THYROID

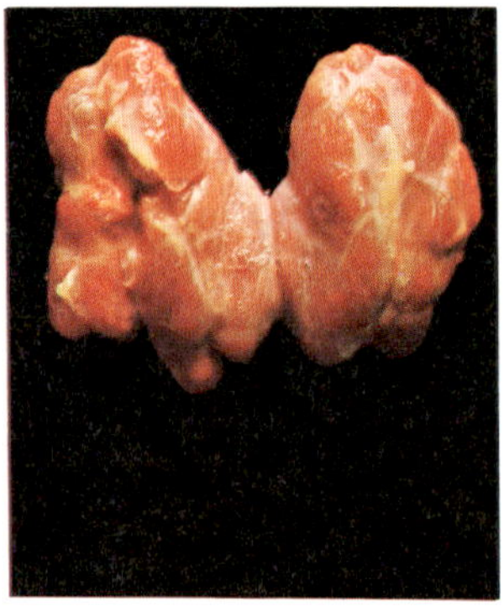

The organ is of normal size, the lobes are approximately symmetrical, and the isthmus is of normal dimensions. A slight abnormality is the presence of fibrous septae that tend to separate the lateral lobes into coarse nodules. Normally each lateral lobe has roughly the shape of a pyramid and the external surface is devoid of such septae.

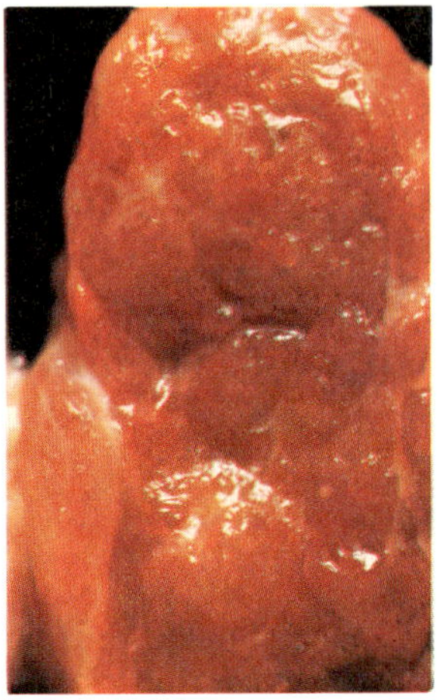

Section reveals a fleshy red cut surface over which fibrous septae divide the tissue into small pseudo-nodules.

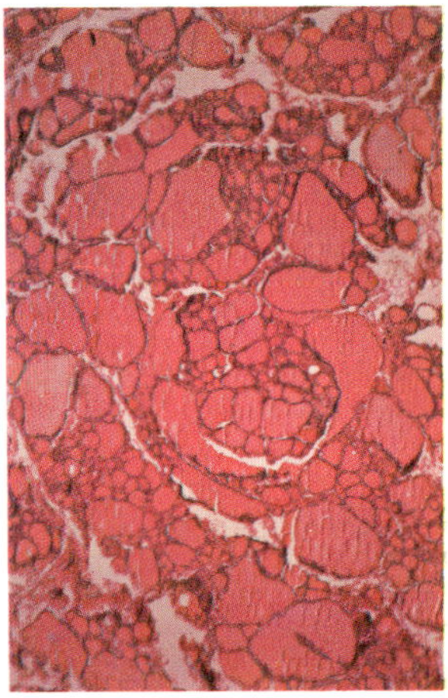

Low power examination reveals a dispersion of glands of approximately equal size.

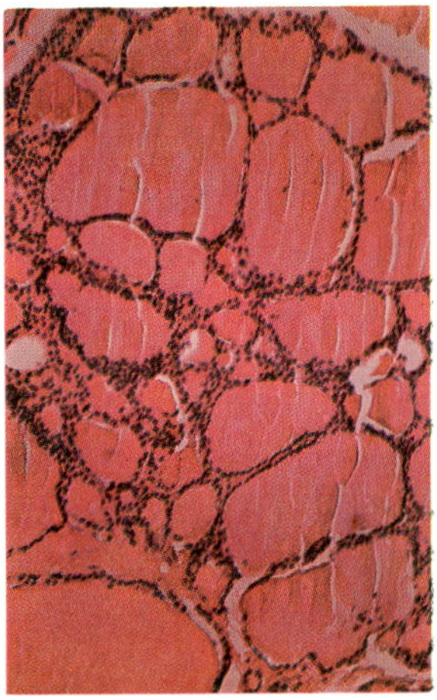

At higher power the gland is composed of small and moderate-sized follicles that are evenly distributed and uniformly filled with clear pink colloid. The lining epithelial cells are cuboidal, the gland margins are smooth and round, and the interstitial tissue is sparse and devoid of leukocytes.

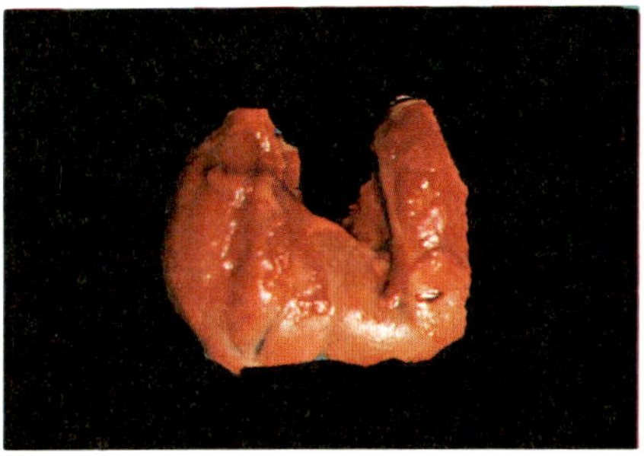

The thyroid is slightly asymmetrical and moderately enlarged. No other gross changes are evident.

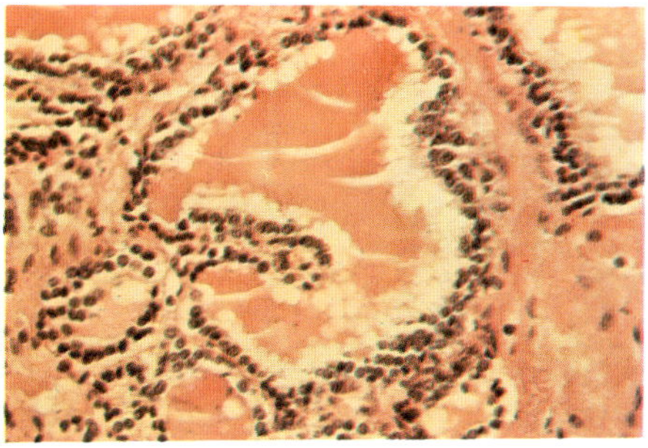

At low power the glands display columnar lining cells, papillary infolding of them, and scalloping of the colloid at the peripheral margins of the follicles. These changes, when diffuse and combined with colloid depletion, are the characteristic histologic features of hyperthyroidism.

The myocardium reveals widespread foci of necrosis with an associated light leukocytic infiltration. The infiltrating cells are lymphocytes, monocytes, in addition to a few segmented granulocytes.

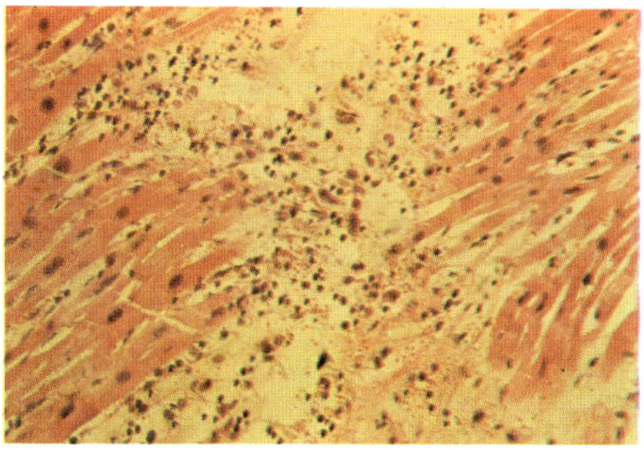

The hepatic tissue also reveals widespread foci of necrosis with leukocytic infiltration. The cells are lymphocytes, monocytes, and occasional neutrophilic granulocytes.

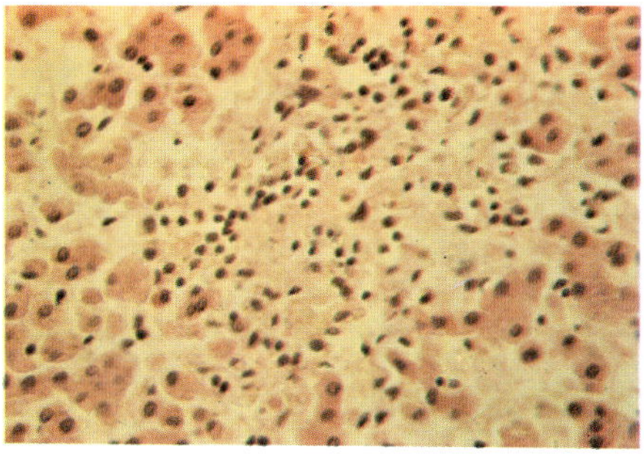

GRAVES' DISEASE

CLINICAL ACCOUNT 5834

The patient was a white female 43 years old who was admitted to the hospital because of fever, joint pain, and vomiting. One week previously fever and sore throat developed. Shortly later there were lassitude, weakness, and aching of the legs. Two days before admission arthralgia of the shoulders, wrists, knees, and ankles began. There was no redness or swelling of the joints.

The temperature was 104 degrees F., respirations 28, pulse 130, and blood pressure 140/60. The patient was toxic, trembling, dehydrated, and undernourished. The eyes did not protrude. The thyroid was symmetrical and twice enlarged. The heart, lungs, and abdomen were not remarkable.

The urine revealed 4 plus protein, many bacteria, and occasional casts. The hemoglobin was 10.8 Gm., hematocrit 39, and leukocytes 13,100 with 70 segmented granulocytes, 11 band cells, 13 lymphocytes, and 6 monocytes. The blood cholesterol was 92 mg. The cephalin flocculation was 2 plus at 24 hours and 3 plus at 48 hours. The protein-bound iodine was 9.2 mcgm., and the tri-iodothyronine uptake was 53 per cent.

During the hospital course the temperature remained above 102 degrees F., and occasionally spiked to 105 degrees F. The pulse varied from 110 to 140. The hemoglobin steadily declined to 6.3 Gm., and the leukocytes rose to 21,000 with a neutrophilia. Jaundice developed; the total serum bilirubin was 7.1 mg. with 6.8 mg. unconjugated. On the eleventh hospital day 8 drops of Lugol's solution were given every 8 hours. The patient was excessively restless and desperately ill. She died on the fourteenth hospital day.

Autopsy examination revealed hyperplasia of the thyroid, which weighed 50 Gms., acute fibrinous epicarditis, focal acute myocarditis, focal hepatic necrosis, focal degeneration of smooth and skeletal muscle, and hyperplasia of the spleen (230 Gms.). Grossly the thyroid was twice normal size and symmetrical in contour. The cut surface was firm, moist, red, and fleshy.

THE ENTITY

The lesion of hyperthyroidism is diffuse epithelial hyperplasia. This is manifested by an increase in the number of acini, which are small and irregular, a scalloping of the colloid margins, and a papillary infolding of the lining cells which become tall and columnar. This produces enlargement of the gland and reflects hyperfunctioning of it. The hypermetabolic state is characterized by nervous excitability, tremors, tachycardia, palpitation, moistness of the skin, and excessive production of heat so that there is insensitivity to cold. Wasting is gradual as nutrition fails to keep pace with this state. Also associated, though not regularly present, is protrusion of the eyes (exophthalmos). The cause of this protrusion is not known; it does not correlate with the degree of hyperthyroidism, and the only morphologic change is an increase in the amount of retrobulbar adipose tissue. The clinical features of hyperthyroidism, or Graves' disease, are thus enlargement of the gland and a hypermetabolic state with or without exophthalmos.

The course of the condition may be rapid and fulminant ("thyroid storm"), or it may wax and wane and gradually subside. Treatment consists of ablative measures including removal, irradiation, or functional blocking with drugs such as propylthiouracil.

The cause of the condition is uncertain; it may be due to overproduction of thyroid stimulating hormone by the pituitary.

COLLOID GOITER

CLINICAL ACCOUNT 5982

The patient was a white female 75 years old who developed symptoms of a gastric ulcer. She had been hypertensive for 15 years and diabetic for 10 years. She had also had a goiter for the past 10 years that was untreated.

Physical examination revealed moderate asymmetrical enlargement of the thyroid. The gland was soft and nontender; no bruit was heard.

A barium study disclosed a gastric ulcer and operation revealed that it had eroded into the pancreas. The lesion was excised, the postoperative course was stormy and the patient died on the twentieth postoperative day.

Autopsy examination revealed partial absence of the stomach with a gastro-jejunal anastamosis and an acute peritonitis with subdiaphragmatic and pelvic abscesses. There were also microabscesses (Candida) of the heart and kidneys, thromboemboli of both pulmonary arteries, and hyalinization of the islets of Langerhans consistent with diabetes mellitus. The thyroid weighed 170 Gms.

THE ENTITY

Goiter means enlargement of the thyroid. The three common types are diffuse colloid, nodular colloid, and toxic goiter associated with hyperthyroidism and exophthalmos.

Diffuse colloid goiter is a uniform enlargement due to hyperplasia with accumulation of colloid. It is a work hypertrophy caused by insufficient iodine due to excessive need as in adolescence when body development is rapid, or inadequate supply as in the Great Lakes region and the St. Lawrence River Basin where the soil is poor in iodine. When adolescence is completed, or iodine is given, the condition ordinarily disappears. Enlargement of the neck is usually the only clinical sign.

In adult life cycles of hyperplasia and involution may occur, the gland may be affected irregularly, and foci of hyperplasia interspersed with nodules of colloid may result. The latter are often large and bounded by fibrous scars. A nodular goiter thus develops and palpation of the neck reveals asymmetry of the gland. Where colloid accumulates the glands are dilated, the lining cells are flat or cuboidal, and papillary infolding is not seen. Symptoms of this aspect are due to pressure, outwardly to distort the neck and inwardly to compress the trachea and interfere with breathing. The hyperplastic sites cause increased metabolism, the symptoms of which are reviewed under hyperthyroidism. Treatment consists of excision of the enlarged or toxic part.

COLLOID GOITER

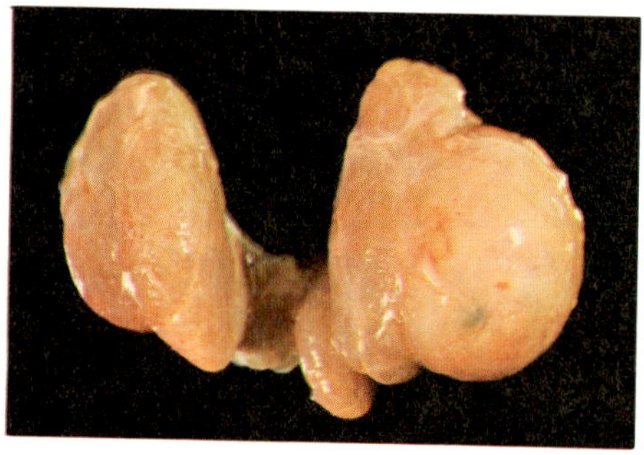

The photograph is taken from the posterior surface to reveal a smooth oval bulging mass in the right lateral lobe.

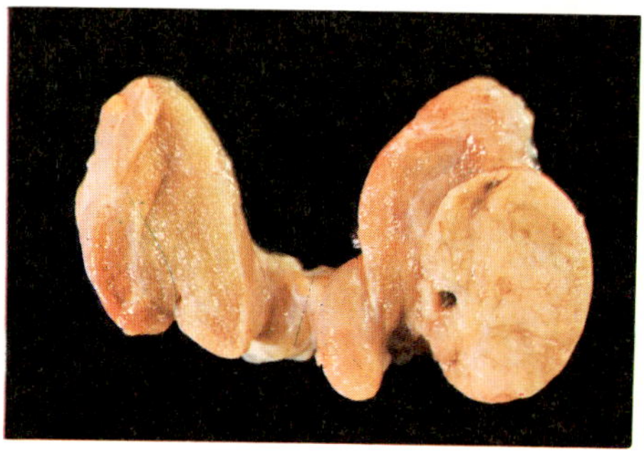

Section reveals a fleshy adenoma that measures 3 cm. in diameter. The capsule is thin, smooth, and intact, and a central brown focus of cystic degeneration is evident.

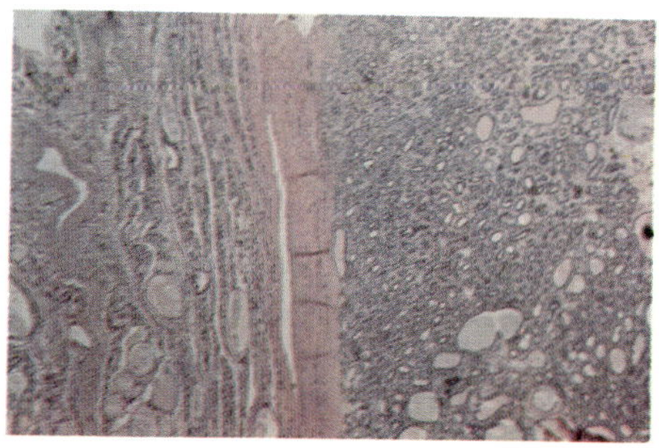

At low power the central fibrous capsule separates the minute closely spaced glands of the adenoma from the larger colloid-filled glands of the adjacent normal thyroid.

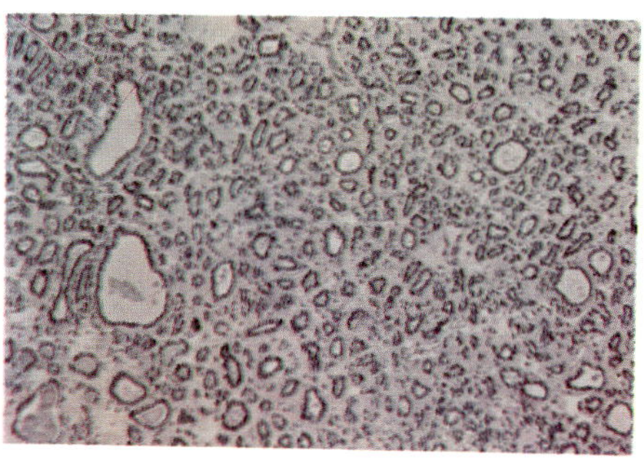

At higher power the small glands of the adenoma are seen. They are regularly small, colloid formation is scant, and the epithelial cells are uniformly cuboidal. No departure from this pattern such as anaplasia or capsular invasion is seen.

ADENOMA OF THYROID

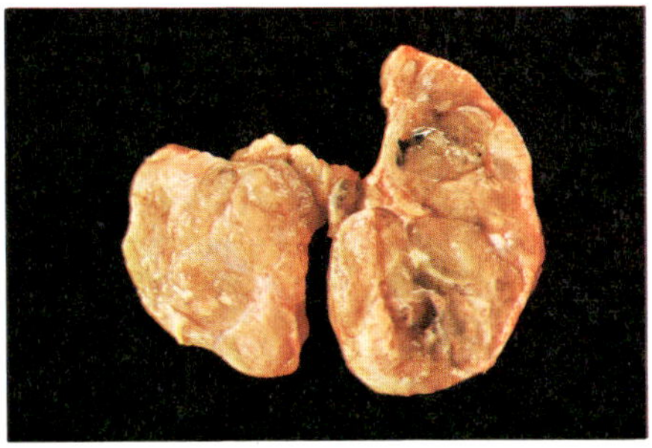

The gland seen here is enlarged, asymmetrical, and coarsely lobulated.

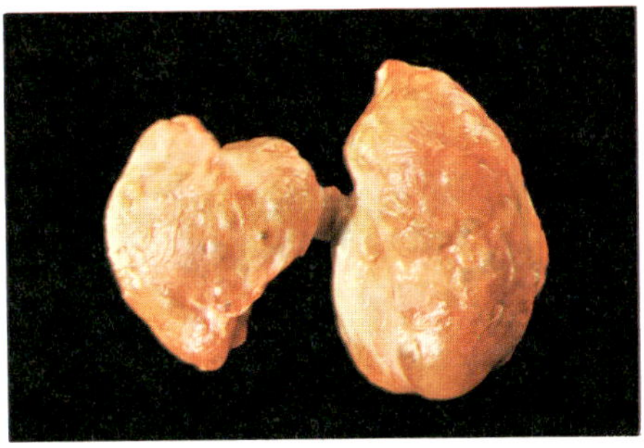

The cut surface reveals large tanks of colloid within dilated follicles that are demarcated by thin bands of dense fibrous connective tissue.

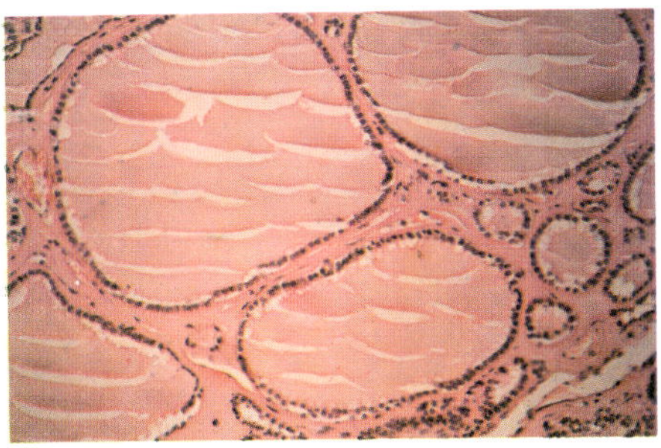

At low power a gland margin is composed of thin strands of fibrous connective tissue and compressed epithelial elements. The follicle consists of markedly dilated glands with smooth contours and lumens that are gorged with clear pink retained colloid.

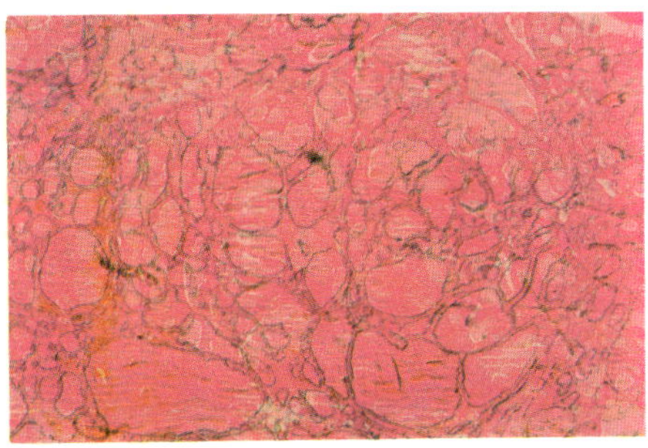

Higher power reveals that the gland margins are smooth, papillary infolding is absent, the lining cells are low cuboidal or flat, and lumen is distended with colloid that shows no marginal scalloping.

ADENOMA OF THYROID

CLINICAL ACCOUNT 5926

The patient was a Negro male 44 years old who was admitted to the hospital because of ankle swelling and shortness of breath of one-week duration. He had been in renal failure for many months and had undergone peritoneal dialysis several times. He was thought to have chronic membranous glomerulonephritis. A weight gain of 7 pounds had taken place during the week prior to admission.

The patient was emaciated and puffy-faced. The temperature was 98.2 degrees F., respirations 20, pulse 80, and blood pressure 160/110 mm. Hg. Physical findings included rales at both bases, enlargement of the heart, a reducible right inguinal hernia, and pronounced pitting edema of the extremities.

The urine was yellow, cloudy, and alkaline. There was a 2 plus proteinuria; the sediment revealed 10 leukocytes per high power field. The hemoglobin was 6.2 Gm., hematocrit 18 per cent, and leukocytes 11,900 with a slight neutrophilia. The blood urea nitrogen and serum creatinine were 99 and 10.6 mg. per 100 ml.

Peritoneal dialysis was performed. Paracentesis removed 1100 ml. of ascitic fluid. An ischiorectal abscess developed and was drained. Massive edema of the scrotum developed and the skin sloughed. He remained afebrile. His sensorium deteriorated, and he died after two weeks in the hospital.

Autopsy examination revealed hypertrophy of the heart (560 Gms.), edema of the right and left lungs, empyema of the right pleural space, acute suppurative prostatitis, ischiorectal abscess, and marked chronic glomerulonephritis. The thyroid weighed 48 Gms.

THE ENTITY

The most common neoplasm of the thryoid is the adenoma. These are round, encapsulated, and small or large. They differ from the normal adjacent tissue by their altered histologic pattern. The two principal types are follicular, which are common, and papillary, which are not. Follicular adenomas form glands, are benign, and are subclassified according to various histologic features although the clinical importance of this is not great (1). The subclassification includes fetal, microfollicular, macrofollicular, embryonal, and oxyphil or Hurthle cell types. In contrast papillary adenomas are uncommon, form finger-like projections that extend into the gland lumens, and resemble papillary carcinomas which appear similar except for capsular invasion and extension into blood vessels.

Most adenomas grow slowly and are clinically silent. When larger than 1 cm., a nodule may be palpated in the neck. When hemorrhage occurs, sharp pain may result. As this subsides and the blood is absorbed, foci of cystic degeneration form within the adenoma. When hormone is produced, thyrotoxicosis may arise. Most adenomas function, take up radioactive iodine, and thus differ from most carcinomas which do not (2).

1. Hazard, J.B., and Smith, D.E., Editors. The Thyroid. International Academy of Pathology Monograph. The Williams and Wilkins Company, Baltimore, 1964.
2. Williams, R.H., Editor. Textbook of Endocrinology. W.B. Saunders Company, Philadelphia, 1968.

CARCINOMA OF THYROID

CLINICAL ACCOUNT 6196

The patient was a white female 75 years old who had been hypertensive for the past 10 years and had experienced angina pectoris for the past 5 years. For some months she had also had shortness of breath, dyspnea on exertion, 2-pillow orthopnea, nocturia, and ankle edema which disappeared in the morning. On the night before admission she had severe pain in the left anterior chest that radiated to both shoulders and was not relieved by nitroglycerine.

The temperature was 98.6 degrees F., pulse 150, respirations 32, and blood pressure 92/60 mm. Hg. Rales were audible over the lower posterior lung fields. The heart was enlarged to the left, the rhythm was regular, and no murmurs were heard. The abdomen was protuberant; no masses were palpated. There was no fluid wave. There was no ankle edema.

The urine was not remarkable except for 15 leukocytes and many epithelial cells and hyaline casts in the sediment. The hemoglobin was 12.9 Gm., hematocrit 41, and leukocytes 9,000 with a normal differential count. An electrocardiogram disclosed atrial fibrillation. The patient was digitalized, the heart rate decreased, and a harsh systolic murmur radiating to the neck and axilla was then heard. The serum glutamic transaminase and lactic dehydrogenase were normal. The blood urea nitrogen was 42 mg. per 100 ml. A chest x-ray indicated pulmonary hyperemia, pleural effusions, and cardiac enlargement. On the fourteenth hospital day dyspnea became pronounced and the patient died.

Autopsy examination revealed hypertrophy of the heart (475 Gms.), rheumatic disease of the aortic valve with stenosis, nondeforming rheumatic disease of the mitral valve, hyperemia of the lungs, pleural effusions (400 ml., right, 350 ml., left), arteriolar nephrosclerosis, carcinoma of the thyroid, carcinoma of the right breast, and a cortical adenoma of the left adrenal. The thyroid weighed 19.8 Gms.

THE ENTITY

Thyroid cancer occurs mainly in adults and affects women three times more often than men. The most common clinical sign is a nodule in the neck. Somewhat more than half fail to take up radioactive iodine. The lesion is a unilateral pale brownish gray unencapsulated nodule that slowly enlarges. Microscopic involvement of the opposite lobe is common. Most thyroid cancers are papillary or follicular, some are medullary with amyloid stroma, and least common are undifferentiated carcinomas. The differentiated cancers (papillary and follicular) grow slowly and metastasize late. Treatment consists of total extracapsular thyroidectomy. The differentiated cancers have a 10 year post-treatment survival rate of about 90 percent. The outlook for medullary cancer with amyloid stroma is only slightly worse. Undifferentiated carcinomas are extremely malignant and spread rapidly.

Cause is related to interference with thyroxine production; the latter inclines the pituitary to produce thyroid-stimulating hormone which causes prolonged epithelial hyperplasia of the gland. Thyroid cancer thus tends to be more common in endemic goiter areas than elsewhere. It also occurs, often after a long latent period, in patients who have had irradiation of the neck. The incidence of thyroid cancer in the United States is about 3 cases per 100,000 population (1).

1. Anglem, T.J., and Meissner, W.A. Cancer of the thyroid and parathyroid, in Cancer, A Manual for Physicians, Fourth Edition, American Cancer Society, Massachusetts Division, p. 47, 1968.

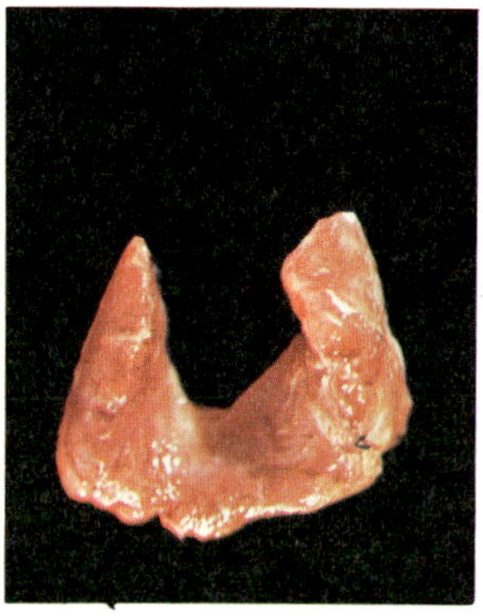

The photograph shows the posterior surface, from which it can be seen that there is a slight enlargement of the right lobe.

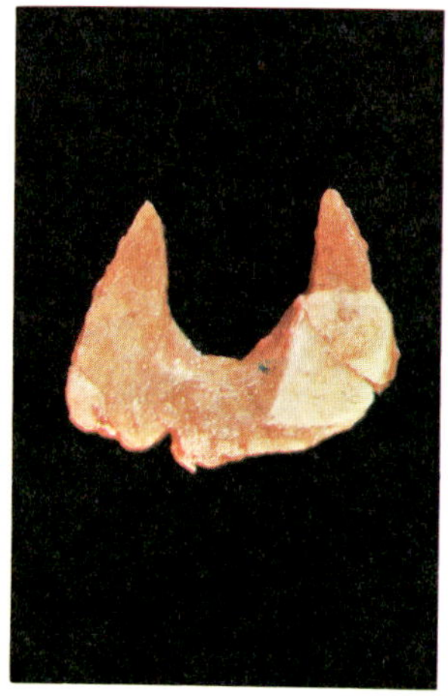

Section discloses a sharply demarcated pale pinkish gray nodule occupying the lower portion of the right lobe. The tissue of this nodule is firm and differs in texture from the spongy resilient nature of the opposite lobe.

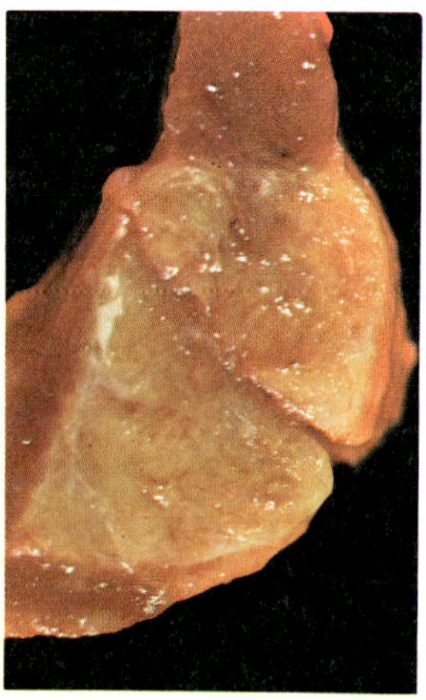

At close up the margin of the tumor is distinct from the normal tissue.

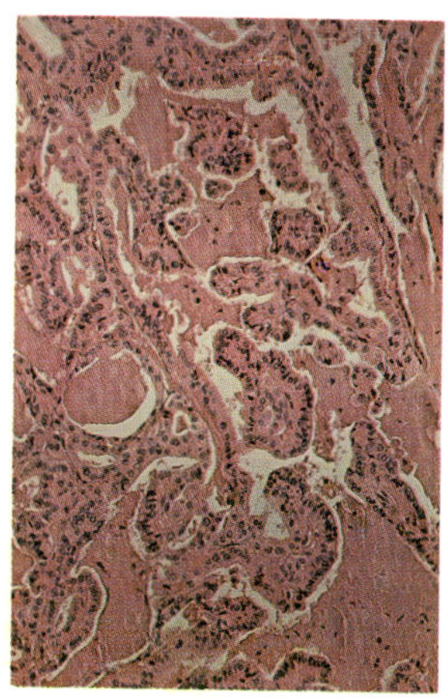

Histologic examination reveals coarse papillary fronds projecting into open spaces and covered with epithelial cells that are large, irregular, and lacking in polarity. Despite this anaplasia, mitotic figures are scarce.

NORMAL ADRENAL

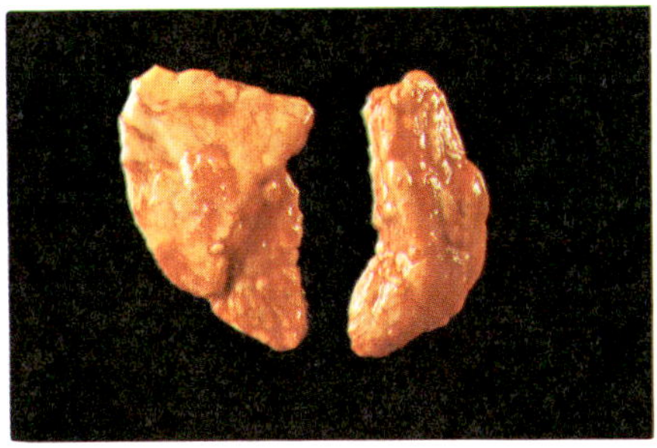

The adrenals are of normal size and shape.

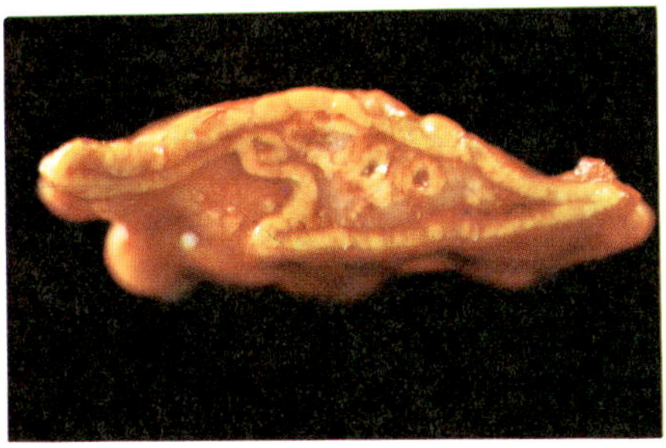

The cut surface displays a yellowish orange cortex of uniform thickness and a light pinkish gray medulla. The color of the cortex is due to the high lipid content of the cortical cells.

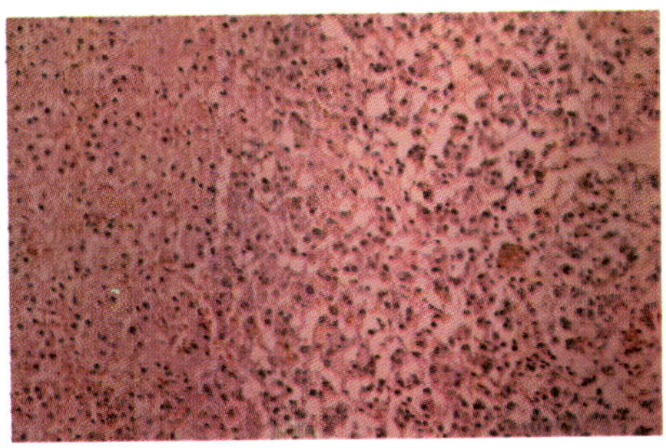

The junction of cortical cells (left) with medullary cells (right) is shown. The latter are smaller, polygonal, and more deeply basophilic.

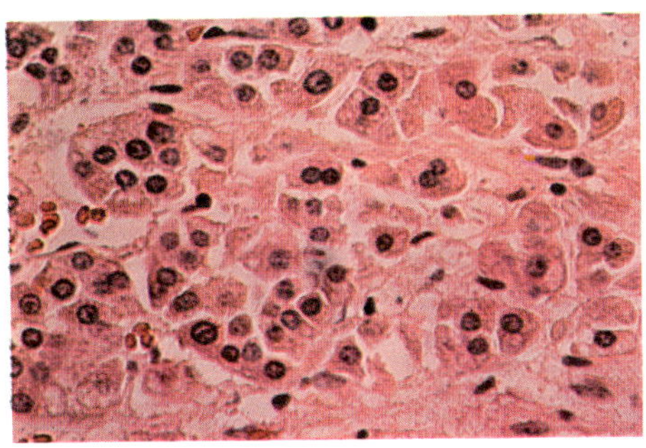

At higher power the cortical cells are seen to be densely eosinophilic with moderately large basophilic approximately round nuclei.

NORMAL ADRENAL

CLINICAL ACCOUNT 6210

The patient was a white female 86 years old who "passed out" and was brought to the emergency room of the hospital. Examination revealed ventricular fibrillation. Defibrillation was performed. The patient was well developed and well nourished. She was known to have had atrial fibrillation for the past 10 years. Physical examination was not remarkable except for cardiac enlargement, slight hepatomegaly, and one plus pitting edema of the ankles. The blood and urine were not remarkable except for two plus albumin in the latter with 20 to 30 leukocytes in the sediment. The patient died after five hours in the hospital.

Autopsy examination revealed hypertrophy and dilatation of the heart (500 Gms.), a recent infarct of the posterior wall of the left ventricle, and edema of the right and left lungs. Except for a recent infarct of the right kidney, additional diagnoses were of incidental interest.

THE ENTITY

Normal adult adrenals weigh 5 to 7 Gm. each. Oxygenated blood is supplied by the phrenic artery (superior), aorta (middle), and renal artery (inferior). Venous blood drains via the heavily muscled central vein. Each adrenal is composed of an outer cortex and an inner medulla. The cortex synthesizes over 30 steroids from cholesterol precursors and is necessary for life; it is composed of an outer zona glomerulosa, a middle zona fasciculata, and an inner zona reticularis. The middle zone comprises 80 per cent of the total cortical volume. The z. glomerulosa secretes mineralocorticoids (aldosterone) which regulate sodium, chloride, potassium, and hence water balance. An excess causes edema; a deficiency causes Addison's disease. The z. fasciculata secretes glucocorticoids (cortisone) which convert amino acids to glucose, suppress inflammation, lyse lymphocytes, and cause eosinophiles to disappear. An excess causes Cushing's disease. The z. fasciculata and reticularis secrete androgens and some estrogens; an increase causes virilism.

The medulla is of neural origin and consists of pheochromocytes which secrete adrenaline and noradrenaline. These catecholamines exert an emergency function by causing blood pressure to rise and liver glycogen to be converted to blood glucose.

Each gland is enclosed within a thin fibrous capsule although extracortical nodules of cortical tissue are common. These are small, multiple, unencapsulated, and not known to be the source of tumor formation or functional disturbance (1).

1. Smith, J.C. Anatomic Alterations of the Adrenal Cortex. Urology 69:339, 1953.

ADENOMA OF ADRENAL CORTEX

CLINICAL ACCOUNT 5981

The patient was a Negro female 42 years old who lost consciousness, had a convulsion, and was admitted to the hospital. The informant stated that she had been hypertensive for the past 5 years and that she had recovered from a myocardial infarction. The date of this was not given. Physical examination disclosed decerebrate rigidity and indicated a recent cerebrovascular accident. The cerebrospinal fluid was blood-tinged. An electrocardiogram was consistent with an old myocardial infarction. On the day after admission the patient died.

Autopsy examination revealed hypertrophy of the heart (475 Gms.), an aneurysm of the left ventricle, and an overlying acute fibrinous pericarditis. The ventricular aneurysm contained a mural thrombus. There were also a recent thrombus of the right internal carotid artery, and a recent infarct of the cerebrum. The lungs disclosed bronchopneumonia, and the right adrenal revealed a cortical adenoma. The right adrenal weighed 8.5 Gms.

THE ENTITY

Adenomas of the adrenal cortex are common, single, soft, round, encapsulated, and usually 0.5 to 4.0 cm. in diameter. The cut surfaces are bright yellow flecked with brown. Microscopically the cell arrangement is variable with arcades suggesting zona glomerulosa and columns suggesting zona fasciculata. Pleomorphism is not conspicuous. Nonfunctioning and functioning adenomas are indistinguishable. Small extracortical nodules are extremely common (1), and large cortical adenomas weighing several hundred grams are most uncommon (2).

Most cortical adenomas are nonfunctioning. Functioning adenomas in middle age secrete aldosterone which causes polyuria, polydipsia, hypokalemia, alkalosis, and hypertension (Conn's syndrome). The patient may also experience muscle weakness and periodic paralysis. Excision is curative. Functioning adenomas in children, and occasionally in adults, may secrete androgens and cause virilism in both sexes. Such adenomas usually measure 7 to 8 cm. in diameter; excision is curative.

1. Smith, J.C. Anatomic alterations of the adrenal cortex. Urology 69:339, 1953.
2. Smith, J.C. Large nonfunctioning adrenal adenoma. Ill. State Med. J. 101:325, 1952.

ADENOMA OF ADRENAL CORTEX

The adrenal contour is distorted by an oval nodule that measures 1.6 cm. in its greatest diameter.

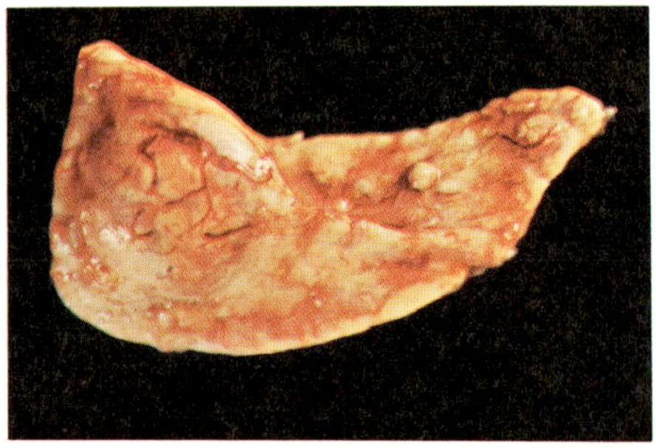

The cut surface discloses a sharply demarcated nodule that is soft and pale yellow. The cut surface otherwise is not remarkable.

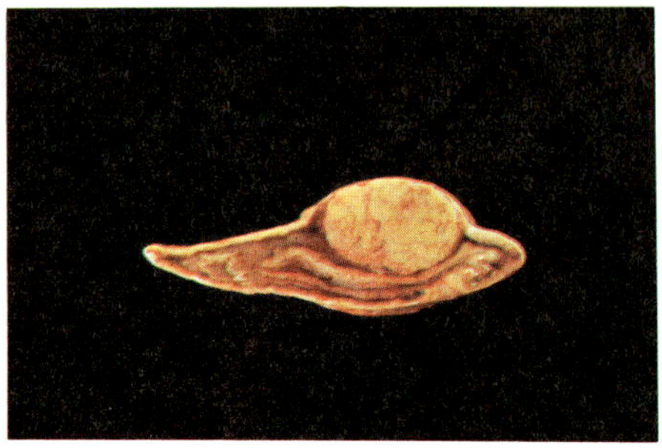

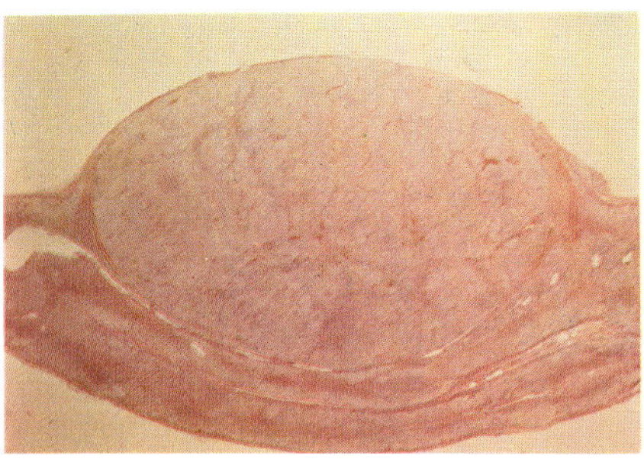

The unmagnified histologic section reveals the discrete border of the cortical adenoma and its relation to the rest of the adrenal.

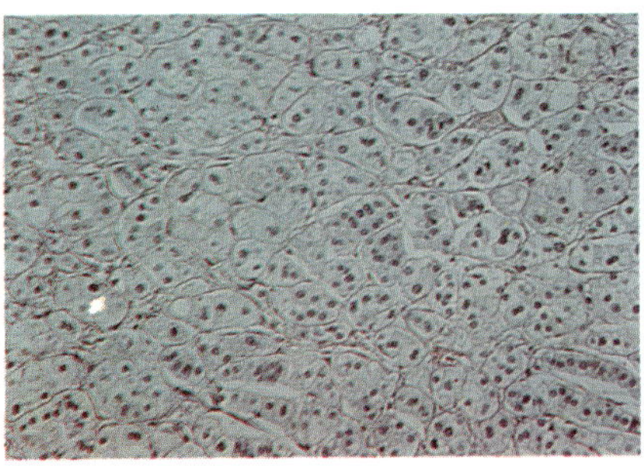

At higher power the cortical cells disclose small central nuclei and empty-appearing cytoplasm. The latter is due to the solvents used in the paraffin embedding process which wash out the cytoplasmic lipids. No mitoses or anaplasia are seen.

MYELOLIPOMA

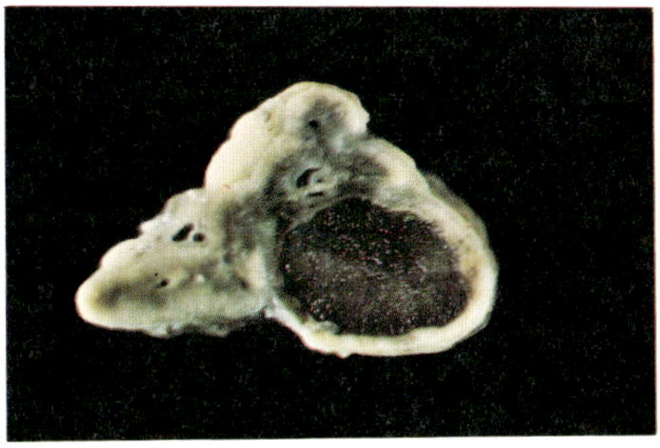

The right adrenal is fixed in formalin; the cut surface discloses a dark reddish brown oval mass in the medulla that is sharply demarcated.

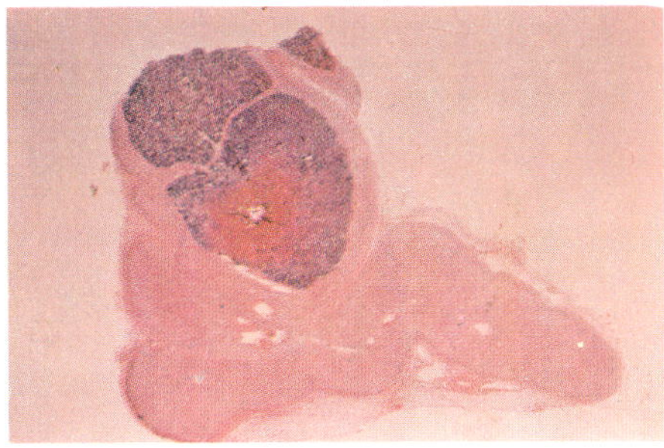

The unmagnified histologic section shows the medullary position of the tumor, its basophilic composition, and a scattering of fat cells. A focus of recent hemorrhage is also evident.

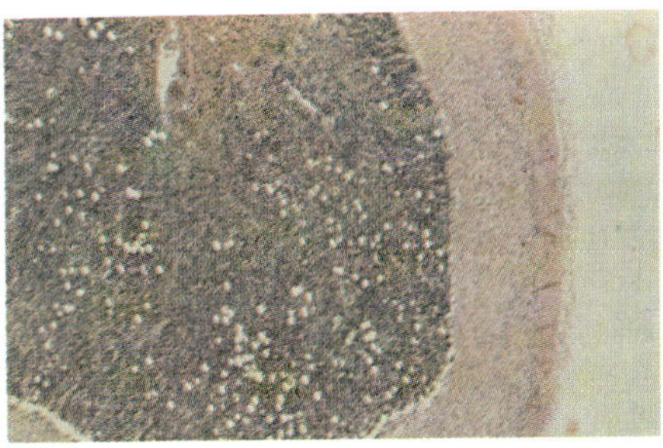

At low power the tumor can be seen to be composed of deeply basophilic hematopoietic cells and empty spaces which represent adipose tissue from which the fat has been dissolved by the embedding process.

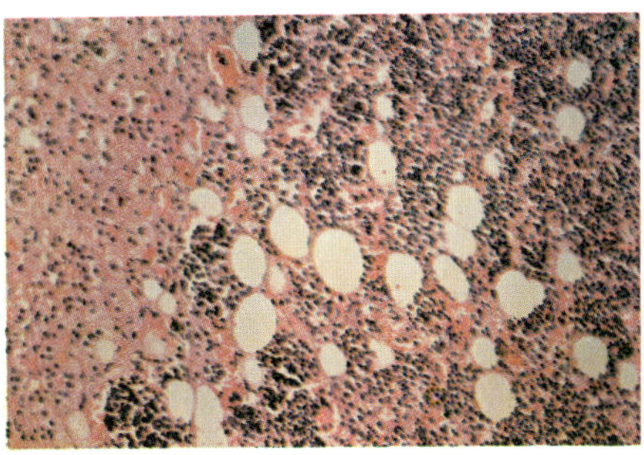

At higher power, both cell types are again apparent. There is no anaplasia.

MYELOLIPOMA

CLINICAL ACCOUNT 5997

The patient was a white female 67 years old who had a carcinoma of the colon resected two years before the present admission. Since then weakness, lassitude, and anorexia had been progressive. In recent days, nausea and vomiting had developed.

The temperature was 98.6 degrees F., pulse 84, respirations 16, and blood pressure 80/60 mm. Hg. The patient was cachectic, and the skin was pale yellow. The abdomen was distended, as were the veins of the abdominal skin. The liver was nodular, and the margin was felt at the level of the umbilicus. There was moderate pitting edema of both lower extremities.

The urine was yellow, cloudy, and acid, and the sediment revealed large numbers of leukocytes. The hemoglobin was 15 Gm., the hematocrit was 44, and the leukocytes numbered 16,500 with a slight neutrophilia. The blood urea nitrogen was 54 mg. The serum alkaline phosphatase was 7 units (0-4*). The total bilirubin was 11 mg.; all direct reacting. The uric acid was 12.6 mg. The total serum protein was 6.3 Gm. with 3.5 Gm. albumin and 2.8 Gm. globulin.

The patient died after ten days in the hospital.

Autopsy examination revealed metastatic carcinoma of the liver; the organ weighed 3400 Gms. The tumor extended from the liver into the hepatic veins and thence into the inferior vena cava to pass through the diaphragm and into the right atrium of the heart. There was residual carcinoma in the abdominal scar occasioned by the colectomy performed two years previously. The adrenals together weighed 14.5 Gms. Additional diagnoses were incidental.

THE ENTITY

Myelolipoma is a rare lesion of the adrenal of no clinical significance that is an incidental finding at autopsy examination. The lesion is approximately round, tends to lie beneath the cortex, is usually sharply circumscribed, and is composed of varying amounts of adipose tissue and myeloid cells of bone marrow. When adipose tissue predominates, the cut surface is yellow and resembles a lipoma; when bone marrow predominates, the cut surface is brownish red and myeloid cells are abundant. The lesion measures 0.5 to several centimeters in diameter. It is not associated with anemia or other functional abnormality and is not an example of extramedullary hematopoiesis. Whether the lesion is a true tumor, an example of metaplasia, or a developmental abnormality is not clear.

*Normal range.

CARCINOMA OF ADRENAL CORTEX

CLINICAL ACCOUNT 6262

The patient was a white male 63 years old who was admitted to the hospital because of weakness, lethargy, and confusion. He had been well until six months previously, when he suffered a pathologic fracture of the left femur. A chest x-ray disclosed a mass in the mediastinum that extended into the right upper lung field. Bronchoscopy, scalene node biopsy, and cytologic examination of aspirated pleural fluid failed to reveal tumor cells. The mediastinal mass enlarged and a superior vena caval syndrome developed. After radiation therapy the syndrome subsided. Later, additional x-rays revealed metastases in ribs and in dorsal and lumbar portions of spine. The patient had been told 15 years previously that he had cirrhosis. Since then there had been several episodes of abdominal swelling.

The patient was cachectic. The vital signs were normal. Physical examination revealed slight enlargement of the liver, a fluid wave in the abdomen, and dilatation of the veins over the abdomen. The spleen was not palpable.

Urinalysis was not recorded. The hemoglobin was 12.6 Gm., the hematocrit was 39 per cent, and the leukocytes numbered 8,000 with a normal differential count. A serologic test for syphilis was negative. A chest x-ray revealed massive enlargement of the mediastinum. An electrocardiogram disclosed low voltage in the main leads. Serum electrolytes, glutamic transaminase, and urea nitrogen were normal. The serum lactic dehydrogenase was 1650 units per 100 ml. The stool was 4 plus guaiac positive. The patient's condition worsened, and he died after nine days in the hospital.

Autopsy examination revealed a carcinoma of the right adrenal cortex, and metastatic carcinoma of the lungs, spine, abdominal wall, left adrenal, and para-aortic, mediastinal, and bronchopulmonary lymph nodes. Bronchopneumonia was pronounced in the upper lobe of the left lung. The liver weighed 1475 Gms., and revealed postnecrotic cirrhosis. No metastases were found in the hepatic tissue. Additional diagnoses were only of incidental interest. The right adrenal measured 10x6x4 cm.

THE ENTITY

Carcinoma of the adrenal cortex is extremely uncommon. It arises in either adrenal, occurs in children and adults, and affects women somewhat more often than men. It is manifested clinically by either a nonfunctioning tumor that is palpable or radiographically demonstrable and causes pain and discomfort in the abdomen, or by a functioning tumor that causes virilization, Cushing's syndrome, or precocious puberty with excess excretion of 17-ketosteroids in the urine. The distribution of nonfunctioning and functioning cortical carcinomas in one tabulation was 81 to 103 (1).

The tumors are large, often weighing several hundred grams, and locally invasive with extension into adjacent veins. The cut surfaces are soft, friable, and yellowish brown mottled with red. Foci of hemorrhage and necrosis are common. Microscopically the tumor cells may show little pleomorphism and be indistinguishable from benign neoplasia, or varying degrees of anaplasia that are characteristic of carcinoma. In both instances, the rate of growth is rapid and widespread metastases form early, especially in lungs, liver, and para-aortic lymph nodes. The tumor is not radiosensitive and survival rates after extirpative surgery are low.

1. Lipsett, M.B., Hertz, R., and Ross, G.T. Clinical and pathophysiologic aspects of adrenocortical carcinoma. Am. J. Med. 35: 374, 1963.

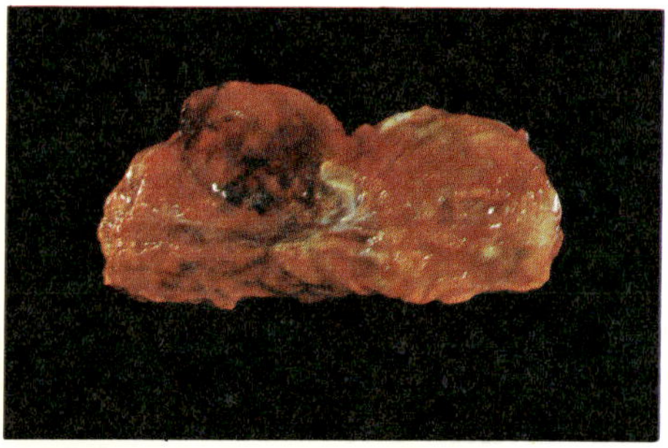

The adrenal reveals marked enlargement and gross distortion of shape.

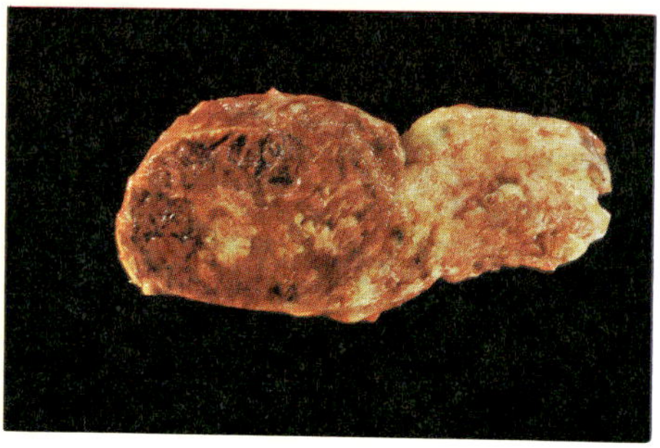

Section discloses extensive tumor that replaces all of the normal structure.

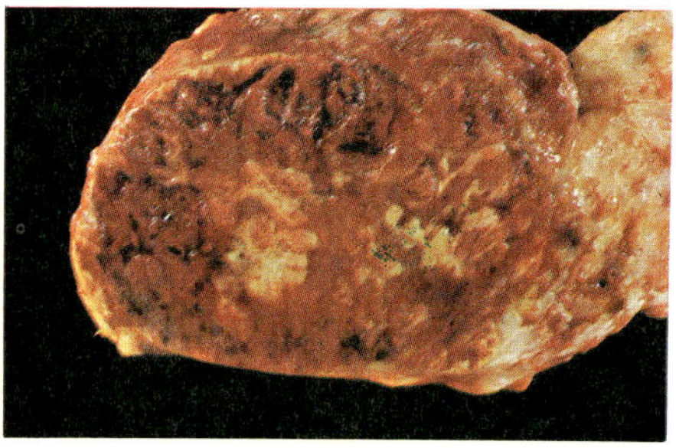

A close-up view reveals hemorrhagic tumor with yellow foci of necrosis.

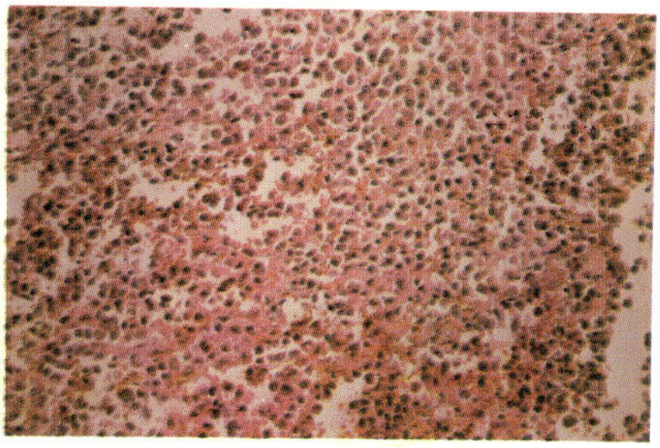

The microphotograph reveals the tumor cells which display a conspicuous enlargement and moderate irregularity of the size of the nuclei. There is less cytoplasm than in normal cortical cells. Nevertheless, anaplasia is slight and mitotic figures are not seen.

The contour is distorted by an oval tumor that is covered by intact cortex.

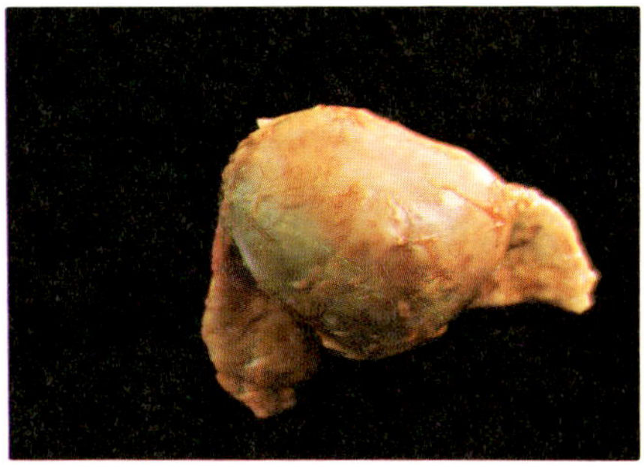

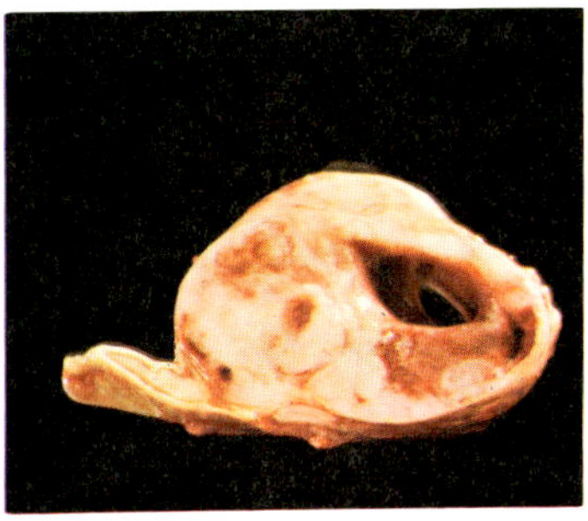

The cut surface reveals a pale gray tumor that is sharply circumscribed and mottled with pink and measures 4 cm. in greatest diameter. A cyst within the tumor is present, and foci of recent hemorrhage are evident. The cortex is intact.

The unmagnified section shows the tumor covered by intact cortex. The tumor margin is sharply delineated.

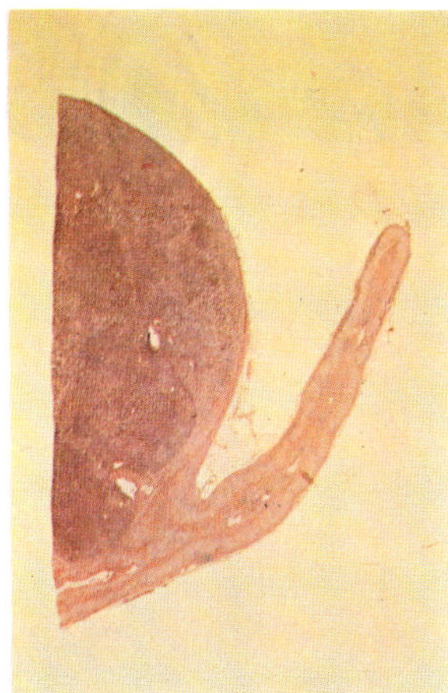

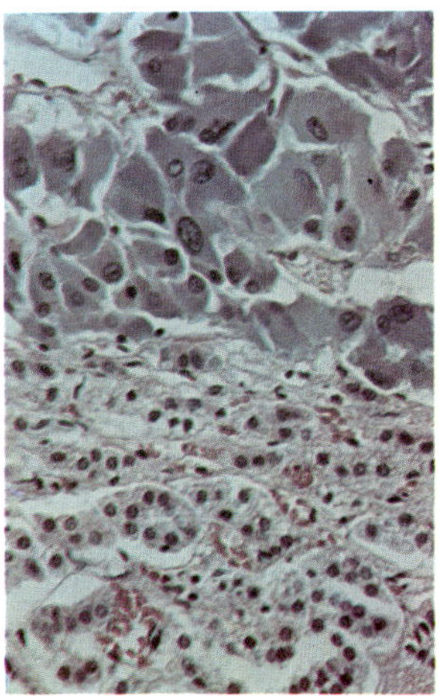

The magnified tissue section shows the junction between the tumor, composed of large cells, and the normal cortex, composed of much smaller cells. The tumor cells are polygonal, with nuclei that display moderate variation in size and shape. No mitotic figures are seen.

PHEOCHROMOCYTOMA

CLINICAL ACCOUNT 5962

The patient was a Negro female 37 years old who had been treated for slight hypertension but was otherwise well until the morning of admission to the hospital. On awakening she experienced a severe headache and became nauseated. She asked for aspirin and was shortly thereafter found lying on the floor unconscious.

The temperature was 98.6 degrees F., respirations 24, pulse 70, and blood pressure 190/100 mm. Hg. The optic discs were blurred, the deep tendon reflexes were hyperactive and symmetrical, and slight spasticity was detected in the lower extremities. No localizing neurologic signs were elicited. A diagnosis of cerebrovascular accident was made and it was held that examination of the spinal fluid would not be necessary to confirm the diagnosis. Shortly later her pulse increased to 190 and her blood pressure rose to 220/140 mm. Hg. After 1 mg. of reserpine the blood pressure fell to 80/60 mm. Hg. and then could not be sustained. The patient died on the afternoon of the day of admission.

Autopsy examination revealed hypertrophy of the heart (375 Gms.), edema of the right and left lungs, arteriolar nephrosclerosis with necrotizing arteriolitis, and a massive recent intracerebral hemorrhage. There was also a pheochromocytoma of the left adrenal. The gland weighed 7.4 Gms.

THE ENTITY

Pheochromocytoma is an uncommon benign tumor of the adrenal medulla that secretes catecholamines, causes hypertension, and is cured by surgical excision. The tumor is ordinarily unilateral, occurs in adults and children, and affects the sexes nearly equally. The catecholamines (adrenaline, noradrenaline) cause hypertension which is often paroxysmal and occasionally sustained. The paroxysms are associated with headache, nervousness, a hypermetabolic state, and often glycosuria. Diagnostic aids include measurement of catecholamines in the urine, pharmacologic tests with adrenergic blocking drugs, and aortography with perirenal insufflation of air. A urinary screening method is available (1).

The tumors are rounded, small or large, sharply circumscribed, and often weigh 100 Gm. The cortex is stretched over the margins, and the cut surfaces vary from pale gray to pinkish brown. Foci of recent hemorrhage and cysts from old hemorrhage are common. The tumor cells (pheochromocytes) are large with coarsely granular cytoplasm and small basophilic nuclei. Scattered large irregular and bizarre nuclei are a histologic feature. Mitotic figures are scarce. Staining methods reveal catecholamines in the cytoplasm of the tumor cells (2). Very uncommonly the tumor may metastasize and is thus malignant, but this cannot be foretold by histologic examination. The tumor is occasionally associated with neurofibromatosis and sometimes occurs in a familial distribution.

1. Wolf, R.L., Mendlowitz, M., Roboz, J., and Gitlow, S.E. New rapid test for pheochromocytoma. JAMA 188:859, 1964.
2. Blaclock, J.W.S., Ferguson, J.W., Mack, W.S., Shafar, J., and Symington, T. Phaeochromocytoma. Brit. J. Surg. 35:179, 1947-48.

NORMAL BRAIN

CLINICAL ACCOUNT 6210

The patient was a white female 86 years old who collapsed at 11:30 a.m. and was brought to the hospital cyanotic and without pulse. An electrocardiogram revealed ventricular fibrillation; this was converted to a supraventricular tachycardia. The temperature was 98.6 degrees F., pulse 92, respirations 24, and blood pressure 138/82 mm. Hg. The neck veins were distended, the lungs were clear, and no cardiac murmurs were heard. The urine was normal except for a 2 plus proteinuria and a 4 plus glucosuria. A second electrocardiogram indicated a recent posterior myocardial infarction. The serum glutamic transaminase and lactic dehydrogenase were normal. Breathing became labored, cyanosis developed, and the patient died five hours after admission to the hospital.

Autopsy examination revealed hypertrophy of the heart (500 Gms.), a recent infarct of the posterior wall of the left ventricle, and edema of the right and left lungs. A small recent infarct of the right kidney was also present. Additional diagnoses were of incidental interest. The brain weighed 1330 Gms.

THE ENTITY

Small branches of the internal carotid and posterior cerebral arteries extend into the lateral ventricles to form the frond-like vascular channels of the choroid plexus. This is covered by a single layer of epithelial cells through which the cerebrospinal fluid is formed by filtration of the plasma. The fluid leaves the lateral ventricles through the foramina of Monro, enters the vertical slit-like third ventricle, and passes backward into a small tube-like channel, the aqueduct of Sylvius, to enter the fourth ventricle at the undersurface of the cerebellum. The fluid then flows out the foramina of Luschka and Magendie to enter the subarachnoid space and circulate over the surfaces of the brain and spinal cord. Small evaginations of arachnoid (Pacchionian granulations) project into the great venous sinuses of the dura, and through these the fluid returns to the blood. Pressure progressively decreases from choroid plexus to cerebrospinal fluid to venous sinuses so that the flow is unidirectional and continuous. The normal pressure is 100 to 200 mm. of water.

The choroidal epithelium disallows the passage of bile, resists the passage of protein and glucose, and promotes the passage of chloride. Hence the cerebrospinal fluid, while clear, colorless, and without odor, is hardly a simple filtrate of the plasma. Its normal constituents are shown below.

	Plasma	Cerebrospinal Fluid
1. Protein	6.0-8.0 Gm.	15-45 mg.
2. Glucose	80-120 mg.	50-80 mg.
3. Chloride	570-620 mg.	700-750 mg.
	100-106 mEq.	120-130 mEq.
4. Leukocytes	5,000-10,000	0-5

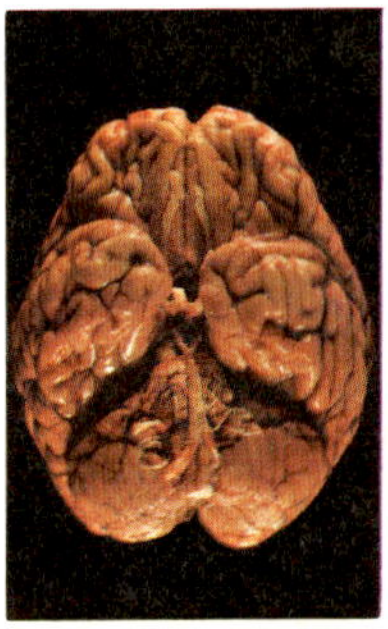

The undersurface shows the cerebral hemispheres to be symmetrical except for blunting of the tip of the temporal lobe on the patient's left. The olfactory tracts are intact. The optic chiasm is not remarkable, although the left temporal lobe obscures a part of it. The pons, medulla, and cerebellum are symmetrical. The vessels at the base of the brain are intact, and there is only slight arteriosclerosis. Cranial nerves emerge from each side of the medulla. There is no herniation of the portions of cerebellum adjacent to the medulla which are known as the cerebellar tonsils.

After fixation, a coronal section reveals intact cortical gray matter and subjacent white matter with the corpus callosum connecting the two cerebral hemispheres. The section is asymmetrical so that the insula of Reil shows only on the viewer's right. The thalamus and basal ganglia are evident; the internal capsule passes between them. The lateral ventricles are symmetrical and of usual size. The choroid plexus is not well seen in either lateral ventricle. The optic chiasm is intact. No abnormality is seen.

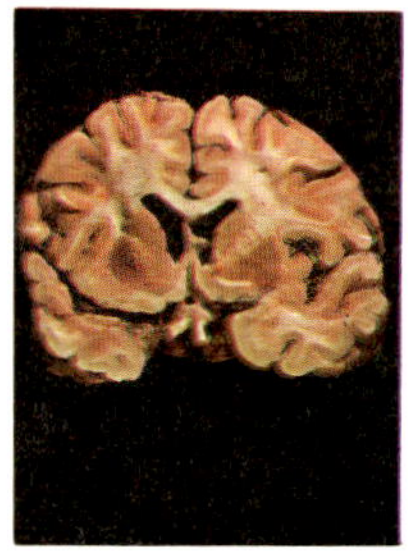

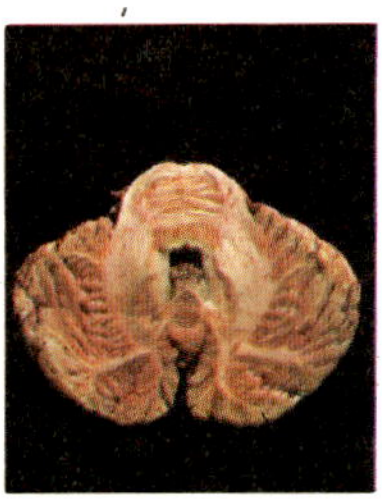

Section through the pons and cerebellum reveals the dark central chamber of the fourth ventricle. Above this are the transverse cortico-cerebellar tracts of the pons raddled with the longitudinal cortico-pontine fibers. The vermis lies in the midline subjacent to the fourth ventricle; the lateral cerebellar lobes extend to each side. The folia of the cerebellum are not remarkable.

The basilar vessels and circle of Willis are shown. At the lower portion of the picture the two vertebral arteries join to form the basilar artery that courses over the anterior surface of the pons. The basilar artery ends by dividing into two posterior cerebral arteries that nourish the posterior portions of the cerebral hemispheres. The single vessel on the viewer's left is the superior cerebellar artery. Its counterpart on the opposite side is missing. Delicate posterior communicating arteries connect the posterior cerebral with the large internal carotid arteries that immediately extend laterally to become the middle cerebral arteries. The latter also give off the anterior cerebral arteries which nourish the frontal lobes and are connected by an anterior communicating vessel. A vascular circle is thus formed.

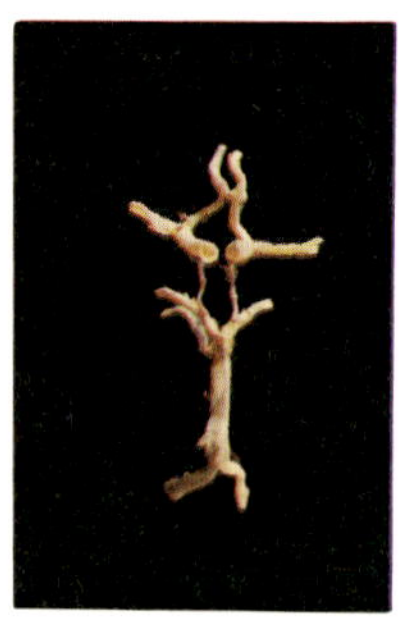

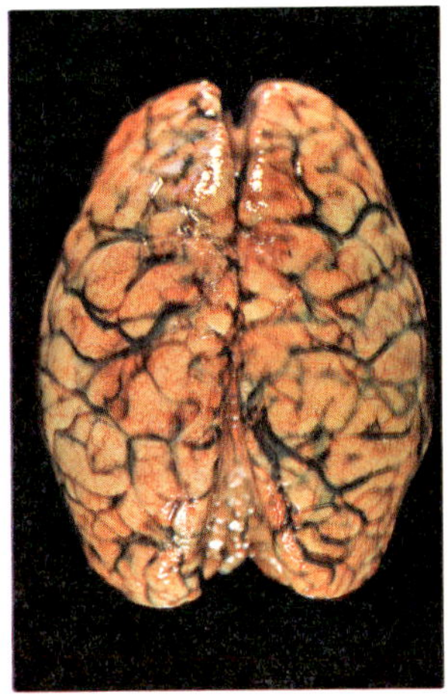

Hyperemia of the meninges and edema of the cerebrum are evident on the superior surface of the brain.

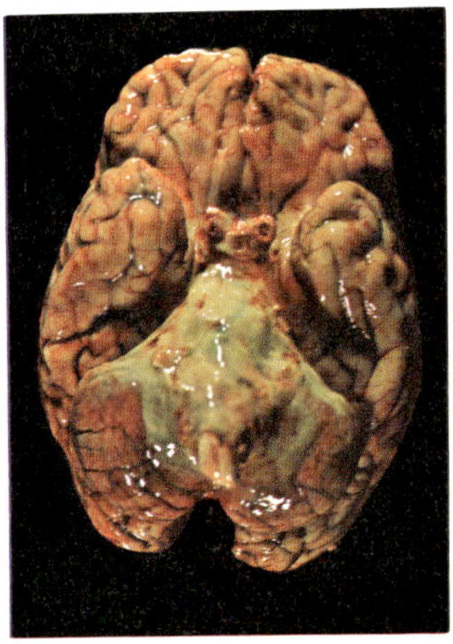

The undersurface shows the thick opaque pale greenish gray exudate characteristic of pneumococcal meningitis.

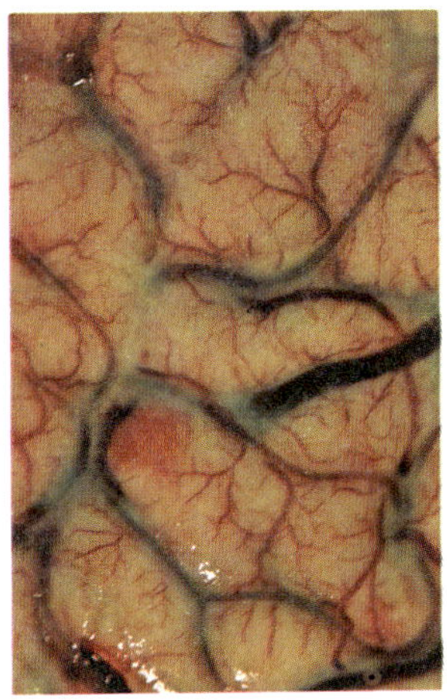

A close-up of the surface shows the pale greenish gray exudate lying in the meninges adjacent to veins.

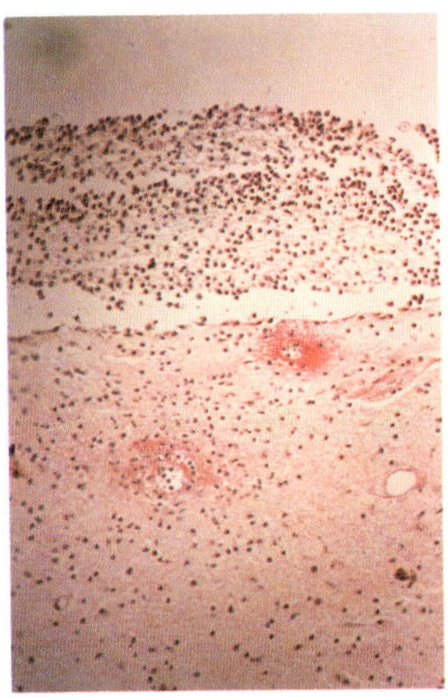

Neutrophils in abundance within the pia-arachnoid constitute the exudate.

PNEUMOCOCCAL MENINGITIS

CLINICAL ACCOUNT 458

The patient was a Ugandan female 25 years old who was well until four days before coming to the hospital. At that time she developed fever and headache. These persisted, and on the day before admission she complained of a stiff neck. The patient was taken to a dispensary where she was thought to have cerebral malaria and was given intramuscular chloroquine. Instead of improving, she became semicomatose and was transferred to the hospital.

The patient was emaciated, comatose, and desperately ill. The temperature was 39 degrees C., pulse 100, respirations 34, and blood pressure 120/80 mm. Hg. Physical examination was not remarkable except for a stiff neck, pupillary responses to light and accommodation that were sluggish, and deep tendon reflexes that were hypoactive. The patient died on the day of admission before laboratory data could be secured.

Autopsy examination revealed acute suppurative meningitis consistent with pneumococcal infection.

THE ENTITY

Acute suppurative meningitis is often caused by meningococci, *Hemophilus influenzae*, or pneumococci. These organisms originate in such conditions as nasopharyngitis, middle ear infection, paranasal sinusitis, or acute upper respiratory infections. The symptoms are chills, fever, nausea, vomiting, and headache. The signs are stiffness of the neck, backward fixation of the neck (opisthotonus), pain on extension of the leg while supine with thighs flexed (Kernig's sign), and involuntary drawing up of the knees on forward flexion of the head (Brudzinski's sign). Diagnosis is established by examination of the spinal fluid, which reveals increased pressure, large numbers of leukocytes, decreased sugar, and positive culture for bacteria.

With antibacterial therapy the inflammatory process ordinarily resolves and the patient recovers. When resolution fails and fibrosis follows, cranial nerves may be bound in the connective tissue and strabismus, blindness, deafness, or facial weakness may result. When foramens or fluid channels are blocked, internal hydrocephalus may develop. With meningococcemia, massive hemorrhage may take place in the adrenals and death may follow abruptly. This is the essence of the Waterhouse-Friderichsen syndrome.

HEMOPHILUS MENINGITIS

CLINICAL ACCOUNT SLH-A-126

The patient was a Mexican male infant 10 months old who was well until three days before admission to the hospital. At that time he became irritable and on the next day began to vomit. He was unable to retain food during the two days before admission. A slight fever was noted during this illness. There had been no diarrhea or known exposure to contagious disease.

The temperature was 103 degrees F. by rectum, pulse 110, and respirations 34. The ears, eyes, mouth, and scalp were not remarkable. The lungs and heart were normal. The abdomen was not unusual except for increased peristalsis. Neurologic examination was normal.

The hemoglobin was 6 Gm., erythrocyte count 2.06 million, and leukocyte count 14,650 with a moderate neutrophilia. On the evening of the day of admission the patient had a convulsive seizure. Physical examination then revealed slight nuchal rigidity and sustained bilateral ankle clonus. The spinal fluid disclosed 14,000 leukocytes per cmm., most of which were segmented granulocytes, and a protein of 138 mg. per ml. Culture revealed *Hemophilus influenzae*. The patient developed respiratory distress and died after four days in the hospital.

Autopsy examination revealed acute suppurative meningitis and bronchopneumonia of the right lung with abscess formation in the upper lobe. Except for focal atelectasis of the left lung, additional diagnoses were incidental. The brain weighed 800 Gms. Culture of the meninges revealed colonies of *Hemophilus influenzae*.

THE ENTITY

Acute suppurative meningitis is often caused by meningococci, *Hemophilus influenzae,* or pneumococci. These organisms originate in such conditions as nasopharyngitis, middle ear infection, paranasal sinusitis, or acute upper respiratory infections. The symptoms are chills, fever, nausea, vomiting, and headache. The signs are stiffness of the neck, backward fixation of the neck (opisthotonus), pain on extension of the leg while supine with thighs flexed (Kernig's sign), and involuntary drawing up of the knees on forward flexion of the head (Brudzinski's sign). Diagnosis is established by examination of the spinal fluid, which reveals increased pressure, large numbers of leukocytes, decreased sugar, and positive culture for bacteria.

With antibacterial therapy the inflammatory process ordinarily resolves and the patient recovers. When resolution fails and fibrosis follows, cranial nerves may be bound in the connective tissue and strabismus, blindness, deafness, or facial weakness may result. When foramens or fluid channels are blocked, internal hydrocephalus may develop. With meningococcemia, massive hemorrhage may take place in the adrenals and death may follow abruptly. This is the essence of the Waterhouse-Friderichsen syndrome.

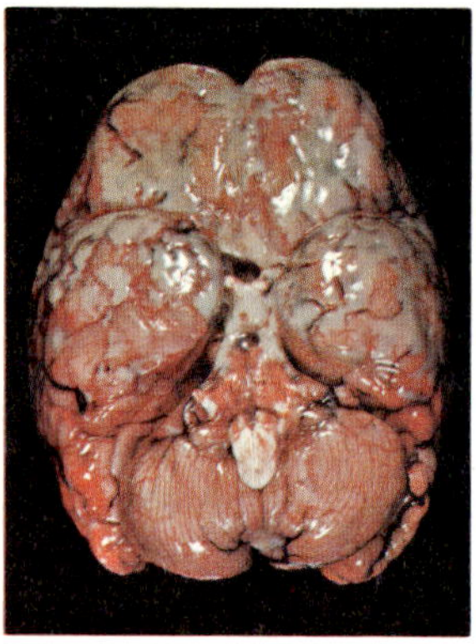

The meninges of the brain are covered with a thick opaque pale greenish gray exudate. The exudate is actually within the pia-arachnoid so that the surface is glistening and the subdural space is clear.

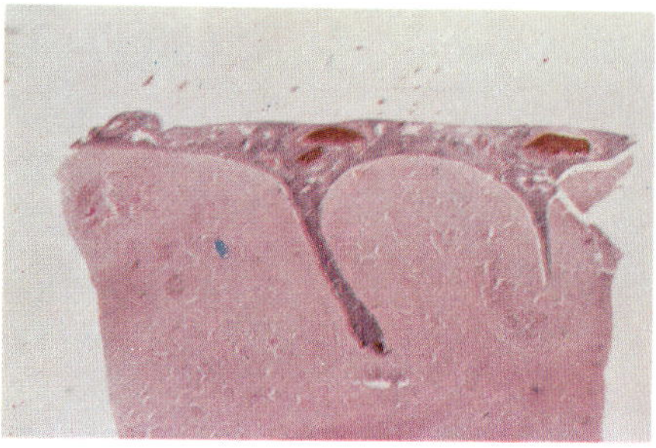

In the unmagnified histologic section the basophilic exudate may be seen to lie within the pia-arachnoid and to penetrate to the deepest levels of the intergyral sulci.

Left: At low power the exudate over the surface of the cerebrum is shown with a sharp delineation from the cerebral tissue below and the pial margin above. Neutrophils of course escape from the pial surface and account for the cellularity of the spinal fluid in acute meningitis. **Right:** The photograph discloses the thick exudate filling an intergyral sulcus. Leukocytes follow the arteries and veins into the cerebral tissue from these sulci, and the cells are found in the Virchow-Robins lymph spaces that surround small vessels. Except for the surface, leukocytes within the cerebral tissue itself are uncommon.

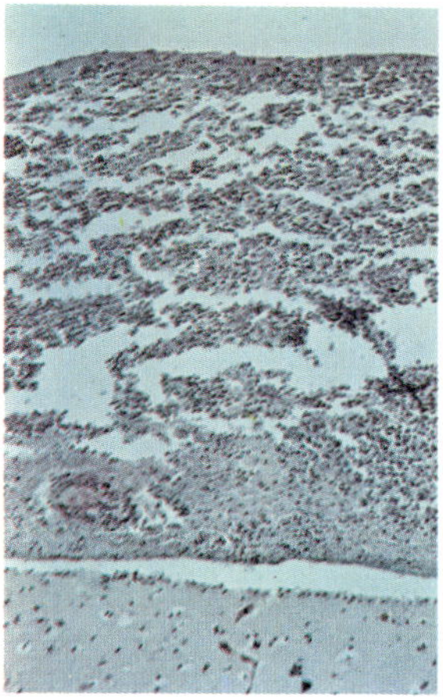

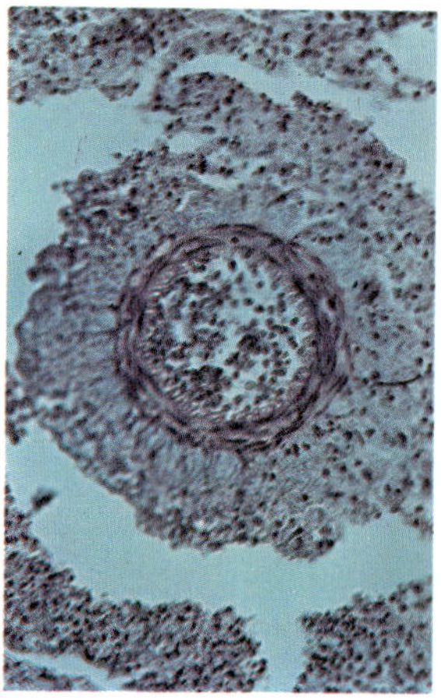

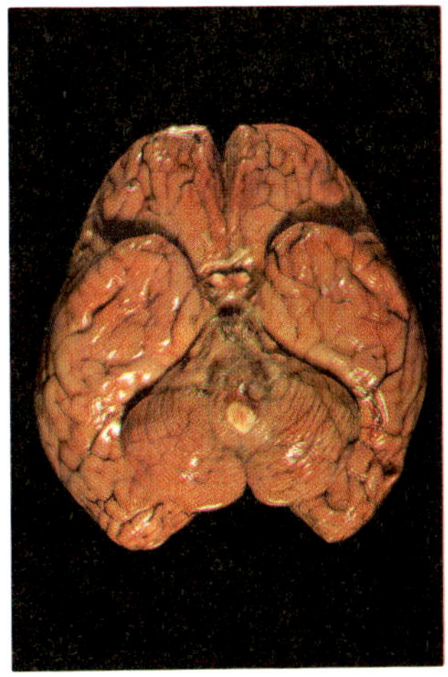

Undersurface of brain; the meninges are clouded near the region of the medulla.

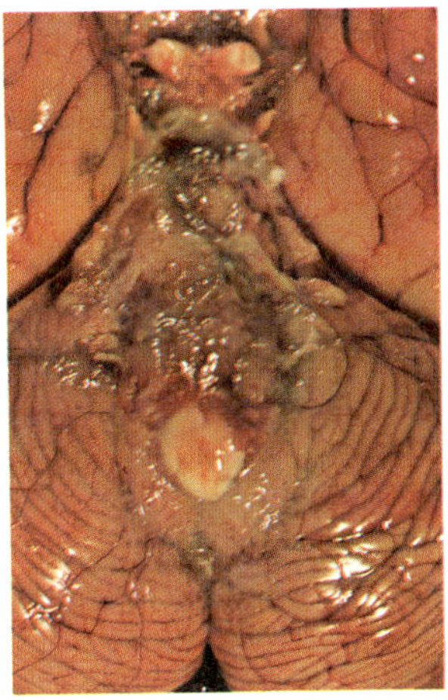

Close-up shows the gray wet gelatinous thickening of the meninges about the medulla and on the undersurface of the pons.

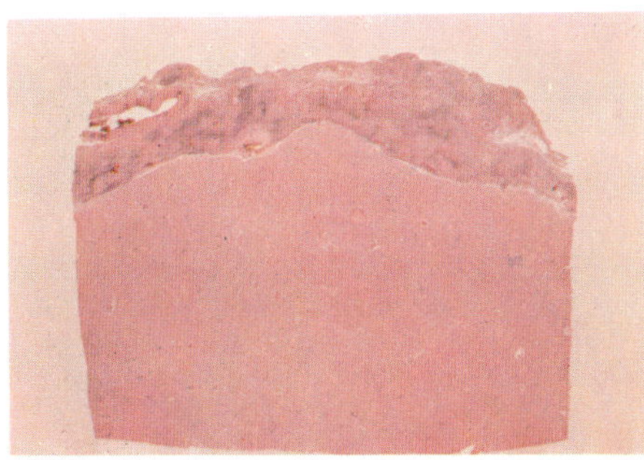

Scanning power cross section of pons with meninges at base. The pia-arachnoid is infiltrated with leukocytes; tubercles are numerous.

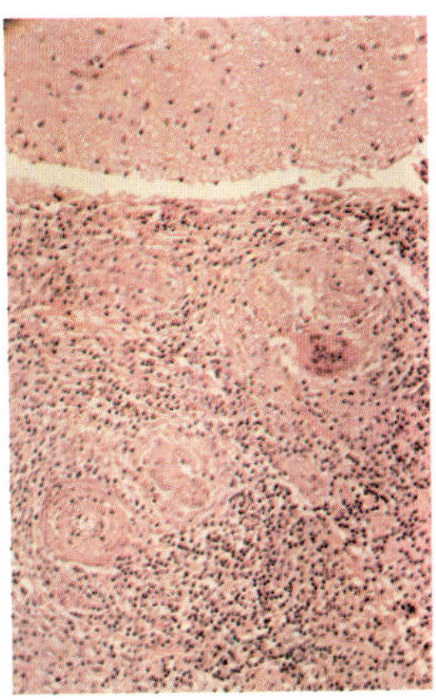

Pons above, meninges below with tubercle formation and Langhans' multinucleated giant cells.

TUBERCULOUS MENINGITIS

CLINICAL ACCOUNT 435

The patient was a black male child 1½ years old who was well until three months before entering the hospital. At that time he developed whooping cough and was given various treatments as an outpatient. One month later convulsions developed, and these occurred three to four times daily. The convulsions gradually became less frequent and were replaced by generalized tremors. One week before admission the child became drowsy, the neck was stiff, and all feedings were followed by vomiting. The temperature was 36.5 degrees C., pulse rate 90, respiratory rate 14, and systolic blood pressure 170 mm. Hg. The patient was emaciated, the expression was vacant, and the neck was held in a retracted position. The chest and abdomen were not remarkable. All deep tendon reflexes were inactive. A Kernig's sign was not elicited. The urine and blood were normal. The spinal fluid was clear, slightly xanthochromic, and revealed 300 cells per cmm. of which 80 per cent were lymphocytes. The spinal fluid protein was 900 mgs. per 100 ml. The child lapsed into coma and died on the day after admission to the hospital.

The main autopsy diagnoses were acute tuberculous meningitis and fibrocaseous tuberculosis of the apex of the right lung.

THE ENTITY

Tuberculous meningitis occurs principally in children and often follows an upper respiratory infection such as measles or whooping cough, which are presumed to lower resistance and allow the infection to flourish. The meningitis is usually secondary to miliary tuberculosis. In about 10 per cent of cases, however, no miliary spread is found, and in these patients, careful examination of coronal sections of the brain often reveals a subcortical tuberculoma which has ruptured onto the cerebral surface. The exudate of tuberculous meningitis has three gross characteristics: it is pale gray in color, gelatinous in consistence, and localized over the base of the brain. The thick nature of the exudate and the basal localization tend to block the tentorial opening, the foramina of Luschka and Magendie, and the foramen magnum. As a consequence, cerebrospinal fluid cannot move upward through the tentorial opening, outward through the foramina of the fourth ventricle, or downward through the foramen magnum to the spinal cord. If the infection develops before the fontanelles have fused, internal hydrocephalus may become pronounced. The basilar inflammation also causes a tuberculous arteritis, especially of the anterior and posterior cerebral arteries, and these vessels often become thrombosed with infarction of the cerebral tissue. Death is attributable to obstruction of the flow of the cerebrospinal fluid, and, less often, to infarction of the brain.

Clinically the patients are usually febrile and shown signs of meningeal inflammation. The cerebrospinal fluid reveals a moderate pleocytosis with a predominance of lymphocytes. In addition, the protein is raised, and the chloride and glucose are low. The reduced chloride is nonspecific; the lower glucose is characteristic. The diagnosis is established by the finding of tubercle bacilli in the pellicle that forms in the freestanding cerebrospinal fluid. The course, without treatment, gradually worsens, coma eventually supervenes, and death occurs after an illness of about three weeks' duration.

ACUTE POLIOMYELITIS

CLINICAL ACCOUNT SLH-A-12

The patient was a white female 8 years old who felt well until 36 hours before admission to the hospital, when she developed headache, fever, and vomiting. The headache was over the vertex, the fever was 102 degrees F., and the vomiting occurred twice and was nonprojectile. The patient also complained of a sore neck and difficulty in swallowing. During the night the neck pain increased. On the morning of the day of admission the headache persisted, vomiting recurred twice, and the patient complained that her neck was stiff. She refused food, and the temperature rose to 104 degrees F.

The pulse was 120 per minute. The eyes showed a "suggestion of lateral nystagmus," the neck was rigid, and the lungs were clear. Cranial nerve function was intact. The deep tendon reflexes were normal. No motor or sensory loss was detected. The Kernig sign was negative.

The urine revealed 2 plus proteinuria and 4 plus bacteriuria. The hemoglobin was 12.8 Gm., and the leukocyte count was 7,400 with a slight neutrophilia. The spinal fluid was clear and disclosed 367 cells per cmm. of which 290 were segmented granulocytes and 77 were lymphocytes.

On the day after admission right facial paralysis developed. Difficulty in swallowing persisted. On the next day chest expansion diminished and the function of cranial nerves V, VII, and XI was decreased. The patient became drowsy and could not talk. Stupor developed. On the fourth day cyanosis was evident, the pulse was 140, and the respirations were 8 to 10 per minute. The patient died of respiratory failure after five days in the hospital.

Autopsy examination revealed acute polioencephalomyelitis with focal acute myocarditis and hemorrhagic bronchopneumonia of the left lung. The right and left lungs weighed 90 and 230 Gms., respectively.

THE ENTITY

Poliomyelitis is caused by an extremely small neurovirus which consists of a spherical RNA core enclosed within a protein envelope. Differences in the envelope distinguish three strains, of which the first (Lansing) is epidemic. The disease appears to occur naturally only in man. The virus resides in the gut of carriers, infection takes place by ingestion of contaminated food, and the housefly may serve as a vector for the agent.

The ingested virus localizes in the gut, a viremia follows, and many tissues including the myocardium are affected. In most, nothing more happens, but in a few the nervous system is affected, especially the medulla and anterior horns of the spinal cord. At these sites the ganglion cells show chromatolysis with loss of Nissl substance, infiltration with neutrophilic segmented granulocytes, and later, phagocytosis of neuronal debris. If the patient recovers, gliosis gradually follows.

The incubation period is 7 to 10 days. The onset is characterized by fever, headache, vomiting, lassitude, and muscle pain. The spinal fluid shows an elevation of pressure, an increase of protein, and a cell count of 100 to 200 per 100 ml. of which most are lymphocytes and some are neutrophils. Muscle weakness develops and progresses to complete paralysis. Cervical and thoracic cord involvement paralyzes the phrenic nerve and weakens the thoracic muscles so that respiratory failure is a common cause of death.

One attack confers life-long immunity. Prevention is achieved by injection of a formol-killed virus or ingestion of an attenuated-live virus.

ACUTE POLIOMYELITIS

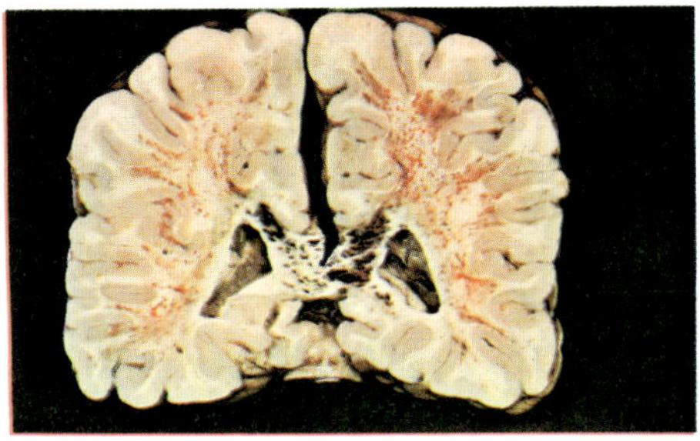

The cut surface of cerebrum reveals small hemorrhages throughout the white matter.

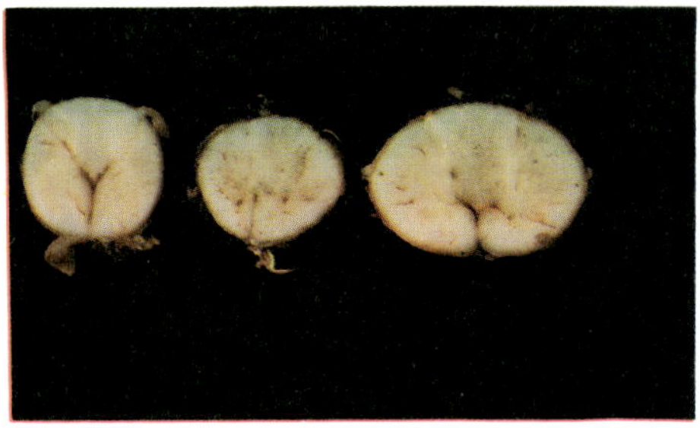

The cut surface of spinal cord shows edema and petechiae.

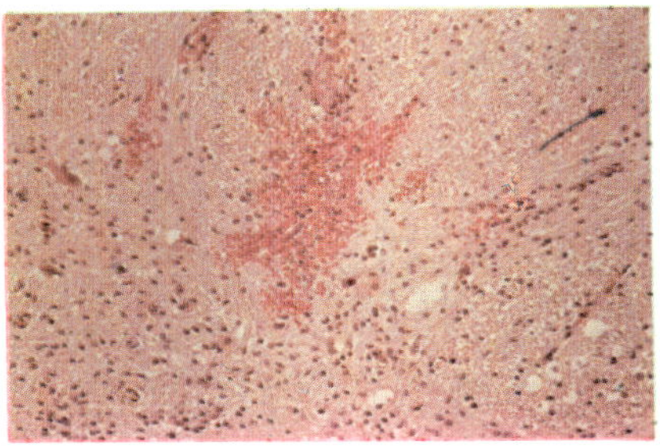

A microsection reveals a small recent hemorrhage in the spinal cord.

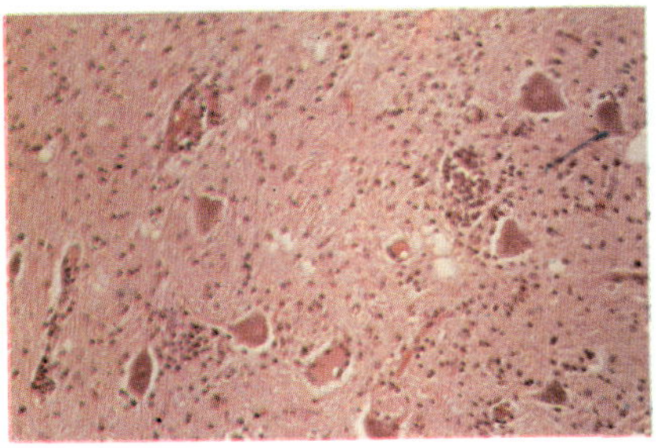

At higher power, degeneration of anterior horn ganglion cells (motor nuclei) and infiltration with microglial cells become evident.

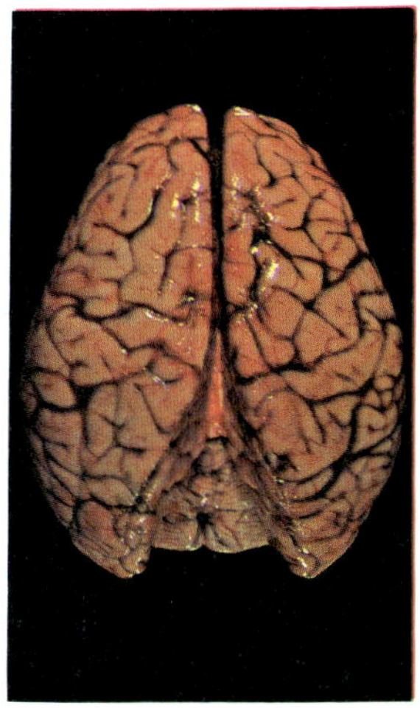

Superior surface of brain showing hyperemia of meninges and moderate cerebral edema.

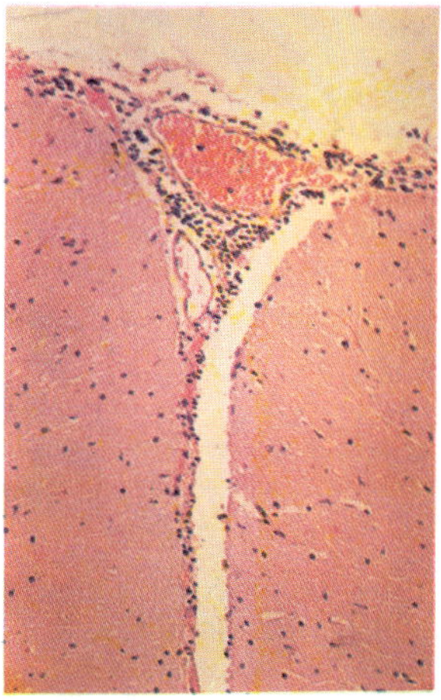

Microsection of cerebrum showing leukocytes in meninges.

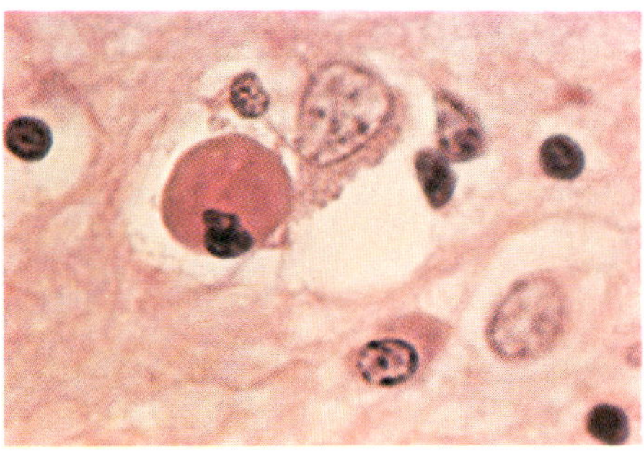

Morula cell in cerebral tissue.

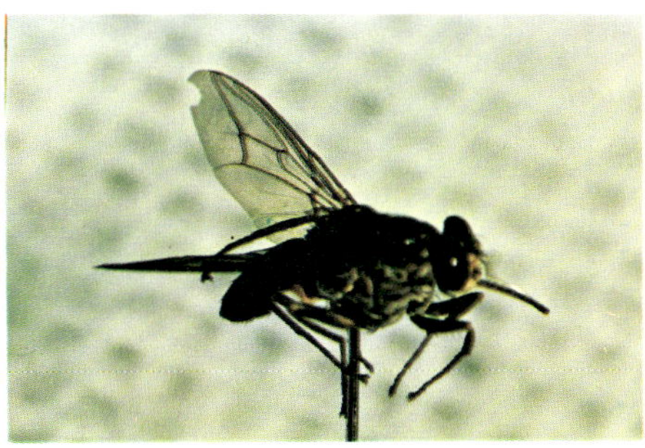

Tsetse fly which transmits trypanosomes. All 22 species of *Glossina* have a coarse proboscis (covered by sheath), meat cleaver vein pattern in wings, and overlapping wings when standing.

TRYPANOSOMIASIS

CLINICAL ACCOUNT 482

The patient was a 13-year-old Ugandan male who was well until four months before entering the hospital, when he felt chilly, became drowsy throughout the day, and began dropping things from his hands. Two months later he developed a fever, became confused, and threw stones at people and cars. Questioning disclosed irrelevant answers, general confusion, loss of concentration, and visual hallucinations. Examination revealed drowsiness, proptosis of the eyes, widespread lymphadenopathy, and a palpable spleen. Neurologic function was normal.

The hemoglobin was 10 Gms., and leukocyte count 6,400, with 51 lymphocytes, 37 neutrophils, and 8 eosinophils. The sedimentation rate was 97 mm. per hour (Westergren). A serologic test for syphilis was negative. The urine was normal and the stool revealed hookworm ova. The cerebrospinal fluid disclosed 255 mononuclear cells, normal sugar and protein, and no trypanosomes. The clinical impression was schizophrenia or trypanosomiasis.

On the third hospital day the patient fell, cut the occipital portion of his scalp, and became unconscious. Craniotomy failed to reveal a subdural hematoma. The patient was found dead in bed on the fifth hospital day.

The brain, spleen, and lungs weighed 1370, 300, and 450 Gms. each, and the remaining organ weights were normal. The gross tentative autopsy diagnoses were meningeal hyperemia consistent with trypanosomiasis, frontal lobe ecchymoses consistent with recent trauma, hookworm disease, splenomegaly, and aspiration pneumonia.

THE ENTITY

Sleeping sickness is a relentlessly progressive infection of the central nervous system caused by trypanosomes that are carried by tsetse flies. The organisms are *Trypanosoma gambiense* and *T. rhodesiense*, and the flies are species of *Glossina* (*G. palpalis* and *G. morsitans*). In cattle a similar disease known as nagana is caused by *T. brucei*. These conditions are seen only in sub-Saharan Africa (1).

After ingestion of organisms in a blood meal, the trypanosomes migrate to the salivary glands of the tsetse fly, which become infective in 20 days. When transmitted to the human, a furuncle forms at the tsetse bite. Fever follows and lymphadenopathy develops, especially in the posterior neck (Winterbottom's sign). Indifference, apathy, and intellectual deterioration follow. The organisms may be found in the blood or spinal fluid. The course lasts months to years, and death is usually due to secondary infection. Death may be due to cardiac failure, especially in *T. rhodesiense* infections.

The trypanosomes first reside in the reticuloendothelial tissues and later localize in the heart and brain. The cardiac lesion is a pancarditis with lymphocytes, plasma cells, and histiocytes infiltrating the tissue from epicardium to endocardium. The valves are unaffected. In the brain the meninges are hyperemic and slightly thickened, the exudate consists of lymphocytes and plasma cells, and penetration extends into the cerebral tissue in the Virchow-Robin perivascular spaces. A characteristic feature is the morula cell which is a plasma cell derivative in which the cytoplasm is distended with globules of Russell bodies. It is found in both the meninges and brain. Trypanosomes are not seen in the tissues. The condition is thus a chronic and gradually progressive meningo-encephalitis.

1. Hutt, M.S.R., and Wilks, N.E. African Trypanosomiasis, in Pathology of Protozoal and Helminthic Diseases, p. 57, Williams & Wilkins Co., 1971.

RECENT INFARCT, PONS

CLINICAL ACCOUNT 6166

The patient was a Negro male 69 years old who was admitted to the hospital because of aphasia and weakness of the left arm and leg. He had been well until six months previously, when discomfort in the chest was diagnosed as arteriosclerotic heart disease because of premature ventricular contractions. For the past three days he had experienced anorexia, occasional vomiting, and gradual clouding of the sensorium. On the evening of admission he was aphasic, with muscle weakness in the extremities on the left.

The temperature was 98.6 degrees F., pulse 100, respirations 20, and blood pressure 150/50. Physical findings included 3 plus deep tendon reflexes on the left, 1 plus on the right, and a positive Babinski reflex on the left. There was no papilledema or nuchal rigidity.

The urine was yellow, cloudy, pH 6, and specific gravity 1.012 with a 2 plus reaction for glucose and negative tests for albumin and acetone. The sediment revealed 3 leukocytes and a rare epithelial cell; there were no casts or erythrocytes. The hemoglobin was 6.9 Gm., hematocrit 25, and leukocytes 11,800 with a normal differential count. The blood sugar and blood urea nitrogen were 100 mg. and 23 mg. respectively. The cerebrospinal fluid was normal. A radio-isotope scan of the brain was normal. The mental condition of the patient rapidly deteriorated, and death occurred on the third hospital day.

Autopsy examination revealed bronchopneumonia of the right and left lungs. Other diagnoses that were immediately apparent were incidental including a small adenocarcinoma of the cecum. The brain weighed 1125 Gms. and revealed a recent infarct of the pons.

THE ENTITY

The brain constitutes 2 per cent of the body weight, receives 16 per cent of the cardiac output, and utilizes 20 per cent of the oxygen supply. The cerebral tissue is especially vulnerable to oxygen loss. Atherosclerosis and hypertension are common, and collateral vessels are slow to form after injury. Cerebrovascular disease kills or disables more persons than all other organic neurological diseases combined.

The principal lesions are infarction and hemorrhage. The former is more common and less likely to be lethal than the latter. Infarction is caused by atherosclerosis with or without hypertension. The arterial plaque enlarges, the lumen narrows, the blood eddys, the endothelium is injured, and a thrombus forms. Alternatively, hemorrhage in the plaque expands the lesion and occludes the lumen. Less commonly emboli lodge at atheromatous sites from mural thrombi of the left heart, from vegetations of the mitral or aortic valves, or from fatty marrow released at the site of fractured bones. The cerebral tissue swells, dies, and becomes hemorrhagic as vessels leak. Segmented granulocytes infiltrate the site and are soon replaced with macrophages that phagocytize the debris and gradually leave. Marginal gliosis develops, the center liquifies, and the tissue shrinks. Cyst-like cavities containing yellow fluid in a shrunken scar eventually result.

Clinical onset is rapid rather than abrupt, and events are determined by the size of the artery and the location of the infarct. Headache, convulsions, aphasia, paresthesia, paralysis, anesthesia, dysarthria and loss of consciousness may occur. The clinical signs tend to be maximum at the outset and gradually subside, leaving a disability that is permanent. The spinal fluid is devoid of blood and the pressure is usually normal. Prognosis is worsened by prolonged unconsciousness, hypertension, old age, and general debility.

RECENT INFARCT, PONS

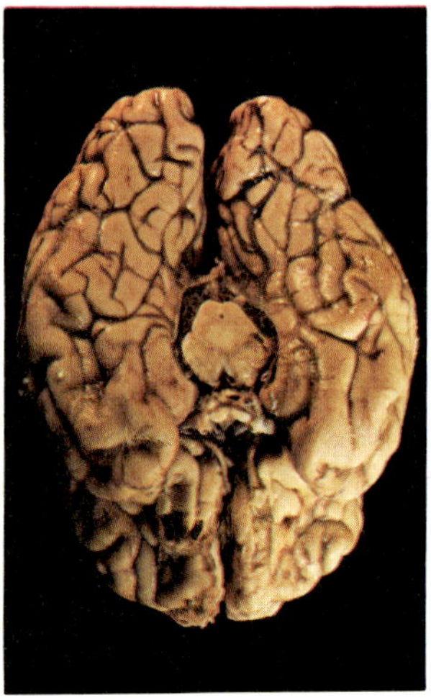

The cerebral undersurface is not remarkable. The brain stem has been transected and the cerebellum removed. The aqueduct of Sylvius can be seen in the lower part of the cut surface of the brain stem.

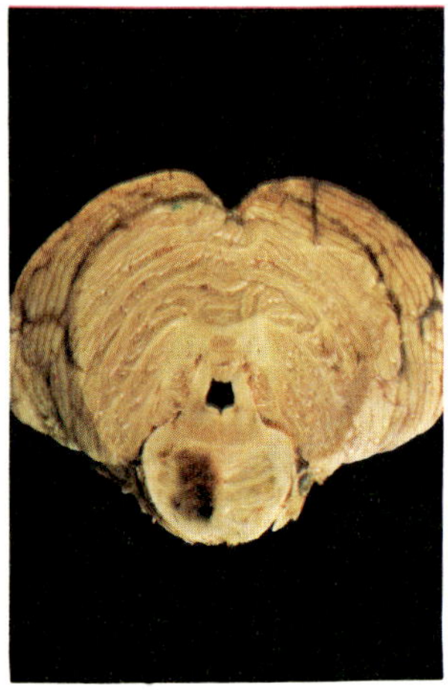

After fixation the cerebellum and pons are sectioned; a recent hemorrhagic infarct on the right side of the pons is revealed.

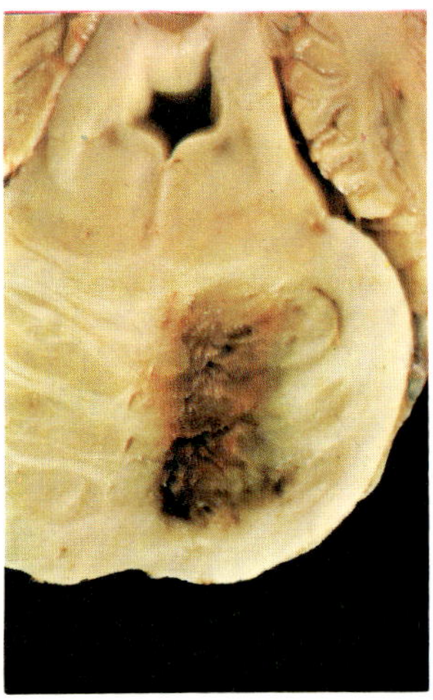

A closer view discloses the destructive nature of the infarct. Necrosis is evident, and the longitudinal and transverse fiber tracts are destroyed by the process.

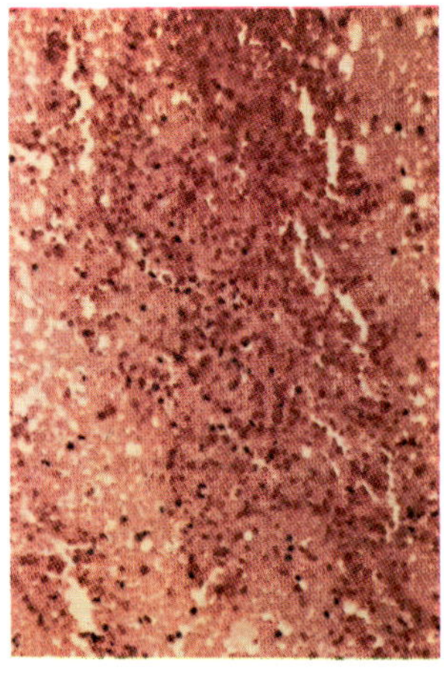

The histologic section reveals necrotic pontine tissue, a scattering of segmented granulocytes, many macrophages, and much extravasated blood.

OLD INFARCT, CEREBELLUM

The left cerebellar lobe is shrunken and discolored.

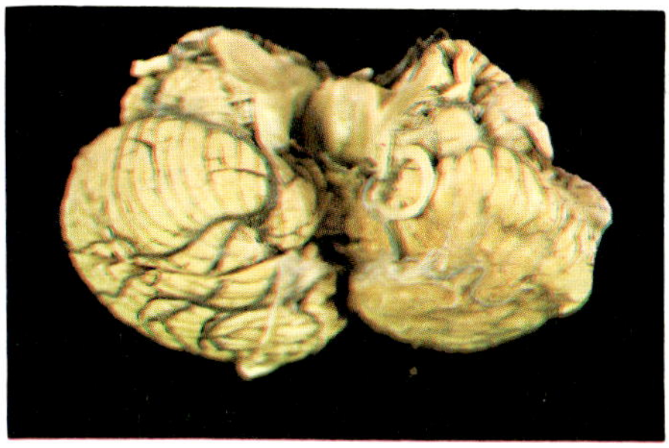

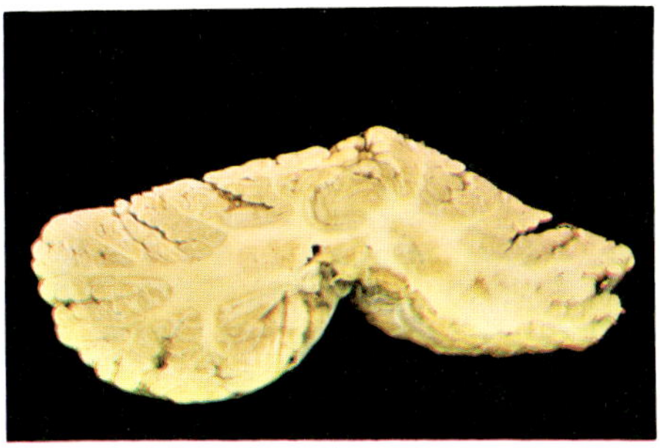

On section, the atrophy and discoloration are localized to the cortical tissue.

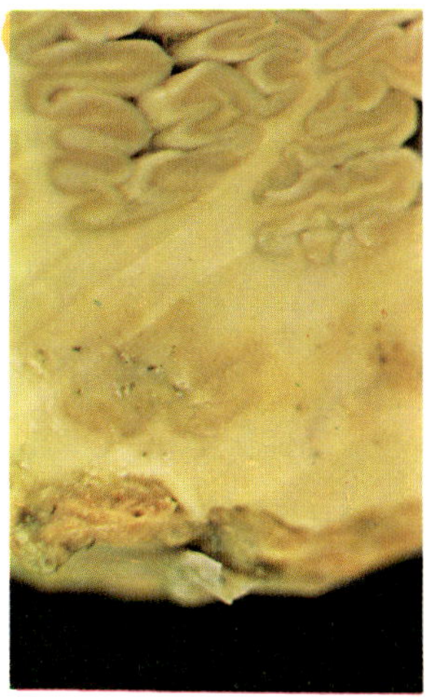

The cortical localization of the process is further evident.

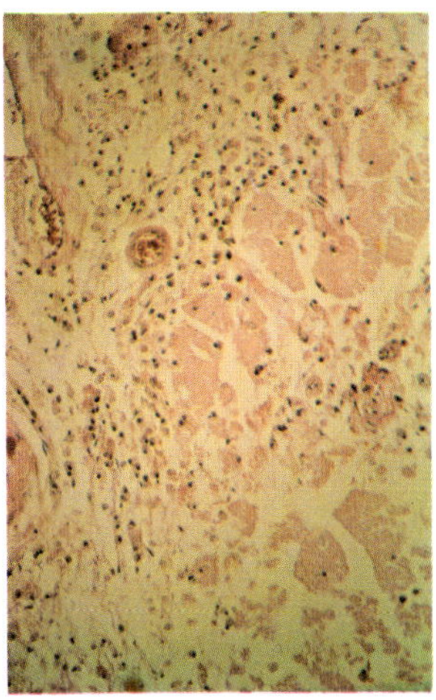

A microsection reveals fragments of necrotic cerebellar tissue and large numbers of macrophages (gitter cells) engulfing the debris.

OLD INFARCT, CEREBELLUM

CLINICAL ACCOUNT 7322

The patient was a white male 72 years old who had been well until one year before admission, when he had a myocardial infarction that was followed by congestive heart failure. He was found collapsed on the day of admission. The temperature was 38.1 degrees C., pulse 90, respirations 12, and blood pressure 90/60 mm. Hg. Physical examination revealed neck vein distension, rales over both lung fields, cardiac enlargement to the left, and pronounced edema of the extremities. The blood urea nitrogen was 83 mg. per 100 ml., and the electrocardiogram disclosed a posterior infarct of uncertain age. Urinary output decreased, the temperature rose, and the patient died after three days in the hospital.

Autopsy examination revealed hypertrophy of the heart (725 gm), an old infarct of the myocardium, and pronounced atherosclerosis of the coronary arteries. There were also bronchopneumonia of both lungs, passive hyperemia of the liver, arteriolar nephrosclerosis, and a small carcinoma of the right kidney. The brain disclosed atherosclerosis of the cerebral vessels and an old infarct of the left lobe of the cerebellum.

THE ENTITY

Vascular disease of the brain is the most common cause of neurologic disability. Twenty-five per cent of autopsies reveal vascular lesions, although most are without clinical manifestations. Two-thirds are due to atherosclerosis, one-third to embolism (1).

Atherosclerosis affects especially the vessels at the base of the brain, and the intimal proliferation and lipid deposits are prone to occur at the ostia of vascular branches. This gradual process causes slowing of blood flow by luminal stenosis or sudden obstruction by thrombus formation. Partial or total ischemia results. The brain is especially vulnerable to ischemia because of its dependence on oxidative metabolism, its high metabolic rate, and its low glycogen reserve.

The effect of ischemia is localized tissue necrosis termed infarction. Infarcts are most common in the cerebral hemispheres, less common in the brain stem and cerebellum, and rare in the spinal cord. The infarcts are "anemic," i.e., pale, edematous, and poorly demarcated. Some, however, display hemorrhage and become dark red. After a slight marginal infiltration with segmented granulocytes, the tissue undergoes liquefactive necrosis (dissolves), and the debris is carried away by an abundance of macrophages. Over the ensuing weeks, astrocytes proliferate to form a glial scar, and the necrotic site is converted to a cyst-like space. When extremely small, this may consist of nothing more than perivascular defects, especially in the basal ganglia, called "lacunes." When larger, the atrophy and cyst formation may alter the contour of the cerebral ventricles. When huge, the cyst-like cavity may extend from ventricle to cortex with only meninges to fill the defect (porencephaly).

Clinical manifestations include temporary attacks, often lasting less than a day, that consist of aphasia, hemiparesis, hemianesthesia, or visual defects when located in the cerebrum, and dysarthria, diplopia, and weakness of the legs when located in the brain stem. Recurrence of temporary attacks are common and many go on to permanent attacks within one to three years. Permanent attacks, i.e., "strokes," are abrupt in onset, are often briefly preceded by confusion, unsteadiness or dizziness, and cause paralysis that is irreversible. The nature and degree of the neurologic deficit indicates the size and location of the lesion.

1. Robertson, D.M., and Dinsdale, H.B. The Nervous System. The Williams and Wilkins Company, Baltimore, 1972.

SACCULAR ANEURYSM

CLINICAL ACCOUNT 7362

The patient was a white male 36 years old who had been well until six months before admission to the hospital, when he began having headaches that had become worse during the month preceding admission. On the day of admission the headache became severe abruptly and was associated with nausea, dizziness, and double vision. He promptly became comatose. The blood pressure was 180/120 mm. Hg. The right pupil was larger than the left, the optic fundi were normal, and decerebrate posturing of the extremities was noted. Motor and sensory function were normal, the Babinski reflex was negative, and bilateral ankle clonus was elicited. The leukocyte count was 19,400 per cmm. with a slight neutrophilia. A carotid arteriogram revealed an aneurysm of the right internal carotid artery near the posterior communicating vessel. The spinal fluid was tinged with blood. On the tenth hospital day a craniotomy was performed, and a clip was placed on the base of the aneurysm. On the next day the patient died.

THE ENTITY

Berry aneurysms are small saccular outpouchings of intracranial arteries that occur on the circle of Willis at the sites of vessel bifurcation. Nearly 90 per cent arise on the anterior portion of the circle of Willis, principally from the internal carotid, middle cerebral, and anterior communicating arteries. In 20 per cent the aneurysms are multiple. Most measure less than 1 cm. in diameter. The wall is thin, the opening to the parent vessel is wide, and thrombi tend to occupy those over 0.8 cm. in diameter. The aneurysms are occasionally embedded in the cerebral tissue. They are the most common arterial aneurysms of man, and have been found in 7 per cent of routine autopsies (1). These aneurysms are attributed to a congenital defect of the muscle layer at the sites of arterial bifurcation.

Rupture of a berry aneurysm is the most common cause of spontaneous subarachnoid hemorrhage in man (2). The patients are 40 to 70 years old, about equally male or female, and often hypertensive. The aneurysms that rupture usually measure more than 0.5 cm. in diameter. The hemorrhage extends over the base of the brain and frequently bursts outward through the arachnoid to form a subdural hematoma, or inward into the cerebral tissue to reach the lateral or third ventricles which become filled with blood. The patients experience sudden excrutiatingly severe headache that is followed quickly by disorders of consciousness and the rapid development of frank coma. About 20 per cent die of the first hemorrhage; those that survive and are untreated may expect a second hemorrhage within four weeks with a mortality of about 40 per cent. Few give clinical signs of aneurysm (headache, ptosis, diplopia, blurring of vision) before rupture takes place.

1. Stehbens, W.E. Aneurysms and anatomical variation of cerebral arteries. Arch. Path. 75:45-64, 1963.
2. Locksley, H.B. Hemorrhagic strokes. Med. Clin. N. Am. 52: 1193-1212, 1968.

SACCULAR ANEURYSM

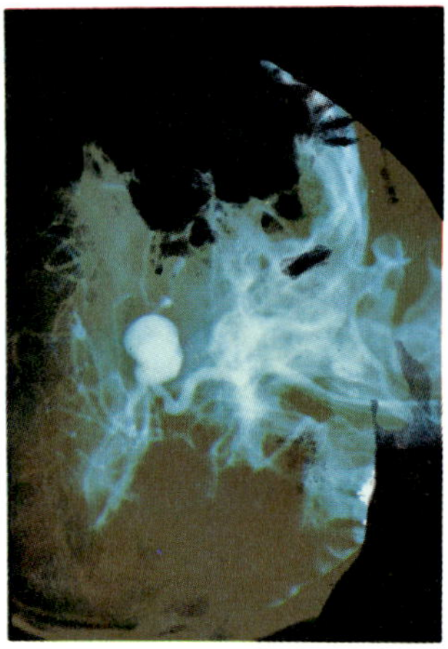

Arteriogram with opaque material identifying size and position of the aneurysm.

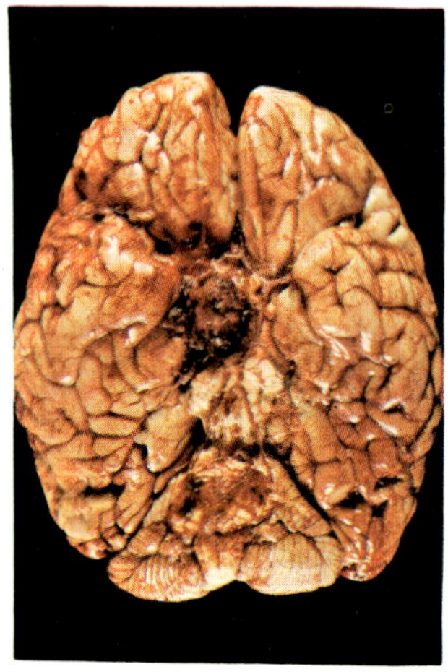

Undersurface of brain with aneurysm on circle of Willis.

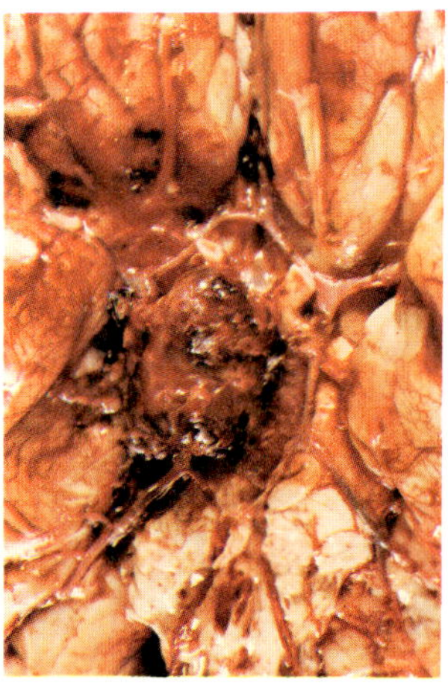

Close-up showing aneurysm.

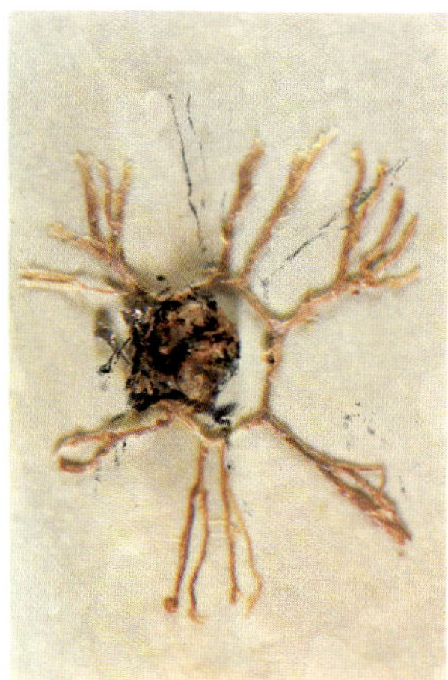

Aneurysm dissecting away from cerebral tissue; the structure is filled with thrombus.

SACCULAR ANEURYSM

Superior surface of cerebrum disclosing widespread subarachnoid hemorrhage.

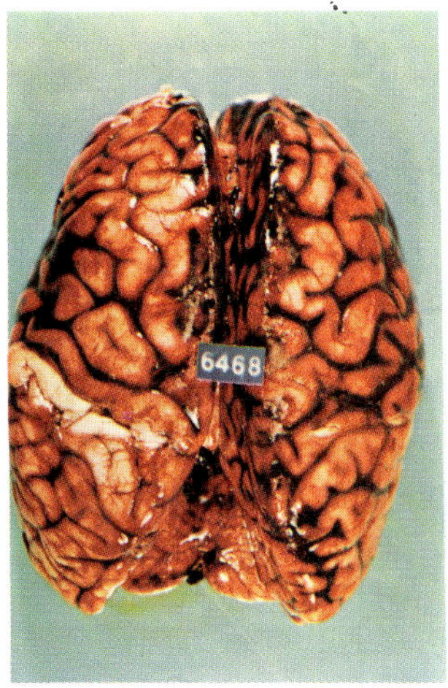

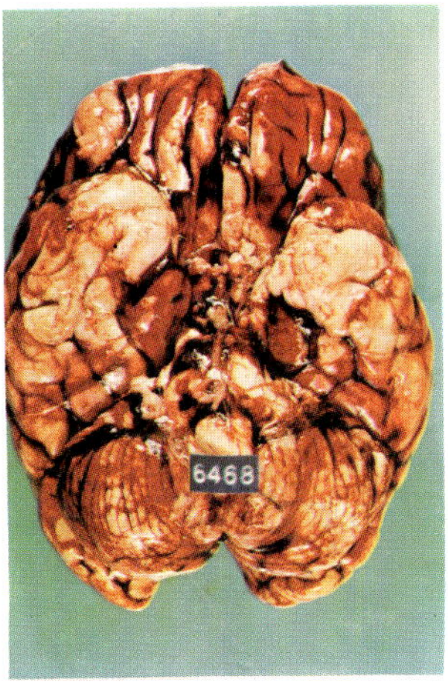

The undersurface also displays extensive subarachnoid hemorrhage; aneurysm not easily discernible.

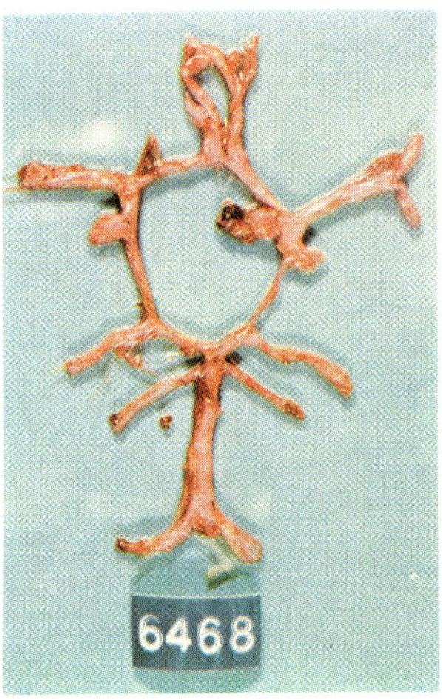

After dissection of the circle of Willis, the ruptured and empty aneurysm is clearly evident.

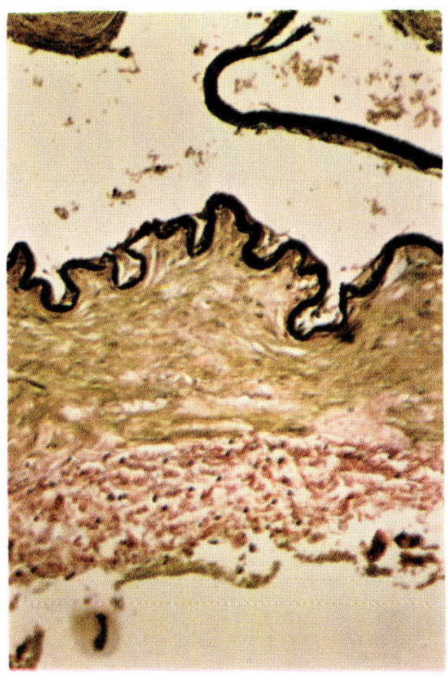

The Verhoeff stain reveals elastic fibers in the wall of the aneurysm.

SACCULAR ANEURYSM

CLINICAL ACCOUNT 6468

The patient was a white male 28 years old who had been in good health until he suddenly collapsed while playing baseball. Examination revealed him to be comatose, with a pulse of 120 and a blood pressure of 50/0 mm. Hg. Deep tendon reflexes could not be elicited, and there was no response to painful stimuli. Cardiac fibrillation developed and resuscitative measures were started. The patient died on the following day.

Autopsy examination revealed marked edema of the lungs, moderate atherosclerosis of the coronary arteries, and a saccular aneurysm of the left anterior cerebral artery. The aneurysm had ruptured, and there was extensive recent subarachnoid hemorrhage and marked brain edema. Additional diagnoses were incidental.

THE ENTITY

Berry aneurysms are small saccular outpouchings of intracranial arteries that occur on the circle of Willis at the sites of vessel bifurcation. Nearly 90 per cent arise on the anterior portion of the circle of Willis, principally from the internal carotid, middle cerebral, and anterior communicating arteries. In 20 per cent the aneurysms are multiple. Most measure less than 1 cm. in diameter. The wall is thin, the opening to the parent vessel is wide, and thrombi tend to occupy those over 0.8 cm. in diameter. The aneurysms are occasionally embedded in the cerebral tissue. They are the most common arterial aneurysms of man, and have been found in 7 per cent of routine autopsies (1). These aneurysms are attributed to a congenital defect of the muscle layer at the sites of arterial bifurcation.

Rupture of a berry aneurysm is the most common cause of spontaneous subarachnoid hemorrhage in man (2). The patients are 40 to 70 years old, about equally male or female, and often hypertensive. The aneurysms that rupture usually measure more than 0.5 cm. in diameter. The hemorrhage extends over the base of the brain and frequently bursts outward through the arachnoid to form a subdural hematoma, or inward into the cerebral tissue to reach the lateral or third ventricles which become filled with blood. The patients experience sudden excrutiatingly severe headache that is followed quickly by disorders of consciousness and the rapid development of frank coma. About 20 per cent die of the first hemorrhage; those that survive and are untreated may expect a second hemorrhage within four weeks with a mortality of about 40 per cent. Few give clinical signs of aneurysm (headache, ptosis, diplopia, blurring of vision) before rupture takes place.

1. Stehbens, W.E. Aneurysms and anatomical variation of cerebral arteries. Arch. Path. 75:45-64, 1963.
2. Locksley, H.B. Hemorrhagic strokes. Med. Clin. N. Am. 52: 1193-1212, 1968.

HEMORRHAGE OF BRAINSTEM

CLINICAL ACCOUNT 7530

The patient was a black male 38 years old who had been well until two months before admission, when depression, loss of concentration, and irritability developed. These progressed and in the week before admission dysarthria, weakness of the right side, and drooping of the right cheek also were noted. Physical examination revealed slight hemiparesis on the right, hyperesthesia of the right hand, and ankle clonus on the right. The cranial nerves were intact, there was no papilledema, and the deep tendon reflexes were symmetrical. X-ray studies of the brain indicated a large mass in the left frontoparietal region. Bilateral papilledema developed. On the thirteenth hospital day a craniotomy revealed a glioblastoma, and a left subtotal lobectomy was performed. Later on that day the patient died.

Autopsy examination revealed a glioblastoma of the left cerebral hemisphere, a defect of the left frontal lobe, edema of the cerebrum, and a recent hemorrhage of the pons.

THE ENTITY

Primary hemorrhage within the brain usually occurs in adults who are hypertensive and have arteriosclerosis of their small cerebral vessels. The vessels also reveal minute thin-walled dilatations (Charcot-Bouchard aneurysms), and rupture is presumed to occur at a weakened site (1). The high arterial pressure then pumps blood into the soft cerebral tissue. The onset usually takes place during a time of exertion when the blood pressure is especially high. The clinical manifestations include sudden intense headache and massive flaccid paralysis. The patient collapses and coma soon follows. With hemorrhage into the cerebrum, life may persist for a few days, but with hemorrhage below the tentorium, death occurs within hours from impingement of the medulla into the foramen magnum.

Primary intracerebral hemorrhage is usually massive, single, one-sided, and fatal. About 70 per cent begin in the basal ganglia with spread into the adjacent white matter of the cerebral hemisphere, 20 per cent arise in the pons or midbrain, and 10 per cent originate in the cerebellum. The blood dissects into the cerebral tissue, pushes it aside, and forms a solid hematoma that occupies half or more of the hemispheric volume. Externally the side affected reveals swelling with broad gyri and narrow sulci, while internally the ventricular system is compressed, distorted, and pushed toward the opposite side. Herniation about the falx and tentorium gives rise to pressure grooves in the cerebral tissue. Rupture of the hematoma into the ventricular system on the inside, or externally into the subarachnoid space, is extremely common. Both cause the spinal fluid to become bloody. Most patients die before a tissue reaction develops. With survival, however, the tissue reaction consists of marginal edema, leukocytic infiltration, macrophage accumulation, and eventually marginal gliosis with the formation of a cavity lined by macrophages pigmented with hemosiderin. Less than 10 per cent survive.

1. Robertson, D.M., and Dinsdale, H.B. The Nervous System. The Williams & Wilkins Co., Baltimore, 1972.

HEMORRHAGE OF BRAINSTEM

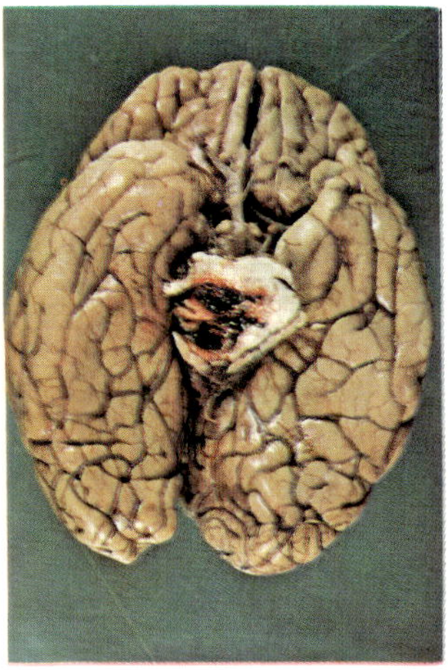

The undersurface of the brain reveals diffuse blood staining of the meninges and solid hematoma extending outward from the fourth ventricle and at the side of the pons.

Section of the brainstem discloses massive recent hemorrhage of the pons.

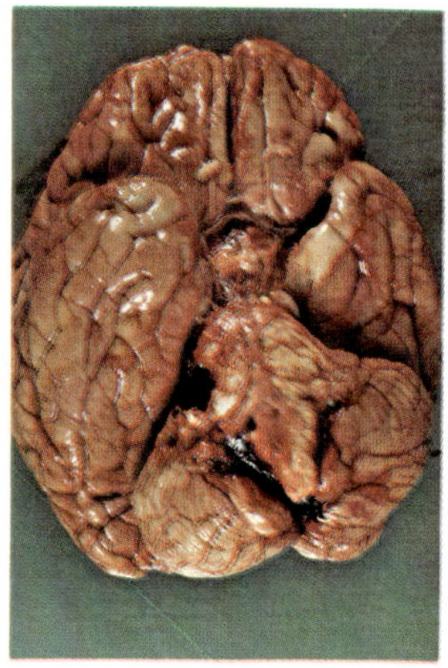

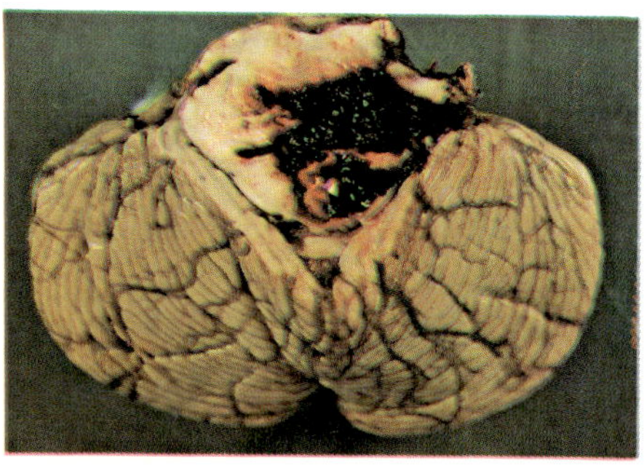

A closer view reveals the massive intrapontine hemorrhage.

The low power microsection shows the abrupt margin of the hematoma and adjacent tissue.

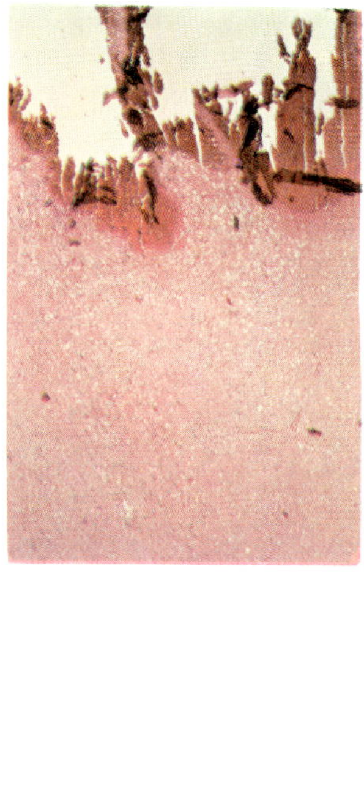

OLD INFARCT, CEREBRUM

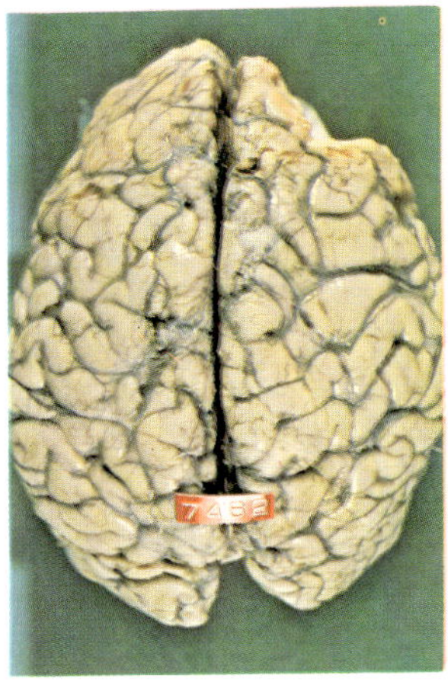

The superior surface reveals a pronounced focal loss of tissue from the right frontal lobe.

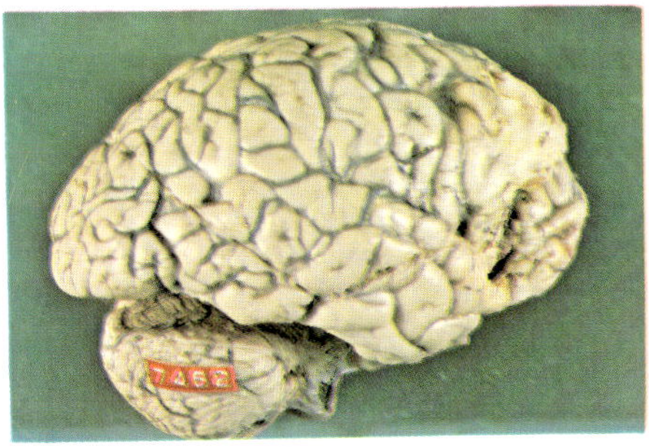

From the side, atrophy and brown discoloration are evident over the site of the lesion.

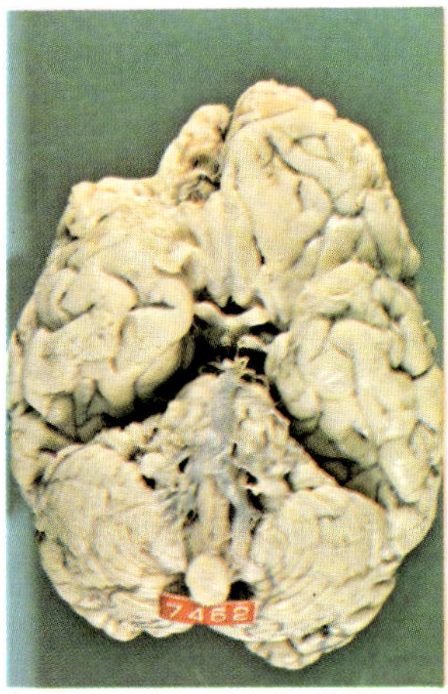

The undersurface reveals the pronounced tissue loss.

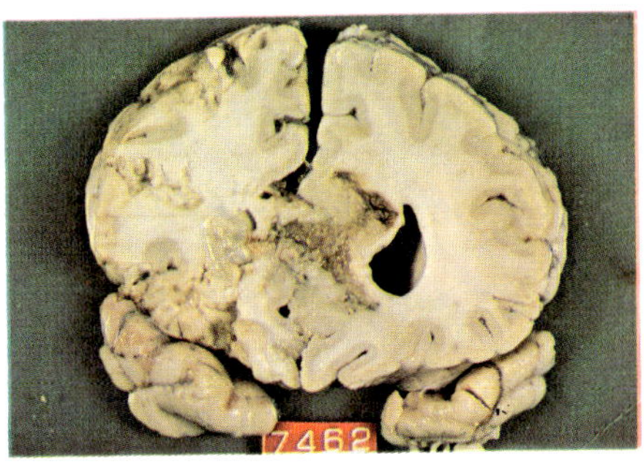

Section reveals that the infarct has extended deeply into the right hemisphere and across the midline to the medial aspect of the left cerebrum.

OLD INFARCT, CEREBRUM

CLINICAL ACCOUNT 7462

The patient was a white female 67 years old who had been well until four months before hospital admission, when her family noted the onset of personality changes. These were followed by double vision, dizziness, and occipital headaches. Examination revealed a right fourth cranial nerve paralysis, ptosis of the left eyelid, edema of both optic nerve heads, a steady gaze nystagmus, and a slow wave complex on the encephalogram. Disorientation developed.

On the eighth hospital day a frontal craniotomy was performed and a nonresectable tumor was identified. Steroids and radiation therapy were given. The patient died after 66 days in the hospital.

Autopsy examination revealed a glioblastoma multiforme of the frontal lobes of the cerebrum, focal fibrosis of the pituitary, bronchopneumonia of the left lung, and an old infarct of the cerebrum.

THE ENTITY

Vascular disease of the brain is the most common cause of neurologic disability. Twenty-five per cent of autopsies reveal vascular lesions, although most are without clinical manifestations. Two-thirds are due to atherosclerosis. one-third to embolism (1).

Atherosclerosis affects especially the vessels at the base of the brain, and the intimal proliferation and lipid deposits are prone to occur at the ostia of vascular branches. This gradual process causes slowing of blood flow by luminal stenosis or sudden obstruction by thrombus formation. Partial or total ischemia results. The brain is especially vulnerable to ischemia because of its dependence on oxidative metabolism, its high metabolic rate, and its low glycogen reserve.

The effect of ischemia is localized tissue necrosis termed infarction. Infarcts are most common in the cerebral hemispheres, less common in the brain stem and cerebellum, and rare in the spinal cord. The infarcts are "anemic," i.e., pale, edematous, and poorly demarcated. Some, however, display hemorrhage and become dark red. After a slight marginal infiltration with segmented granulocytes, the tissue undergoes liquefactive necrosis (dissolves), and the debris is carried away by an abundance of macrophages. Over the ensuing weeks, astrocytes proliferate to form a glial scar, and the necrotic site is converted to a cyst-like space. When extremely small, this may consist of nothing more than perivascular defects, especially in the basal ganglia, called "lacunes." When larger, the atrophy and cyst formation may alter the contour of the cerebral ventricles. When huge, the cyst-like cavity may extend from ventricle to cortex with only meninges to fill the defect (porencephaly).

Clinical manifestations include temporary attacks, often lasting less than a day, that consist of aphasia, hemiparesis, hemianesthesia, or visual defects when located in the cerebrum, and dysarthria, diplopia, and weakness of the legs when located in the brain stem. Recurrence of temporary attacks are common and many go on to permanent attacks within one to three years. Permanent attacks, i.e., "strokes," are abrupt in onset, are often briefly preceded by confusion, unsteadiness or dizziness, and cause paralysis that is irreversible. The nature and degree of the neurologic deficit indicates the size and location of the lesion.

1. Robertson, D.M., and Dinsdale, H.B. The Nervous System. The Williams and Wilkins Company, Baltimore, 1972.

MENINGIOMA

CLINICAL ACCOUNT 6157

The patient was a white male 62 years old who was admitted to the hospital because of low back pain of three months' duration that radiated to the perineum, suprapubic region, and left testicle. A transurethral prostatectomy had been performed, and a prostatic abscess was drained. Over the past two months there had been a weight loss of 10 pounds. Recently the patient had noted a sensation of bowel obstruction. Past history revealed that a myocardial infarction had occurred nine years earlier and that the patient was presently under treatment for angina pectoris.

Physical examination was not remarkable except for nodularity over the right side of the prostate. The deep tendon reflexes were normal, and there were no neurologic complaints.

The urine was normal. The hemoglobin was 11.6 Gm., hematocrit 36.5, and leukocytes 57,400 with 76 segmented granulocytes, 17 band cells, 3 lymphocytes, 3 monocytes, and 1 eosinophile. The serum alkaline phosphatase was 8.0 units per 100 ml. On the fifth hospital day a pelvic abscess was drained through a suprapubic incision. Tissue removed at that time revealed a malignant tumor of uncertain type. On the twelfth hospital day the patient felt weak, and later that day he unexpectedly died.

Autopsy examination revealed a sarcoma of the lower ileum that had metastasized to the mesenteric lymph nodes. The tumor had spread through the bowel wall to form a pelvic abscess that was undergoing organization. There were also edema of the left lung and a recent infarct of the myocardium of the left ventricle. The liver was hyperemic and weighed 2400 Gms. The spleen disclosed acute hyperplasia and weighed 425 Gms. The urinary bladder, prostate, and colon were not remarkable.

THE ENTITY

Meningiomas are benign slowly growing connective tissue tumors that arise from the meninges. They comprise about 15 per cent of all intracranial tumors. They occur in adults of 20 to 60 years, more frequently in men than women (2:1). They arise over the convexity of the brain (50%), especially in the parasagittal region, and on the undersurface, especially over the sphenoid ridges (20%), olfactory grooves (10%), and cerebellopontine angles (5%). They are firm, nodular, pale gray, and sharply circumscribed without encapsulation. The cut surfaces reveal coarse interlacing fibrous bundles. Five histologic types include meningothelial, fibroblastic, mixed, angiomatous, and sarcomatous. The last comprises only 1 to 2 per cent of the total. Most are mixed and biologically similar so that histologic typing is not especially useful (1).

Symptoms begin gradually and often last two years before diagnosis. They include headache, visual disturbance, focal seizures, external swelling and paresthesia, in that order. Cure is achieved by surgical removal.

1. Earle, K.M., and Richany, S.F. Meningiomas. Med Ann. Dist. Columbia 38:353, 1969.

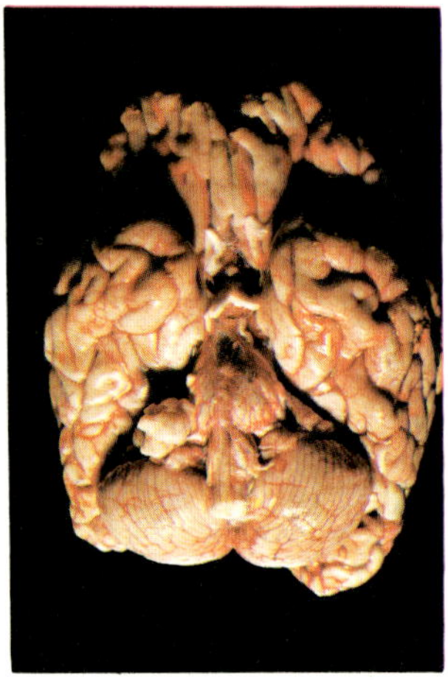

On removal of the brain, a firm pale gray nodular tumor mass is found in the right cerebellopontine angle.

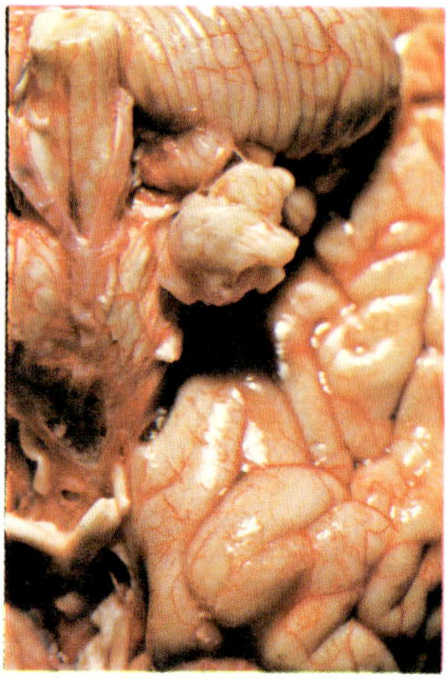

A close up shows the detail of the tumor in the cerebellopontine angle.

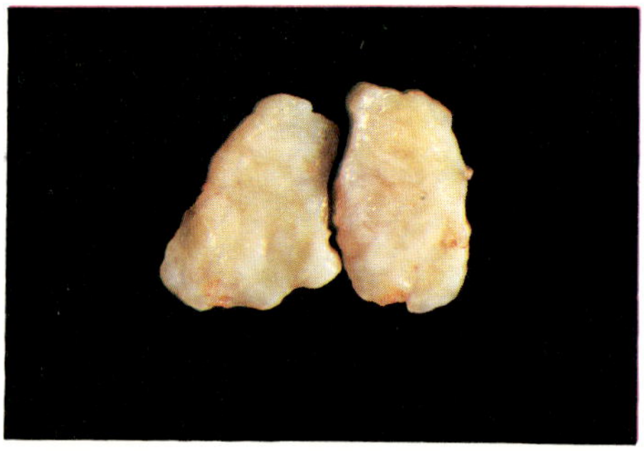

The cut surface is tough and pale gray.

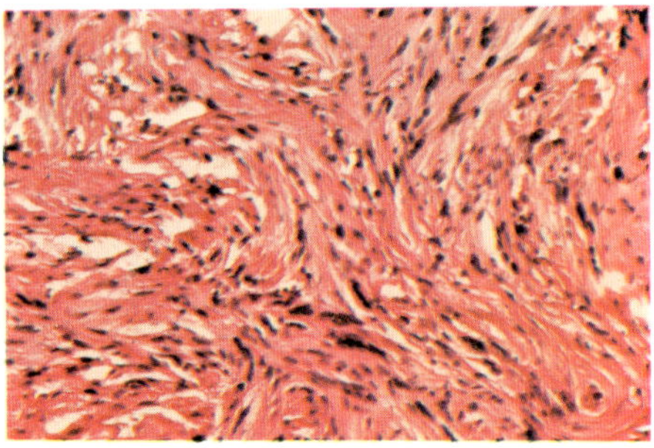

Histologic examination reveals interlacing bundles of connective tissue. The nuclei display hyperchromatism and moderate variation in size. Mitotic figures are nevertheless scarce and this is true for all meningiomas except for those few that undergo malignant transformation and become sarcomas. The meningioma illustrated here is fibroblastic in histologic type.

GLIOBLASTOMA MULTIFORME

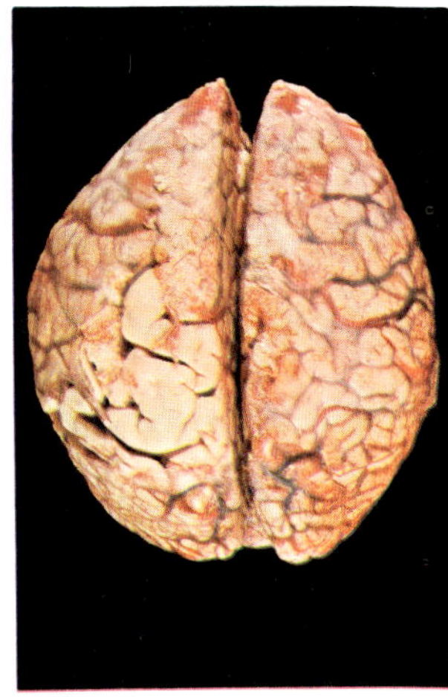

The superior cerebral surface shows asymmetry with enlargement of the left hemisphere.

Transverse section reveals a pale gray poorly demarcated tumor mass that expands the white matter, compresses the lateral ventricle, and causes disproportion of the two cerebral hemispheres.

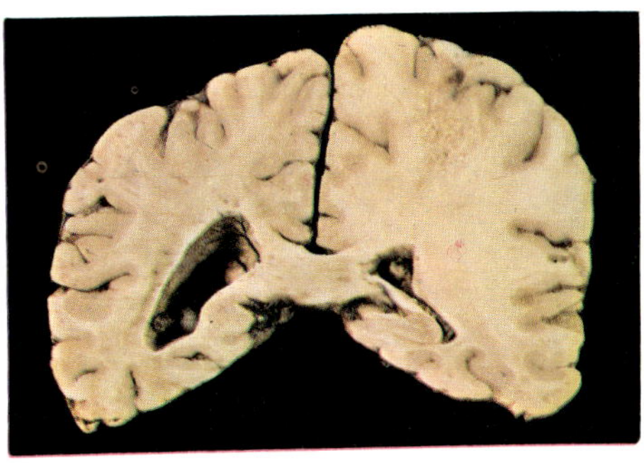

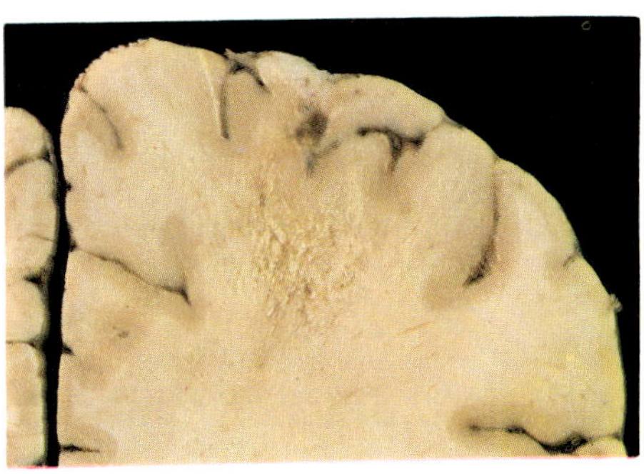

A close-up view reveals central necrosis in the tumor mass and emphasizes the poor demarcation between the tumor and the adjacent white matter.

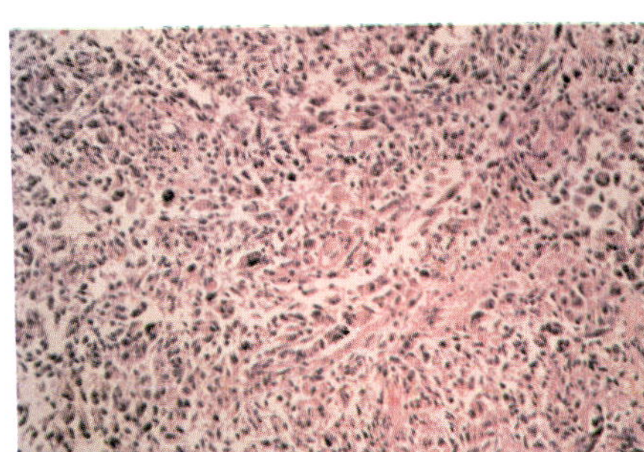

A microsection displays pronounced anaplasia with irregular cell and nuclear size, marked hyperchromatism, and frequent mitotic figures.

GLIOBLASTOMA MULTIFORME

CLINICAL ACCOUNT 7348

The patient was a white male 61 years old who had been well until eight months before entering the hospital. At that time he noted weakness of his right hand. Over subsequent weeks this weakness spread to his entire right side and was accompanied by a regression of mentation. Six months before admission biopsy revealed a glioblastoma multiforme of his right cerebral hemisphere. Focal radiation therapy was given and the patient improved. Two months before admission, weakness recurred and was accompanied by dizziness and headache.

The vital signs were normal. Physical examination was not remarkable except for neurologic function; i.e., the right side was weak, the Romberg test was positive, and the deep tendon reflexes on the right were increased. In addition, the patient forgot words, could not write, could not subtract, and could not hold a train of thought. Cranial nerve and sensory function were physiologic.

The blood and urine were normal. A left carotid arteriogram and a brain scan revealed left parietal changes consistent with recurrent tumor. The patient's condition progressively deteriorated, and he died after two months in the hospital.

THE ENTITY

About half of all primary intracranial tumors are gliomas. The gliomas are classified according to their cell of origin and consist of the astrocytomas, the oligodendrogliomas, and the ependymomas. All are malignant. The great majority of gliomas are astrocytomas, and while some grow with extreme slowness, others are among the most malignant of all human tumors. In order to accommodate this spectrum, a classification of malignancy is used. Grade I astrocytomas are the least malignant, the tumor cells most nearly resemble normal astrocytes, and the mean survival period from the onset of symptoms is about eight years (1). In contrast, Grade IV astrocytomas are composed of highly anaplastic cells, invasion of cerebral tissue is rapid, and the mean survival time is 11 months.

Gliomas tend to occur in children and young adults. In children, astrocytomas arise in the cerebellum, grow slowly, and often become cystic. In adults, astrocytomas arise in the corpus callosum. Grade I tumors are pale gray, poorly demarcated, and occasionally cystic. Grade IV tumors are markedly edematous, focally necrotic, and conspicuously hemorrhagic. All of the astrocytomas form a single tumor mass in the cerebral tissue, and none metastasizes outside of the brain.

While signs and symptoms depend on the site of the tumor and the rate of its growth, clinical manifestations reflect principally increased intracranial pressure and functional loss of destroyed cerebral tissue.

1. Robertson, D.M., and Dinsdale, H.B. The Nervous System, The Williams and Wilkins Company, 1972.

MEDULLOBLASTOMA

CLINICAL ACCOUNT SLH-A-198

The patient was a white girl 8 years old who had been well until six weeks before hospital admission. At that time she awoke one morning and vomited. This condition persisted, and within two weeks she was vomiting after every meal, failing to retain food, and losing weight. The vomiting was unrelieved by a sedative. An upper gastrointestinal x-ray examination was normal. The vomiting abated for one week. It then recurred and was accompanied by paroxysms of severe pain in both ears that made the patient scream. Slight dizziness developed, and on the day before admission blurred vision in the right eye was noted.

The vital signs and physical examination including neurologic function were normal. The blood and urine were normal. An electroencephalogram disclosed a paroxysmal abnormality of grand mal type without localization. The spinal fluid was clear and revealed only increased pressure and slight elevation of protein. The patient became unconscious and died after 10 days in the hospital.

Autopsy examination revealed a medulloblastoma of the cerebellum, edema of the cerebrum, and bronchopneumonia of the right and left lungs.

THE ENTITY

Medulloblastoma is the commonest malignant tumor of the brain in children. It originates in the cerebellum usually before the age of 14 and frequently before the age of 5 years. It is more common in boys than girls. It arises from the midline vermis which forms the roof of the fourth ventricle. It grows rapidly, obstructs the fourth ventricle early, and spreads widely in the subarachnoid space to implant on all of the meningeal surfaces of the brain and spinal cord. The tumor is reddish gray, moderately firm, and sharply circumscribed. Microscopically the growth is densely cellular with scant stroma and few blood vessels. The tumor cells resemble lymphocytes, being small, uniform in size, and deeply basophilic. A tendency to form pseudorosettes is noticeable (radial arrangement of tumor cells about small blood vessels). Mitotic figures are numerous. The tumor arises from embryonic medullary epithelium (1).

Clinical manifestations reflect increased intracranial pressure and consist of headache, morning vomiting, and staggering gait. Physical examination reveals pronounced papilledema. Hydrocephalus may develop. Therapy consists of surgical unblocking of the fourth ventricle and the subsequent use of radiation, to which the tumor is uniquely and extremely sensitive. These measures extend survival, but the tumor is incurable and death takes place 4 to 12 years after the beginning of treatment.

1. Wright, G.P., and Symmers, W. St. C. Systemic Pathology, Vol. II, p. 1247, 1967.

MEDULLOBLASTOMA

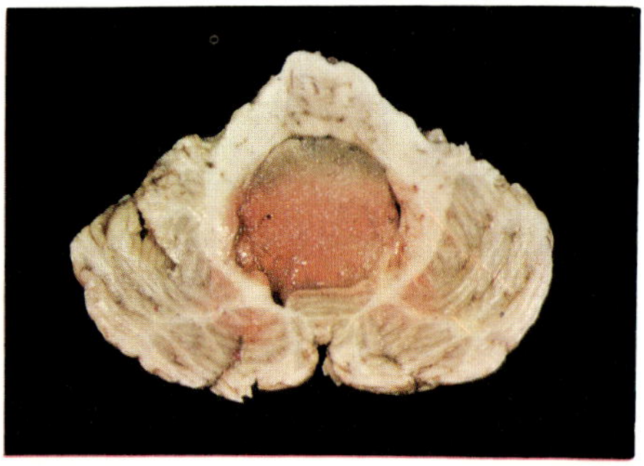

The cut surface of the cerebellum reveals the soft discrete round tumor mass that characteristically occupies the midline vermis.

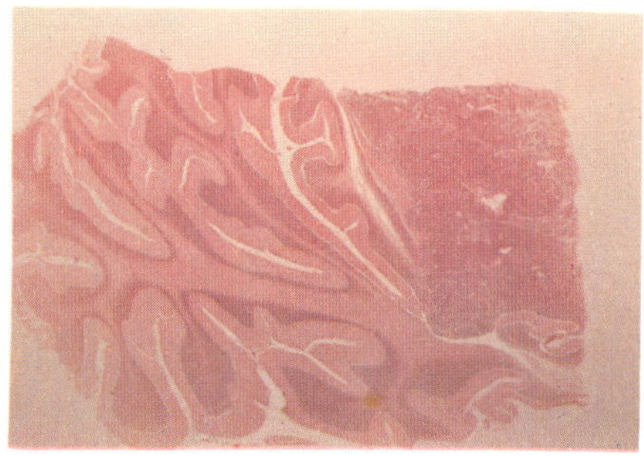

At scanning power the encroachment of the tumor on the cerebellar tissue can be seen.

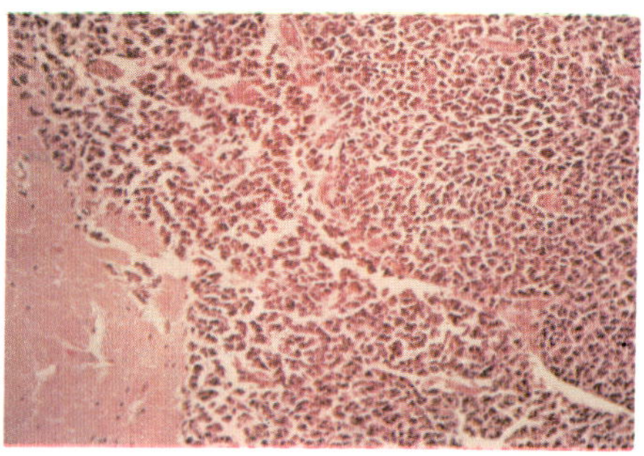

Low power reveals the solid masses of small hyperchromatic cells that infiltrate the tissue.

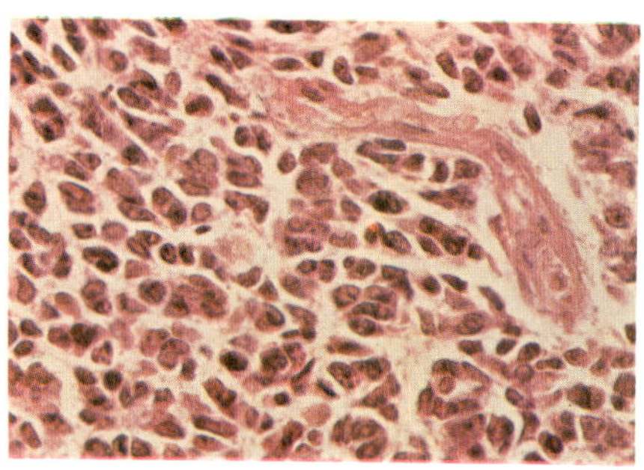

At higher power the uniformity of the cells, their small size, and the hyperchromatism of nuclei stand out.

MENINGIOMA

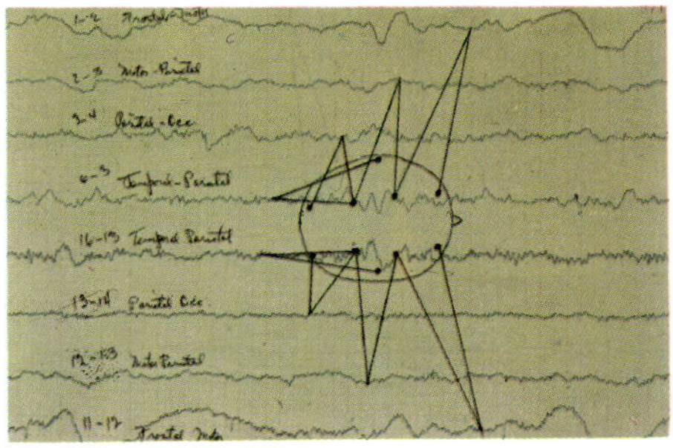

The electroencephalogram described in Clinical Account.

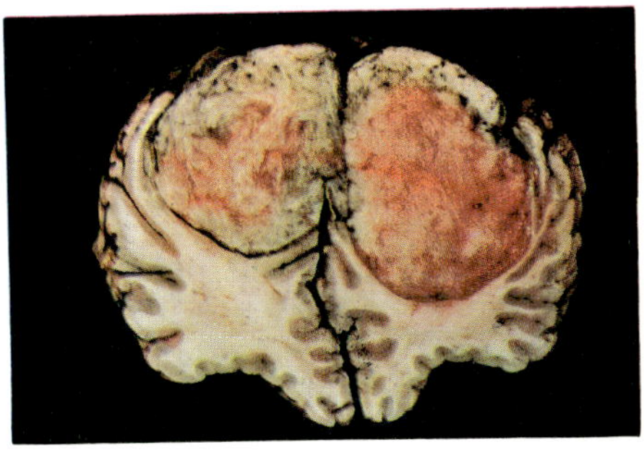

The cerebral cut surface with enormous meningioma extending deeply into both hemispheres. The cut surface is firm, pinkish gray, and coarsely trabeculated. The focal redness is due to lack of fixation.

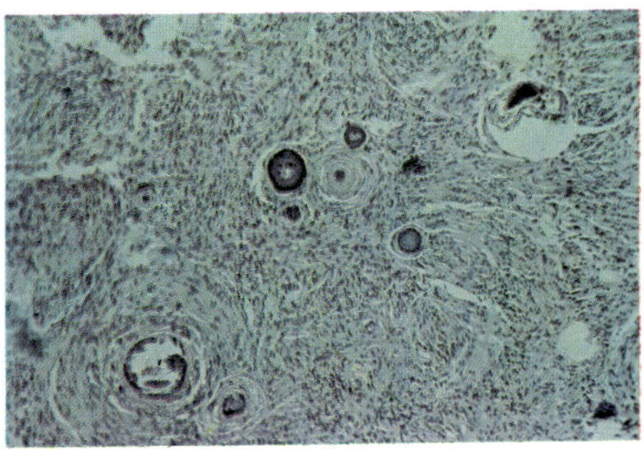

At low power calcified psammoma bodies are seen scattered over whorls of moderately dense fibrous connective tissue.

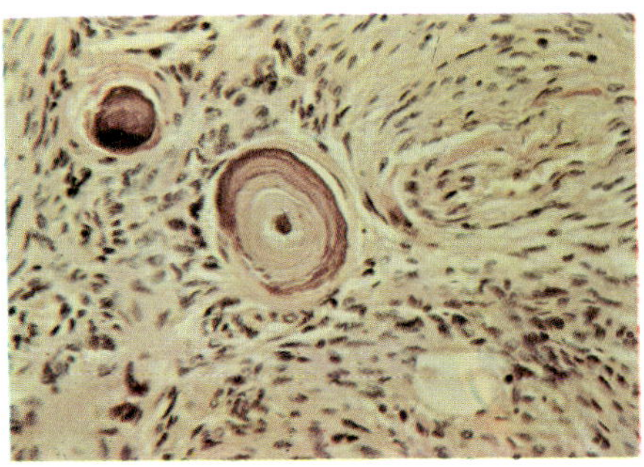

At higher power the details of a psammoma body and the connective tissue nature of the main tumor mass are more clearly evident. The tumor is a fibroblastic meningioma.

MENINGIOMA

CLINICAL ACCOUNT SLH-A-112

The patient was a white male 36 years old who had been well until two months before entering the hospital, when he noted a slowing of his work pace as a tool maker. He stated that he felt "rotten," that what he previously did in two hours now took four days, and that his speech was slow. He appeared depressed.

The vital signs were normal and the physical examination not remarkable except for edema of the optic discs and absence of the right knee jerk. The blood and urine were essentially normal. The spinal fluid was not remarkable. An electroencephalogram suggested a left sided abnormality. A pneumoencephalogram revealed enlargement of the sella turcica; air was not seen in the cerebral ventricles. Radiation therapy was given for a presumed pituitary adenoma; the patient was discharged after 23 days in the hospital.

He returned six weeks later, moribund, incontinent, blind, dehydrated, and unable to eat. There was loss of motor control of all extremities, spastic paralysis of the right arm, and absence of both knee jerks. The pulse was weak and 140. The temperature rose to 106 degrees F., and the patient died after three days in the hospital.

Autopsy examination revealed a large meningioma of the falx and bronchopneumonia of the left lung. The brain weighed 1790 Gms., the sella turcica was dilated, and the chamber was occupied by an atrophic pituitary.

THE ENTITY

Meningiomas are benign slowly growing connective tissue tumors that arise from the meninges. They comprise about 15 per cent of all intracranial tumors. They occur in adults of 20 to 60 years, more frequently in men than women (2:1). They arise over the convexity of the brain (50%), especially in the parasagittal region, and on the under-surface, especially over the sphenoid ridges (20%), olfactory grooves (10%), and cerebello-pontine angles (5%). They are firm, nodular, pale gray, and sharply circumscribed without encapsulation. The cut surfaces reveal coarse interlacing fibrous bundles. Five histologic types include meningothelial, fibroblastic, mixed, angiomatous, and sarcomatous. The last comprises only 1 to 2 per cent of the total. Most are mixed and biologically similar so that histologic typing is not especially useful (1).

Symptoms begin gradually and often last two years before diagnosis. They include headache, visual disturbance, focal seizures, external swelling, and paresthesia, in that order. Cure is achieved by surgical removal.

1. Earle, K.M., and Richany, S.F. Meningiomas. Med Ann. Dist. Columbia 38:353, 1969.

MENINGEAL CARCINOMATOSIS

CLINICAL ACCOUNT 6891

The patient was a black male 70 years old who was admitted to the hospital because of a change in mental status. He had been well until one month previously when the family noted confusion, visual illusions, and instability on walking. During the history-taking, the patient had periods of confusion, momentarily forgetting where he was, and at another time mistaking a television screen for a goldfish bowl.

The vital signs were normal. Physical examination was not remarkable except for staggering to the right on walking and falling forward during the Romberg test. The deep tendon reflexes were active and equal. The Babinski reflex was negative on both sides.

The hematocrit was 43 per cent, the leukocytes numbered 7,200, and the differential count was normal. Lumbar puncture revealed clear fluid with 17 lymphocytes per cmm. The protein and sugar were 57 and 42 mg. per 100 ml., respectively, and the opening and closing pressures were normal. A chest x-ray disclosed blunting of the costophrenic angles, hilar calcifications, and a hazy infiltrate at the right apex. An electroencephalogram was diffusely abnormal, and a brain scan was interpreted as within normal limits. A diagnosis of tuberculous meningitis was considered, and the patient was given streptomycin, aminosalicylic acid, and isoniazid. Smears and cultures of sputum and spinal fluid for pyogenic and acid-fast organisms were negative. Biopsies of liver and bone marrow were normal. The patient lapsed into coma on the fifteenth hospital day and died two days later.

Autopsy examination revealed an alveolar carcinoma of the lung with metastatic tumor in the cerebrum, cerebellum, and leptomeninges.

THE ENTITY

While approximately 5 per cent of patients with cancer develop cerebral metastases, these are almost always multiple and nodular. The least common form of intracranial metastasis is diffuse spread of tumor cells in the meninges without grossly discernible involvement of the cerebral tissue. In such cases the brain is of normal contour and displays only a slight haziness of the meninges. The spinal cord, however, is often seeded, and involvement of cranial nerves is common. The cerebral cut surfaces are not remarkable, the ventricles are not dilated, and the choroid plexus is normal. Carcinoma of the stomach is the usual primary tumor. This is remarkable because gastric cancer otherwise rarely spreads to the brain, whereas carcinomas of the thyroid and kidney which commonly spread to the brain rarely cause diffuse meningeal metastases. Cancers of breast and lung also cause the lesion, but other primary sites are uncommon. Extracranial metastases are often scarce. The metastatic route is uncertain.

The clinical picture is dominated by mental changes, meningeal signs, and cranial nerve palsies that are associated with unusual spinal fluid. The diagnosis is therefore suggested by a middle-aged patient of either sex, with or without a known primary carcinoma, who develops a severe headache, deteriorating mental changes, and facial or oculomotor palsies with visual impairment that may progress to blindness. The spinal fluid is clear, sterile, and characteristically reveals a low sugar level. Tumor cells may be found in the stained sediment. The course is rapid. Only whole-brain radiation has ameliorated symptoms and prolonged life (1).

1. Smith, J.C., Kish, G.F., and Jannotta, F.S. Metastatic meningeal carcinomatosis; report of a case. Med. Ann. Dist. Col. 41: 736-741, 1972.

MENINGEAL CARCINOMATOSIS

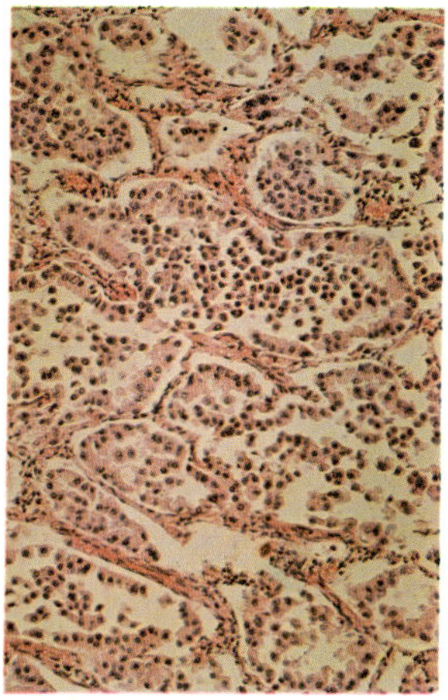

Alveolar pattern of the primary tumor in the lung. Notice that alveoli are not destroyed.

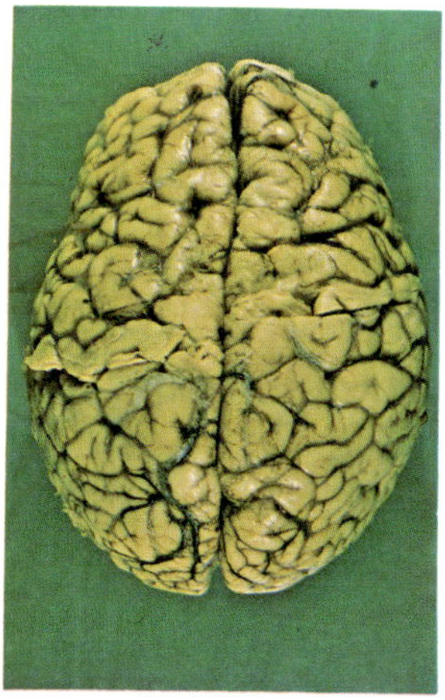

Superior surface of brain. No tumor is grossly evident although tumor cells are widely spread in the meninges.

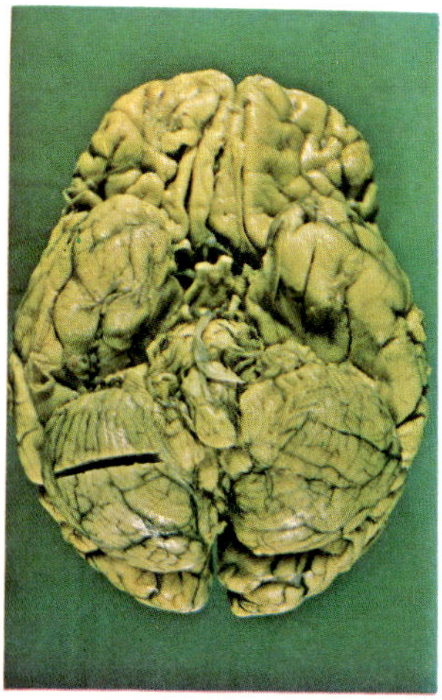

Undersurface of brain; no tumor grossly evident.

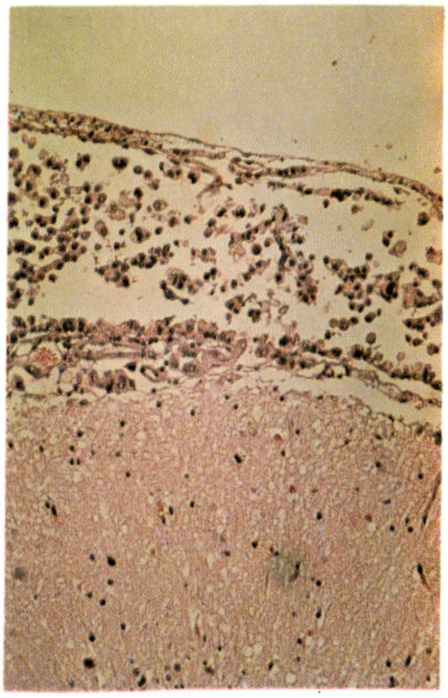

Subarachnoid space of meninges with loose tumor cells scattered throughout.

ADENOMA OF PITUITARY

The red pituitary stalk can be seen in the center of a full and bulging sella turcica.

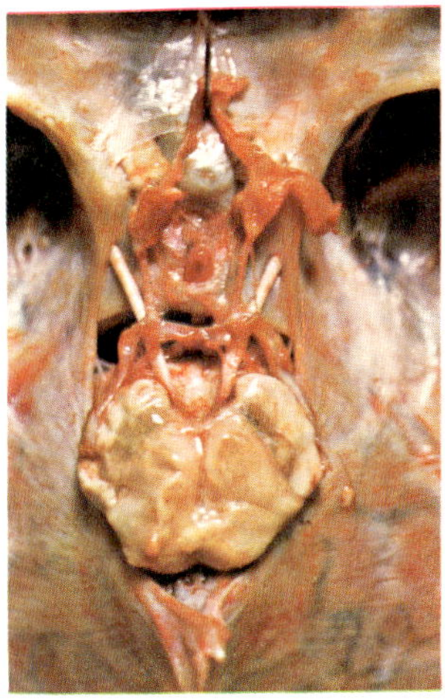

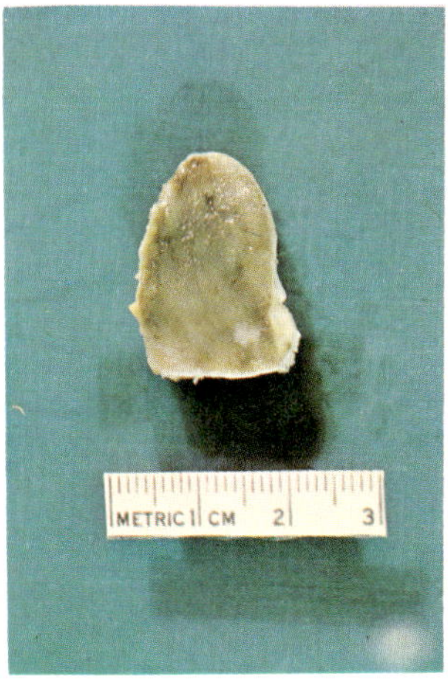

The removed pituitary adenoma after fixation has a pale brownish gray cut surface.

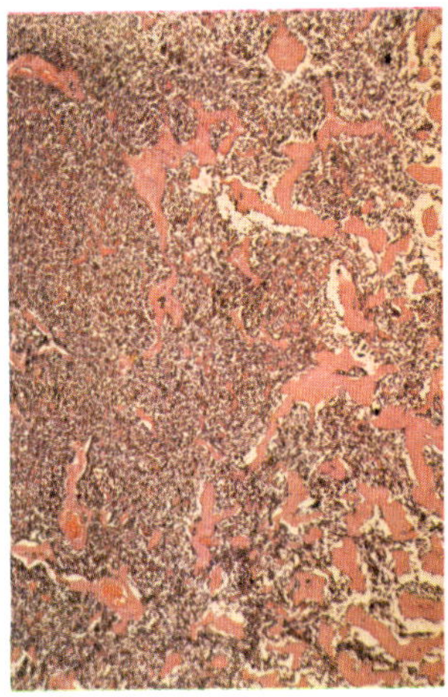

At low power hyaline trabeculae course through the solid masses of epithelial cells.

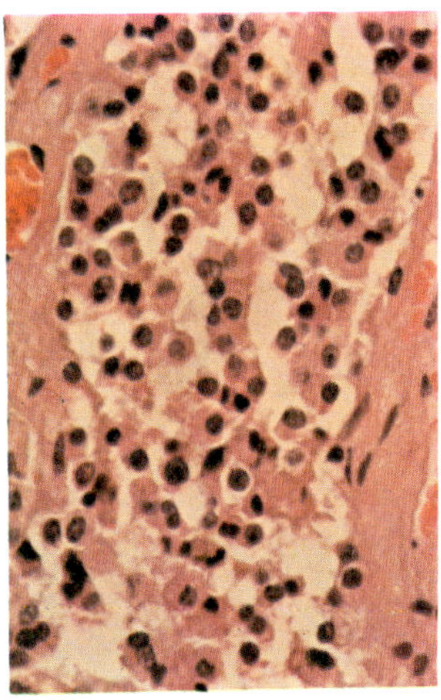

At higher power the cells are uniform in size and shape with cytoplasm that is lacking in eosinophilic or basophilic granules.

ADENOMA OF PITUITARY

CLINICAL ACCOUNT 7063

The patient was a white female 77 years old who entered the hospital because of progressive dysphagia and dysarthria. Her gait became unsteady, she fell repeatedly, and examination revealed facial weakness and atrophy of the shoulder girdle muscles. A diagnosis of amyotrophic lateral sclerosis was made.

Past history disclosed a pituitary adenoma had been diagnosed 22 years previously, and for this radiation therapy had been given on several occasions.

Dysphagia increased so that the patient was only able to eat pureed foods. A feeding gastrostomy was performed. Weakness progressed, respiratory difficulty developed, and the patient died after 33 days in the hospital.

Autopsy examination revealed bronchopneumonia, amyotrophic lateral sclerosis, neurogenic atrophy of skeletal muscle, a parathyroid adenoma, and a chromophobe adenoma of the pituitary.

THE ENTITY

The normal pituitary weighs about 0.6 Gm., and measures 1.5 x 1.0 x 0.5 cm. It is composed of an anterior epithelial lobe which secretes eight hormones, a posterior neural lobe which secretes two hormones, and a rudimentary intermediate lobe. The largest part of the structure is the anterior lobe, which consists of chromophobic, acidophilic, and basophilic cells. These are named for their cytoplasmic granules which selectively take up eosin (acidophils), hematoxylin (basophils), or neither (chromophobes). The latter may represent degranulated dye-absorbing cells (1).

The common symptomatic lesion of the pituitary is the adenoma. Those of basophilic cells rarely cause symptoms. Those of acidophilic cells are uncommon, secrete growth hormone, and cause gigantism in children or acromegaly in adults. Most adenomas are of chromophobe cells which secrete no hormone and cause symptoms by pressure enlargement of the sella and pressure atrophy of the remaining tissue. The patients are 20 to 50 years of age, the onset is extremely gradual, and the usual symptoms are headache and slowly progressive visual disturbance. These increase as the tumor expands the sella, ruptures through the dural tent (diaphragm), and impinges on the optic chiasm or invades the cavernous or paranasal sinuses.

Examination often reveals signs of hypopituitarism, i.e., atrophy of the sex organs and atrophic skin that is smooth, soft, hairless, pallid, and shiny. In addition, there are often decreased libido in men and infrequent menses in women. The diagnosis is made from these observations together with radiographic disclosure of an enlarged sella. The spinal fluid is usually normal but may contain increased protein. The pressure tends to be raised when the sellar tent is ruptured. The condition needs to be distinguished from the Rathke pouch tumor (craniopharyngioma) which lies above the sella, does not enlarge it, and often causes supracellular calcification that is visible in radiographs of the skull.

1. Catt, K.J. ABC of Endocrinology. Pituitary function. The Lancet 1:827-831, 1970.

HYDROMYELIA

CLINICAL ACCOUNT 6135

The patient was a white male 56 years old who was admitted to the hospital because of fever and severe dyspnea. He had been markedly kyphoscoliotic for years and had a secondary chronic pulmonary insufficiency. His vital capacity was under 600 ml., and his vertebral deformity was presumed to cause a progressive injury of his spinal cord. The latter was manifested by a left hemiparesis and a weakness of his right leg. Cerebral function was unimpaired. On the morning of admission he awoke with a fever and severe respiratory distress. He was immediately hospitalized.

The temperature was 104.5 degrees F., respirations 44, pulse 144, and blood pressure 100/60 mm. Hg. There was a pronounced mid-dorsal kyphoscoliosis, cyanosis of the lips and fingers, and edema of the lower extremities. Respirations were shallow and breath sounds were faint.

The urine was normal. The hemoglobin was 16.2 Gm., the hematocrit was 52, and the leukocytes numbered 10,200 with 87 segmented granulocytes and 13 lymphocytes. A chest x-ray could not be interpreted because of the kyphoscoliosis. Antibiotics were given; the fever persisted and the respiratory distress continued. The patient died on the sixth hospital day.

Autopsy examination revealed marked thoracic kyphoscoliosis, atelectasis of the left lung, and cor pulmonale. Except for the spinal cord, which disclosed hydromyelia, additional diagnoses were incidental.

THE ENTITY

Hydromyelia is a congenital dilatation of the central canal of the spinal cord. It is often associated with meningomyelocele or the Arnold-Chiari malformation (herniation of cerebellar tissue into the foramen magnum). It is non-inflammatory and slowly progressive. The dilatation often extends over the entire length of the cord, the lumen contains clear colorless fluid, and the lining surface is smooth and covered by ependymal cells. As the dilatation progresses, the spinothalamic tracts that cross in the anterior white commissure are compressed and undergo atrophy. Clinical disease begins in adolescence or early adulthood. The classical features are gradual loss of pain and temperature with preservation of touch and pressure. This is first evident in the fingers and hands so that injuries to these parts are common. Later, the anterior horn cells may also be affected so that atrophy of the hands, especially of the thenar eminences, and forearms may become pronounced.

The condition should be distinguished from syringomyelia, which is a proliferation of glial cells in the central white matter of the spinal cord that undergo degeneration and cavity formation. The distinguishing anatomic feature is the glial lining of the cavity and the compression and displacement of the central canal which remains intact. Clinically the two conditions are similar.

HYDROMYELIA

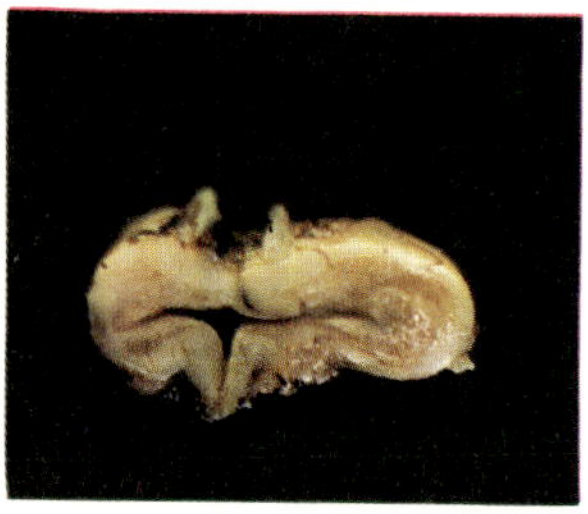

The spinal cord on removal was not remarkable externally except for slight flattening of the contour. Gross sections, however, revealed a central tube-like cavity that extended from the medulla to the cauda equina. The photograph shows the cut surface of the cord with the tube-like central dilatation that is for the most part collapsed.

The unmagnified section of the whole cord reveals the size of the central chamber. The posterior aspect is on the viewer's right; the dilatation extends through the neural tissue on that side. The cleft of the anterior surface is on the viewer's left and branches of the anterior spinal artery are present within that crease.

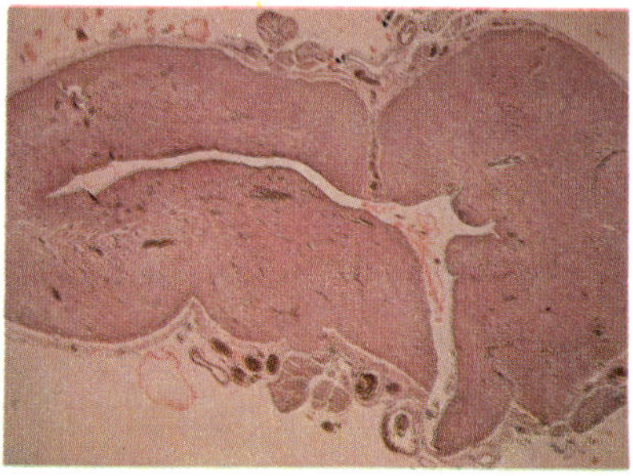

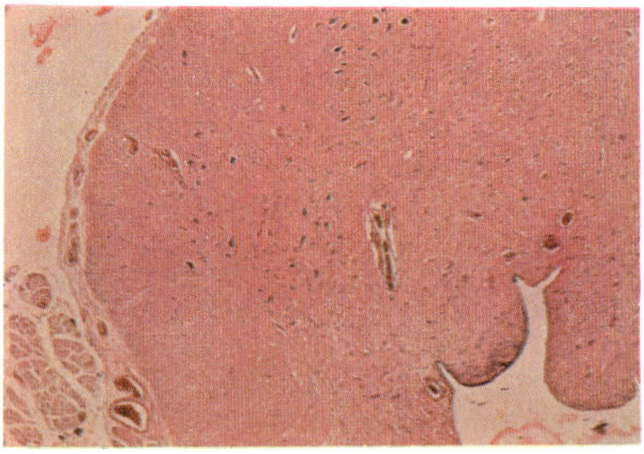

A low power magnification presents the anterior horn region of the cord; only a small number of ganglion cells are present. The most significant observation, however, is that the lining surface of the central chamber is covered by ependymal cells. This signifies that the tube-like chamber is an enormously dilated central canal.

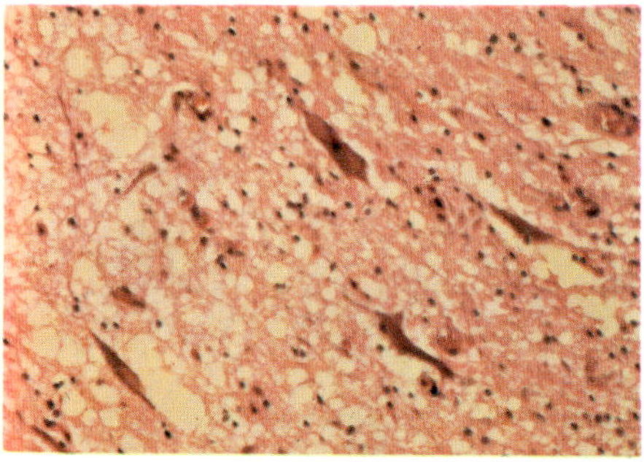

At higher magnification, sparse ganglion cells and atrophy of the adjacent tissue may be made out.

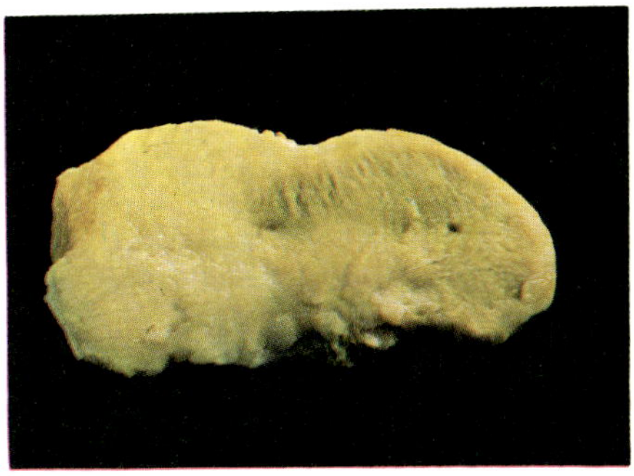

The cut surface of tongue reveals fatty displacement of muscle on the viewer's left as compared with the solid muscle on the opposite side.

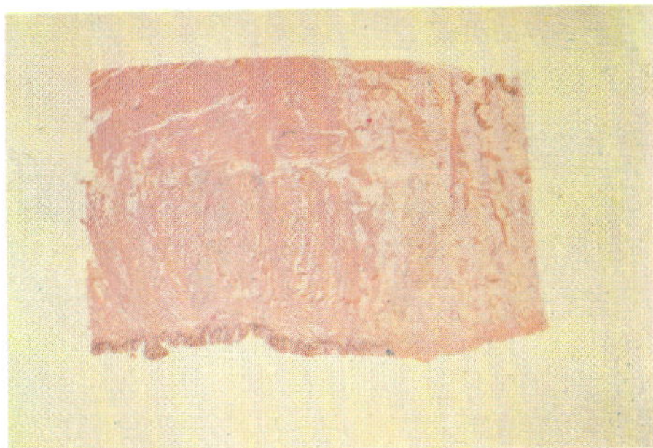

At scanning power the atrophic muscle which is replaced with adipose tissue is abruptly demarcated from the normal muscle.

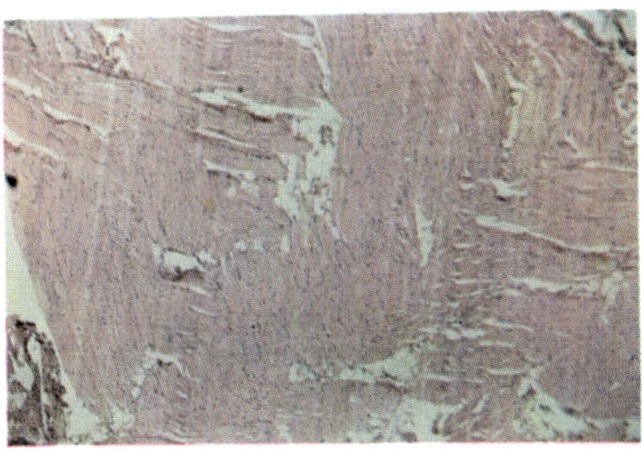

At higher power the normal tongue muscle reveals the coarse bundles that interlace in three directions.

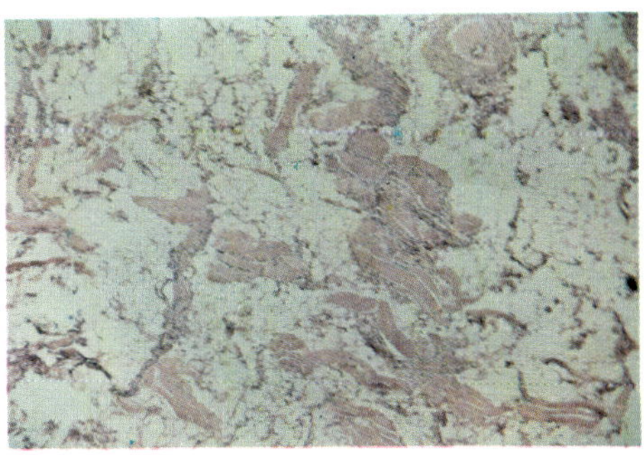

The denervated side at the same magnification reveals only scattered muscle fibers and an abundance of mature adipose tissue.

NEUROATROPHY OF TONGUE

CLINICAL ACCOUNT 5890

The history is available only by hearsay. The patient is reported to have been an adult female who had manifested a clinical syndrome indicating a surgical lesion in the posterior cranial fossa. Some kind of surgical procedure was undertaken; in the performance of that operation, the twelfth cranial nerve was injured on one side. Denervation of half of the tongue followed this hypoglossal nerve injury. Subsequently, neurogenic atrophy of half of the tongue gradually developed. The patient later died of other causes, and autopsy examination revealed the pathologic process of neurogenic atrophy of the tongue as shown in the accompanying photographs.

THE ENTITY

Atrophy is the process of intracellular digestion that causes cells to disappear and organs to shrink. It is acquired and is to be distinguished from congenital abnormalities including failure of an organ to appear (agenesis), failure to progress beyond rudimentary form (aplasia), and failure to achieve normal development (hypoplasia). Atrophy may be physiologic or pathologic. Examples of the former include disappearance of the thyroglossal duct during fetal life, regression of the thymus during infancy, decrease of the lymphoid tissue during adolescence, involution of the uterus after parturition, and regression of the breasts and ovaries after the menopause.

Pathologic atrophy may affect a tissue or the whole body. The latter is associated with chronic infections, carcinomatosis, and starvation (cachexia). It may be due to undernutrition from an impediment to swallowing (esophageal stenosis), a psychologic rejection of food (anorexia nervosa), or an impairment of intestinal absorption (Whipple's disease). In old age, the whole body withers (senile atrophy).

Focal atrophy is caused by disuse, increased pressure, decreased blood supply, inadequate nutrition, or lack of hormonal stimulation. Skeletal muscle wastes rapidly when unused as in fixation (fracture-cast), or motor denervation (severed nerve). Adipose tissue fills in the wasted muscle. Tumors and throbbing aneurysms cause pressure atrophy of adjacent structures. The legs wither with the slow formation of an aortic thrombus (Leriche syndrome). Bed rest causes pressure atrophy of skin and sacral ulceration (decubiti). Duct obstruction (pancreatic, bile, salivary) causes pressure atrophy of the tissue secreting into that channel. Ureteral obstruction causes pressure dilatation of renal pelves with wasting of the nephric tissue (hydronephrosis), and pituitary failure is associated with atrophy of the endocrine organs (Simmond's disease).

After experimental nerve severance, muscle cells undergoing atrophy reveal reduced consumption of oxygen, decreased synthesis of protein, failure of mitochondrial biogenesis, and increased activity of acid hydrolases. Mitochondrial swelling is seen. The process is thus intracellular, metabolic, and associated with increased activity of lysosomes (1).

1. LaVia, M.F., and Hill, R.B., Jr. Principles of Pathobiology Oxford University Press, New York, 1971.